"Pamela makes healthy cooking accessible, easy, and most importantly delicious! She takes your favorite dishes (and ones that are sure to become new favorites) and infuses them with everything your body wants and needs. This is a cookbook that every family needs."

—NIKKI DINKI, COOKING CHANNEL HOST, AUTHOR OF *MEAT ON THE SIDE*

"Pamela Salzman is the guru when it comes to all things healthy cooking! Her recipes are modern, fresh, and full of organic and nutritionally dense foods that nourish the body and taste beyond delicious. Anyone who's looking to up their kitchen game, for better nutrition, more flavor, or just a dose of something new, she's got you covered. Whether you're feeding yourself or your whole family her meals will be a HUGE hit with everyone, even the pickiest of eaters."

—LORI BREGMAN, AUTHOR OF *THE MINDFUL MOM-TO-BE*

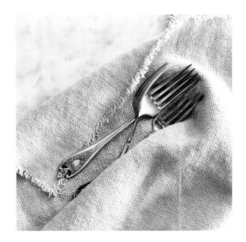

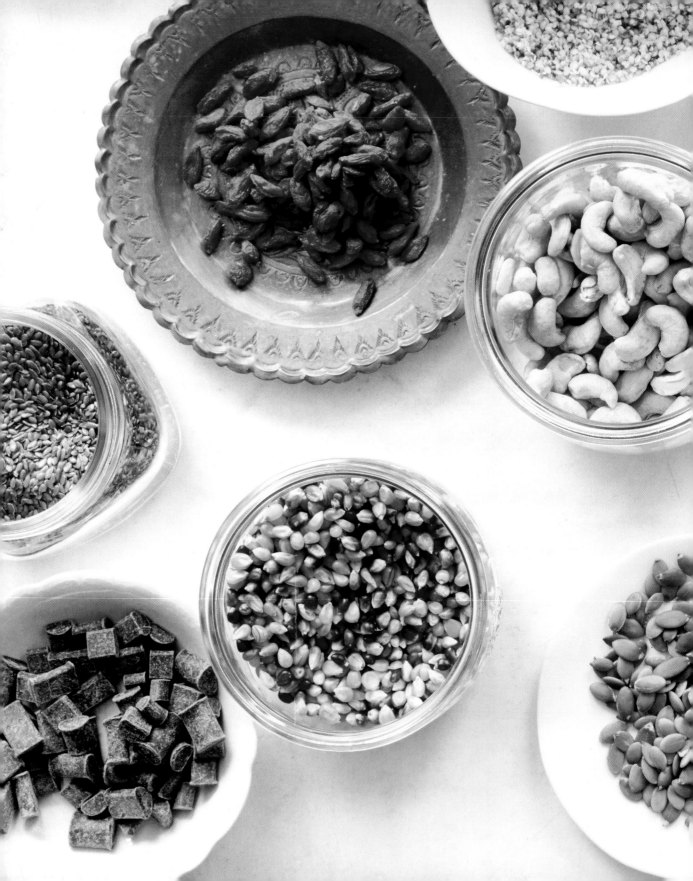

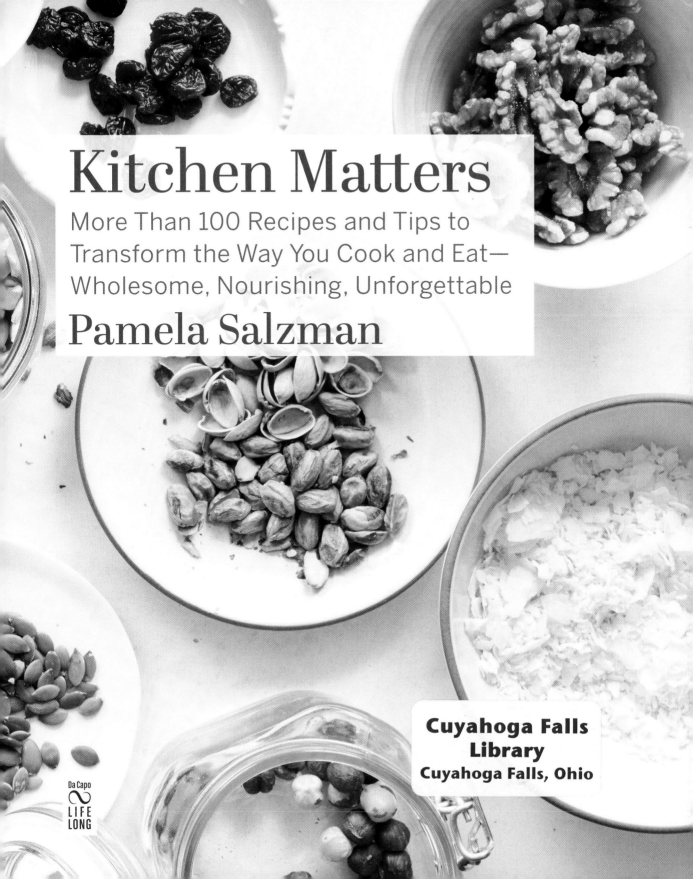

Kitchen Matters

More Than 100 Recipes and Tips to
Transform the Way You Cook and Eat—
Wholesome, Nourishing, Unforgettable

Pamela Salzman

Da Capo
LIFE
LONG

To Daniel, with all my heart

Editorial production by Christine Marra, *Marra*thon
     Production Services. www.marrathoneditorial.net
Book design by Endpaper Studio
Set in Abril and Benton Sans

Cataloging-in-Publication data for this book is available
from the Library of Congress.

First Da Capo Press edition 2017
ISBN: 978-0-7382-1924-0 (paperback)
ISBN: 978-0-7382-1925-7 (e-book)

Published by Da Capo Press, an imprint of Perseus Books, LLC,
a subsidiary of Hachette Book Group, Inc.
www.dacapopress.com

Note: The information in this book is true and complete to
the best of our knowledge. This book is intended only as an
informative guide for those wishing to know more about
health issues. In no way is this book intended to replace,
countermand, or conflict with the advice given to you by
your own physician. The ultimate decision concerning care
should be made between you and your doctor. We strongly
recommend you follow his or her advice. Information in this
book is general and is offered with no guarantees on the part
of the authors or Da Capo Press. The authors and publisher
disclaim all liability in connection with the use of this book.
LSC-C

10 9 8 7 6 5 4 3 2 1

Contents

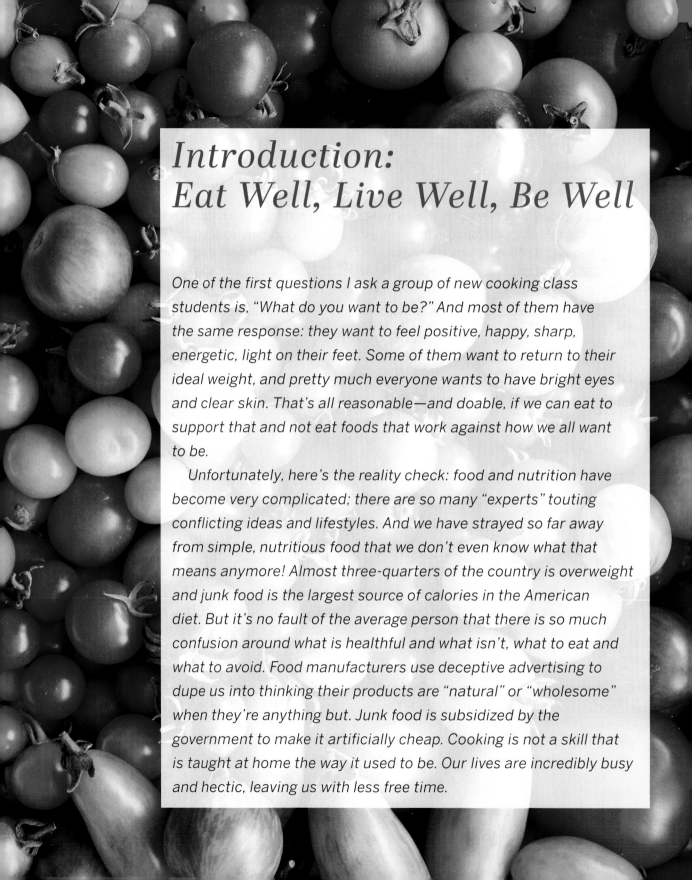

Introduction:
Eat Well, Live Well, Be Well

One of the first questions I ask a group of new cooking class students is, "What do you want to be?" And most of them have the same response: they want to feel positive, happy, sharp, energetic, light on their feet. Some of them want to return to their ideal weight, and pretty much everyone wants to have bright eyes and clear skin. That's all reasonable—and doable, if we can eat to support that and not eat foods that work against how we all want to be.

Unfortunately, here's the reality check: food and nutrition have become very complicated; there are so many "experts" touting conflicting ideas and lifestyles. And we have strayed so far away from simple, nutritious food that we don't even know what that means anymore! Almost three-quarters of the country is overweight and junk food is the largest source of calories in the American diet. But it's no fault of the average person that there is so much confusion around what is healthful and what isn't, what to eat and what to avoid. Food manufacturers use deceptive advertising to dupe us into thinking their products are "natural" or "wholesome" when they're anything but. Junk food is subsidized by the government to make it artificially cheap. Cooking is not a skill that is taught at home the way it used to be. Our lives are incredibly busy and hectic, leaving us with less free time.

I get it. I work full-time and I have three busy kids. But I had a pretty amazing foundation: my parents believed in cooking simple meals from scratch, growing organic vegetables in the backyard, and insisting on dinner together every night. We spent our Sundays surrounded by extended family and bright, vibrant platters of vegetables cooked straight from the garden, warm bowls of rustic pasta with homemade sauce, fork-tender meats, and crisp, colorful salads. I couldn't stay out of the kitchen, whether it was helping with dinner prep or wearing out the pages of the latest *Gourmet* magazine. I taught myself how to cook by observing closely, reading everything I could get my hands on, and getting really messy in the kitchen. Everything we cooked was very simple, but always homemade. But we were certainly not perfect and ate our fair share of (*not* whole-grain) pasta, bread, and (a lot of) cheese. We had normal (sugar-laden) birthday cakes and soda on special occasions. We didn't overthink food.

Getting married and having children was when I changed the way I looked at food. Once I had other human beings to feed, I started to connect the dots between food and nutrition. I went back to school to learn as much as I could about more healthful eating and slowly began to make changes in our pantry, how I cooked, and what we ate. The majority of my friends weren't on the same journey; they had the idea that cooking—be it for one person or twenty—was intimidating. But they were curious, eager to learn, and wanted me to share some of my recipes. Soon, I was giving tips on how to sweeten with dates, swap unhealthy fats for coconut oil, and use lentils in place of ground meat; I shared how I organized my pantry and navigated the farmers' market.

I knew then that I wanted to give other parents a fresh start in the kitchen and to help get their families eating well. My prospective students had one wish—to teach them how I did it. "It" was making three nutritious meals a day for my family, including a very picky son, without a lot of stress. This became the foundation for my cooking classes and my blog and eventually turned into a full-time business.

Over the last decade, I have taught people from all walks of life. I have been in hundreds of home kitchens. I talk to dozens of (mostly) parents every day, fielding questions about everything from picky eaters to allergies to how to boil water (really!). What has become very clear to me is that we all basically want the same thing: we want to live our best lives, be healthy, feel happy, connect with our children and one another.

My students have come to my cooking classes wanting to learn and do better. I have never criticized anyone for what was in her pantry or how many meals she cooked last week. Perfection is stressful, overrated, and unattainable. So, you made a frozen pizza for dinner last night? No big deal. So, you made a frozen pizza every night last month? Then I'm glad you have this book! The important point is that it's what you do most of the time that really matters.

Every individual and every family is unique. There's no judgment anywhere in this book, so don't ever feel bad about doing your best.

I live and teach in Los Angeles, the home of what's the latest, greatest new diet, health craze, and "it" food. In every single class, my students ask my opinion about this diet or that. Personally, I hate diets. Ironically, I can find data to support any diet out there, from Paleo to vegan, but

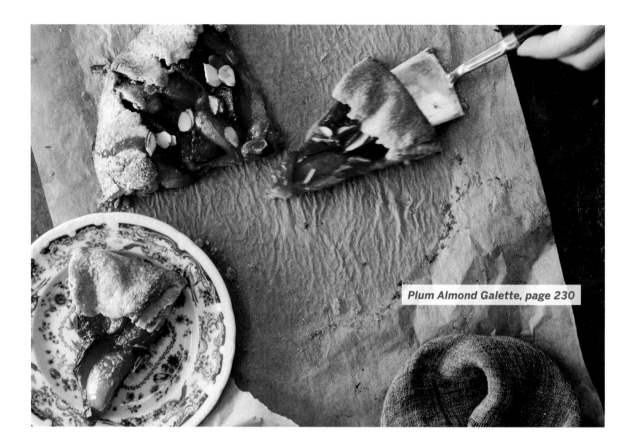

Plum Almond Galette, page 230

that's not what I teach. Whereas I think it's pretty obvious we should be avoiding processed food and chemical-laden junk, there is a whole world of amazing foods you may not have ever eaten or cooked with before. It's so exciting to find new flavors and recipes that are nutritious and absolutely delicious. And I am not talking about turning vegetable pulp from your juicer into a patty—you won't find that here. Instead, you'll find modern, accessible recipes, the majority of which have been taught dozens of times and have been tested on my friends and family.

My kids didn't bounce down the stairs one day asking, "Mom, how come we never have millet in our house?" or "I saw a commercial for kale. Do you think we could try it?" Our unprocessed way of eating was driven by me since I knew that both my health and the health of my family were ultimately my responsibility. I believe with 100 percent certainty that what you eat matters more than anything else. The good news is that you have total control over that. You don't have control over your genetics or the toxins in the environment. But you are the one who chooses what goes in your shopping cart and what goes in your frying pan. I tell my students that we should all try to eat well, live well, be well. They really do work altogether. If you want to be healthy, cooking as much nutrient-dense food as often as you can is a good place to start. Your health matters—and your kitchen matters. And that's what this book is about.

Getting Started

We need to get your pantry and refrigerator stocked with the healthful ingredients that are key to making nutritious recipes. But to get there, the secret is being organized. We'll set up your kitchen so that it is conducive to cooking easily. You'll learn how and why you need to plan your meals for the week. And eventually, you'll learn to prep ahead, which will save you time and make cooking less stressful.

If you feel overwhelmed by all of this, you can and should start small. Make a few pantry swaps or buy one new food to try. If you currently don't cook at all, set a goal of cooking dinner once per week until you can handle cooking twice. Making one small change at a time will help lead to lasting habits down the road.

A LIFE-CHANGING APPROACH TO FOOD

So, what should we eat? At the end of the day, Michael Pollan said it best, "Eat food. Not too much. Mostly plants." And that's what I recommend. The recipes you'll find here will help you eat foods that have anti-inflammatory effects on the body, such as vegetables and legumes, and greatly limit foods that are pro-inflammatory, such as highly processed foods, fried foods, animal products, and sugar. My recipes also have a low-GI focus, which means they will help you severely limit eating such foods as refined carbohydrates and concentrated sweeteners that cause spikes in our blood sugar and lead to the release of a pro-inflammatory, fat-storage hormone called insulin.

Basically, these recipes rely on whole foods. A whole food has just one ingredient—itself—and it exists in the way it came into this world. It hasn't been bleached, deodorized, treated with chemicals, hydrogenated, refined, or combined with additives. Ideally, we should focus on as many whole foods as possible, but there

IN A NUTSHELL, THESE FOODS MATTER IN YOUR KITCHEN:

Fresh, seasonal vegetables, especially dark green leafy vegetables and cruciferous vegetables (e.g., broccoli, cauliflower, cabbage, kale, Brussels sprouts, arugula, radishes, and others)

Whole grains (if you can tolerate them; e.g., brown rice, quinoa, barley, farro, and millet, among others)

High-quality fats (unrefined oils; e.g., olive, avocado, coconut, hemp, and flax)

Legumes

Nuts and seeds

Fresh, seasonal fruit

Anti-inflammatory spices and herbs (especially garlic, turmeric, ginger, oregano, and cinnamon, among others)

Cold-water wild fish and seafood

You'll find these foods incorporated in my recipes, but in smaller portions:

Whole-grain pasta and bread

Unprocessed, organic soy

Free-range organic eggs

Lean, organic poultry and grass-fed meat

Dairy, preferably grass-fed, raw, cultured and/or from goat or sheep milk

Here are two categories I include in my own kitchen, in very small portions:

Natural, unrefined sweeteners

Red wine

I suggest avoiding these at all costs:

Artificial sweeteners

Soda

Refined, industrial seed oils

MSG and its derivatives

Artificial and "natural" colors and flavors

Farm-raised seafood

Conventionally raised meat

Nonfat dairy

Trans fats

are plenty of healthful foods that have been minimally processed, such as olive oil and almond flour. In general, the further you move away from the original food, the less nutritious it is. An orange is a whole food, but most commercial orange juices are not because the pulp (and the fiber) have been removed. To go further down the "food chain," orange Creamsicles don't even resemble the actual fruit and have many undesirable additives.

You're probably wondering about the meat question: high-quality meat has its place at my table, but in small portions. Similarly, a little dairy is fine if you can tolerate it, but I'll explain why it's better to use it as a condiment, and why sheep or goat options are preferred over cow. And is dessert on the menu? Of course! It's a treat and I do my best to use sweeteners that contain nutrients and in much smaller amounts.

COOKING AND EATING WITH POSITIVE INTENTIONS

I can't tell you the number of times I am in the middle of teaching a class with five recipes and a student will say to me, "You're so calm. I would be going nuts right now." And I always reply, "It's just food." Food should provide nourishment, pleasure, and sustenance, not stress and anxiety. Cooking should not generate feelings of fear. Once you set up your kitchen and pantry for success, you can cook anything in this book. You have nothing to prove to anyone. Your dinner is not being photographed or judged. So what if it may or may not look like something in a magazine? Be proud of the fact that you planned a healthful meal, shopped for it, and prepared it with love. The more you cook, the more confident you will become and the easier it will get, just like any skill.

The Well-Stocked Kitchen

If you want to enjoy cooking or at least be efficient in the kitchen, you need to have some basic tools and a strategy. These tips are ones I've learned from cooking in hundreds of homes, with kitchens of all sizes.

COMMON SPACE

Overall, countertops should be free of clutter, lighting should be functional and bright, drawers should be organized by category, keeping likes with likes, and everything should be in an accessible place; otherwise you won't use it. Things that you use once a year can be stored in the garage, but that's no place for your food processor! Make space for the items you use—or would like to use—regularly.

MAJOR APPLIANCES

Oven. Oven temperatures vary wildly. I remember one November when I taught roasted turkey in sixteen Thanksgiving classes. I had the same-size bird, prepared the same way, using the same roasting pan, taken out of the fridge for the same amount of time, and the cooking time varied *one hour* from the slowest oven to the hottest oven!

How do you know if your oven runs hot? Well, if most of the time after you follow a recipe, you're thinking, "Huh. That's so weird. I always burn everything or dry it out," your oven runs hot! But the best way to test the temperature of your oven is to buy a portable oven thermometer that can give you an accurate read. Or have a service technician come and test ("calibrate") it for you.

Regardless, get to know your oven! Know if it cooks faster on the bottom or in the back. And adjust your cooking to reflect that by shortening the cook time or rotating the pan to expose it to equal amounts of heat, if necessary.

TIP: Always check the inside of your oven before preheating it. I have found lots of things in people's ovens that they had forgotten about, including last night's baked potato or this morning's oatmeal, or things they forgot to mention to me, such as their entire collection of baking sheets or their kids' artwork from school!

Stove. I much prefer gas over electric since gas heat adjusts much faster to changes in the dial. But with gas burners you need to keep those openings clean so they light properly.

TIP: If you have a combination range, which has an oven and stove, you should put the fan on if you are using both the oven and stove, to prevent the computer elements from overheating. They are so expensive to replace when they burn out!!

Refrigerator. Make a habit of cleaning out your refrigerator weekly. Quickly wipe down all the shelves and bins and pull to the front the food that needs to get eaten right away so you don't forget about it.

Store likes with likes (e.g., nut butters, jams, cheese, mustards, etc.) to find what you need more quickly. I have found that using a stainless-steel lazy Susan for nut butters and other condiments can really help with organization (lazy Susans can be found very cheaply).

To keep storage spaces clean, line the crisper drawers with washable liners and keep plastic trays for small items, to prevent them from rolling around.

Lastly, you can use your phone to remind yourself to vacuum the refrigerator and freezer vents every three months, to prevent the motors from overheating.

TIP: You can also use this opportunity to menu plan, since your cleaning will help you to know what foods need to get used up pronto. I do my weekly clean on Saturday morning; this helps with my Sunday menu planning.

EQUIPMENT

I have listed equipment here that I believe is helpful to make the recipes in this book and facilitate an enjoyable cooking experience. It's best to keep the inventory of equipment simple. Don't hold on to gadgets that have one use or that you rarely use. Aim for quality over quantity. When I was first married, I started to build my collection of All-Clad pans and Staub cookware slowly one piece at a time, waiting to purchase when I saw a big sale at the store. I have maintained all the same pieces and they still function beautifully.

If you are on a limited budget or you are just starting out, you really only need a couple of good knives and a few pieces of heavy-bottomed, high-quality cookware with which you can do a lot. See the Resources section for specific brands and where to purchase.

Baking Pans. I recommend using baking pans made from glass/Pyrex, ceramic, enameled cast iron, or black baker's steel. Try to avoid nonstick coatings and untreated aluminum, both of which when heated leach into your food.

9- or 10-inch pie plate (2)
8- or 9-inch round cake pan (2)
Standard 12-cup muffin tin + unbleached parchment liners or reusable silicone liners
8-inch square baking pan
8½ x 4½-inch loaf pan
Not necessary, but nice to have if you like to bake:
*   9- or 10-inch springform pan*

Baking Dishes. These are for such things as casseroles, brownies, granola bars, and even roasting a whole chicken. I use Pyrex, ceramic, or enameled cast iron.

9 x 13-inch
7 x 11-inch

Baking Sheets. I use rimmed baking sheets constantly for roasting vegetables, baking cookies, making granola, and so much more. It is very difficult to find heavy, stainless-steel rimmed baking sheets, so I line anything aluminum or nonstick with unbleached parchment paper or silicone baking mats.

I suggest at least two 13 x 18-inch "half sheet" pans and if you have a smaller oven, two 10 x 13-inch "quarter sheet" pans, too.

Blender. A good blender is so useful for making smoothies, nut milk, dressings, and creamy desserts. The stronger your blender, the more creamy and smooth the results will be. If it is in your budget, go for a Vitamix or another high-speed, professional-strength blender. They are worth every penny; they can turn cashews into cream and blitz rock-hard fruit into the smoothest puree. I use mine daily. You don't need both a standard blender and a Vitamix, however.

Coffee Grinder. A small electric coffee grinder is great for grinding seeds (e.g., flax) and spices. It's not an essential tool, but it can come in handy.

Colander and Sieve. Use colanders for draining pasta and veggies; a fine-mesh sieve is what you need for rinsing itty-bitty quinoa or straining stock to be ultraclear.

Cooling Rack. If you ever bake cookies, a wire cooling rack will help them cool properly. These racks are also handy for drizzling doughnuts!

Cutting Boards. You need at least one large cutting board, preferably with grooves on the edges to catch drippings from cooked meat, and a small one for smaller jobs.

I prefer wood, which is naturally antibacterial and won't dull your knives the way plastics do. Wood requires a bit more maintenance, so be sure to dry your boards well before putting them away and every couple of months rub a little coconut oil into the surface.

Food Processor. Your food processor will be your best friend in the kitchen because it makes quick work of such tedious tasks as shredding a dozen potatoes or slicing pounds of onions. You can also use a food processor for pastry dough, pureeing sauces and dips, making homemade nut butter, and sometimes pulsing vegetables. An 11-cup capacity is perfect for most home cooks. If you cook for larger numbers of people, you might find a 14-cup more useful. See the Resources section for the brands I use.

Check out my YouTube video for how to use your food processor. No matter which brand you have, you must keep it in prime real estate in your kitchen, or you will never use it!

Glass Jars and Containers. Unlike plastic storage containers, glass containers don't leach chemicals, are easy to clean, and don't hold onto odors. Glasslock brand containers are a great option for leftovers, and for cut fruit and vegetables. You can store all nuts, seeds, dried fruits, and the like in differently sized glass jars; you can buy them at such places as the Container Store, or you can simply soak the labels off of empty jars from things like nut butter and tomatoes and reuse them for storage. See page 20 for how to freeze in glass containers.

Kitchen Scale. When you need to be accurate, there's no other way than with a kitchen scale. Choose one that can measure in pounds and ounces and can weigh at least up to 5 pounds.

Kitchen Timer. You can use the timer on your phone, but I find that having a dedicated one in the kitchen helps me to use it all the time. If you're a multitasker and cooking more than one thing at a time, a triple timer is a great help to keep you from getting distracted.

Kitchen Towels. Thin towels, such as flour sack towels or herringbone towels, don't leave lint, are inexpensive, and can also double for such tasks as straining yogurt or squeezing the water out of shredded potatoes.

Knives. Hands down, two of the most common questions I am asked are "Which knives should I buy?" and "How often should I get them sharpened?"

Before buying a knife, really hold it to see whether it feels comfortable in your hand. My local Sur La Table allows you to chop vegetables with their knives before buying one. See the Resources section for the brands I use.

You only need four knives to complete your kitchen:
A chef's knife, either a 6-inch or an 8-inch, or both
A 4-inch serrated knife for slicing tomatoes
A paring knife for trimming, poking beets, and coring fruits
A serrated bread knife

TIPS: Please, please, please keep your knives sharp. If you do nothing else I recommend, get your knives sharpened regularly! Prep work will

be so much more fun, easy, and safe with sharp knives. All knives, even expensive ones, need regular sharpening. You can use your honing steel to sharpen your knives at home, but it's still best to take them every six months to a professional. Check your area for cutlery stores or ask your local cookware store if it does sharpening.

Hand wash your knives and dry them right away to make them last longer.

Meat Thermometer. This is nonnegotiable since this is the only way to determine whether your poultry or meat is cooked to the perfect temperature. If you aren't sure your thermometer is accurate, dip the tip of it into a pot of boiling water (put an oven mitt on your hand). If the temperature goes up to 212 degrees Fahrenheit, it's a keeper!

Microplane Grater and Zester. A grater is useful for such things as ginger, Parmesan cheese, and garlic. You can use a finer zester for citrus and nutmeg.

Mixer. A stand mixer is great as it allows you to do other things while it creams butter or beats egg whites. My favorite is the KitchenAid tilt-head stand mixer. Make sure you have the paddle attachment, whisk attachment, and bowl. You can also buy different accessories to make pasta or ice cream, or grind meat. A handheld mixer is fine, but not as efficient as a stand mixer.

Mixing Bowls. Glass nesting bowls are easy to keep clean and easy to store. You need at least one large bowl, one medium-size, and one small.

Nut Milk Bag. If you plan on making nondairy milks frequently, a nut milk bag makes the creamiest nut milk ever. It takes up no space, is very inexpensive, and is reusable for years.

TIP: Keep a second nut milk bag for squeezing the water out of vegetables.

Pepper Mill. You can elevate your cooking simply by swapping freshly ground pepper for pre-ground. Big flavor boost. Trust me.

Pots and Pans. Since untreated aluminum and nonstick cookware can leach aluminum and PTFEs and PFOAs, respectively, into your food at high heat, I only use stainless steel, enameled cast iron, or cast iron. (If you must own a non-stick skillet, look for one with a ceramic coating. They tend to scratch easily, but they are not terribly expensive if you have to replace them frequently.) Here are the basics:

Small: 2-quart saucepan with lid
Medium-size: 3- to 4-quart saucepan with lid
Large: 5- to 6-quart pot with lid
Extra-large: 10-quart stockpot with lid if you want to make a huge amount of stock or chili for a crowd.
Stainless-steel skillets (8-, 10-, and 12-inch)
Dutch oven (7-quart) for pot roasts, soups, and stews

Ruler. If you're like me and terrible at guessing measurements, a standard 12-inch ruler is essential. It can help, whether you need to measure a 2-inch cube of squash or figure out whether your pan is 8 or 10 inches. It's also handy for leveling off flour in a measuring cup.

Slow Cooker. The slow cooker can be a lifesaver. Prep in the morning, press Start, and dinner is done when you get home. You can also use your slow cooker to keep things warm. For example, you can finish a soup at four p.m. and transfer it to the slow cooker on the warm setting until dinnertime. Opt for one with a ceramic or stainless-steel insert rather than nonstick.

Toaster Oven. This is not a necessity for a kitchen to be complete but can be handy for things other than toast. Toaster ovens preheat much more quickly than a wall oven and use less

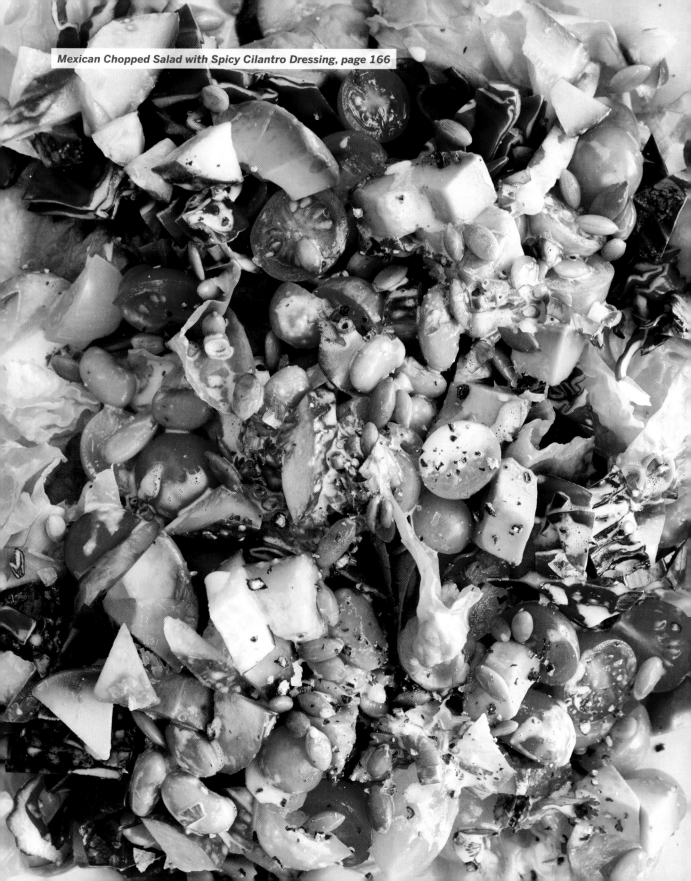

Mexican Chopped Salad with Spicy Cilantro Dressing, page 166

energy. It can be very handy for smaller jobs, such as toasting nuts, and for baking small, flat items, such as a couple of cookies, a frittata, an oatmeal bake, or my Banana-Walnut French toast Casserole (page 50).

Unbleached Parchment Paper. Lining your baking sheets, baking pans, and loaf pans with unbleached parchment paper makes cleanup easy and protects your food from heavy metals and toxins. It also enables you to remove breads and cakes so you can avoid cutting them inside the pan and scratching the pan. (Note that bleached parchment paper may contain a toxin called dioxin, so it's best to use unbleached.) Another option for baking sheets is Silpat reusable silicone baking mats. Silicone does not leach, so it is safe to use in an oven. I have one mat that I use for baking, but not for foods with strong odors, such as fish.

Water Filtration System. Most municipal water is tainted with chlorine, fluoride, and other undesirable toxins. A water filter for the kitchen sink is a great investment; if you can manage, a filtration for the whole house is even better. If you're looking for an inexpensive alternative, a pitcher filter system, such as Brita, is a good place to start. I usually avoid plastic, though.

SMALL TOOLS

Dry Measuring Cups (ones that you can level off). Look for stainless steel with the measurement imprinted into the metal.

Liquid Measuring Cups. Aim for 1-cup, 2-cup, and 4-cup in glass. You can always use your blender to measure larger quantities.

Measuring Spoons. You need at least one set, preferably in stainless steel. It's nice to have a second set if you bake a lot.

Miscellaneous Tools

Can opener
Citrus juicer
Kitchen twine
Metal spatula
Pot holders
Scalloped tongs (buy ones that are self-locking and are stainless steel on the bottom)
Silicone pastry brush (easier to clean than boar's hair and heat resistant)
Silicone spatula
Stainless-steel ladle
Steamer basket
Vegetable peeler
Whisks
Wine opener
Wooden spoons and wooden turners (a.k.a. wooden spatulas)

NICE TO HAVE, BUT NOT NECESSARY

Immersion Blender. You can use a blender to puree soups, but a handheld immersion blender which blends right in the pot is so much more convenient. See the Resources section for the brand I use.

Waffle Iron. You can use a waffle iron to make great hash browns (see the recipe on page 46), cook eggs, and make grilled cheese and peanut butter and jelly sandwiches. Look for a machine that uses a nonlead ceramic coating. See the Resources section for the brand I use.

The Well-Stocked Pantry (and Refrigerator)

One of the most important strategies for avoiding convenience foods and saving money is having a pantry well stocked with basic ingredients. Armed with shelves of the right nonperishables, you can fill in with fresh, seasonal foods and be able to pull together any number of meals, at any time!

Everything listed here can be found at your local Whole Foods Market or health food store, as well as such online sources as Amazon, Thrive Market, and Vitacost. Many you'll only need to buy two or three times a year. For a list of my preferred brands, see the Resources section at the back of the book.

FLOURS

There are many different varieties of flours and ways to use them. For the purposes of this book, I am including the ones you'll find in these recipes. Keep in mind that flours cannot always be used interchangeably, especially when one contains gluten and the other doesn't. The recipes often include suggestions on how to replace the gluten flour.

Other than making pastry dough, I do not use white flour since it is refined, often bleached, and lacking nutrients. If you are new to nonwhite flours, I suggest trying whole spelt or whole wheat pastry flour first. If your budget allows, try experimenting with sprouted flours, which are milled from sprouted grains, contain more nutrients, and may be more digestible.

TIP: Whole-grain flours contain essential fatty acids that can go rancid quickly. Your best bet is to store them in the refrigerator or freezer in an airtight container.

GLUTEN-CONTAINING FLOURS

Whole Spelt Flour. Spelt is a wonderful ancient grain that can be used interchangeably with wheat flour. The gluten in spelt is molecularly different than the gluten in wheat and is more digestible. Some people who are wheat-free, although not necessarily gluten-free, can eat spelt. I also think that spelt tastes a little sweeter than wheat, which makes it great for using in baked goods.

TIP: Spelt flour is more water soluble (i.e., absorbent) than wheat, so you may need to decrease the amount of flour used in a recipe that is sensitive, such as pancakes. Substitution: about one for one for wheat flour.

Whole Wheat Pastry Flour or White Whole Wheat Flour. Both of these flours are milled from whole wheat berries with nothing removed and nothing added back. They contain all the fiber and nutrients from the original grain and they have not been bleached. These whole wheat flours are both lighter in texture than traditional whole wheat flour milled, which can be a little heavy and coarse. They are very versatile and can easily be used in place of white flour in practically any recipe. I use whole wheat pastry flour and white whole wheat flour interchangeably and for most of my baking except pastry, challah bread, and my kids' birthday cakes!

Note: In this book, a few recipes call for oat flour, cornmeal, and blanched almond flour. The other gluten-free flours are only necessary if you need to adapt the remaining recipes to be gluten-free or if you want to experiment further.

King Arthur Gluten-Free Multi-Purpose Flour. This is my go-to premade gluten-free flour blend for gluten-free baking. This product doesn't contain any cornstarch or preservatives and it always works in my recipes in place of gluten flours.

Substitution: You can substitute this one for one in any recipe in this book, but you may need xanthan gum, too.

TIPS: If you are making a gluten-free baked good that needs to rise a little, such as a quick bread, most of the time you need to add xanthan gum to the recipe. Xanthan gum is a gluten-free, plant-based ingredient that can thicken the batter and provide elasticity. It is a component of many gluten-free recipes and blends; you can find it online and in many stores. The package should have instructions on how much to use in what type of recipe.

If you are allergic to xanthan gum, substitute finely ground psyllium husk.

Brown Rice Flour. Stone-ground from brown rice, this flour is often a main ingredient in gluten-free flour blends. Brown rice flour is neutral tasting and slightly nutty, and it can be a little gritty. It can be subbed for gluten flour in sauces and dredging chicken. I like to combine brown rice flour with buckwheat and oat flour in pancake batter for an earthy twist on my standard whole wheat pastry flour.

Substitution: In general, you can substitute ¾ cup of rice flour + ¼ cup of a high-starch flour, such as tapioca flour, for 1 cup of gluten flour in baked goods. For dredging or coating foods, sub one for one.

Buckwheat Flour. Despite its name, buckwheat is not related to wheat at all. In fact it is not even a true grain, but a seed related to the rhubarb family. Buckwheat flour has an assertive earthy flavor. It is high in protein and fiber and can help reduce blood pressure.

Substitution: I recommend combining buckwheat with other flours because of its strong flavor and density, which will inhibit rising. Use it up to one third of a flour blend in a recipe.

Coconut Flour. This grain-free flour is rather dense, heavy, and sweet. You can mix coconut flour with almond flour in grain-free baking, since it is tricky to bake with all coconut flour (due to it absorbing liquid). It contains a lot of fiber and healthy fats with very few carbohydrates.

Substitution: It cannot be substituted for grain or nut flours.

Cornmeal. Cornmeal can come in different "grinds"; the coarser the grind, the more texture your baked good will have. A yellow, medium-grind cornmeal is a good basic. It's best to buy organic since corn is a genetically modified crop. Look for unrefined milled corn products that still contain the fiber-rich bran and germ layers.

Substitution: If you like the texture and flavor of cornmeal, you can sub it in for ¼ cup of flour in any of the pancake recipes.

Finely Ground Blanched Almond Flour and Almond Meal. Almonds are rich in healthy monounsaturated fat and are low in carbohydrates. Blanched almond flour and meal are made from almonds that have had the skins removed. But flour and meal are different, and not always interchangeable. Almond flour is very fine, almost dusty, and is recommended for baking cakes, quick breads, and muffins. Almond meal is coarser and heavier, nice in a crisp topping.

Substitution: It cannot be substituted for grain flours.

Oat Flour. This is one of my favorite flours because of oat's sweet and nutty flavor as well as its high levels of fiber and protein; of course I also love it because it creates a nice, tender crumb. Oat flour is the only flour that can be found with and without gluten, depending on where the oats were grown and in what facility they were processed. Look for specially labeled "gluten-free" oat flour if you are gluten-sensitive, or make your own oat flour by taking old-fashioned rolled oats (use a gluten-free brand, if necessary) and blending them in a food processor until they turn into flour.

Substitute: You can replace wheat flour with oat flour up to 20 percent of the amount in the recipe.

FATS

Good quality fats are part of a healthful diet. You need good fats to fuel the brain (which is made up of 60 percent fat), lubricate the joints, and provide long-lasting energy. Fat also helps us absorb the fat-soluble vitamins A, D, E, and K. The key is choosing the most healthful kinds of fats and knowing how to work with them.

Unrefined and organic fats are best to use whenever possible. Refined oils almost always rely on heat or nasty chemical solvents to strip them of flavor, color, and fragile fatty acids. The result is a neutral-tasting oil that can withstand higher heat, but it is damaged, and its nutrients compromised in place of a whole lot of free radicals that promote inflammation in the body and damage your cells.

Oils are susceptible to oxidation (compounds are broken down and free radicals are formed) from light, heat, and air. Buy oils in dark glass bottles whenever possible. Store them in a cool, dark place, such as the pantry (although you'll want to store fragile nut and seed oils, as well as butter in the fridge).

Here are the unrefined fats/oils I use for cooking and baking (I've listed the specific brands I use at the back of this book):

Organic, Cultured Unsalted Butter. I use butter, a saturated fat, in baking and very occasionally in cooking. Buy unsalted butter so that you can control the amount of salt in a recipe, and because unsalted butter is fresher than salted (salt acts as a natural preservative, so salted butter lasts a lot longer on the shelf). Cultured means that there have been strains of bacteria put back into the pasteurized cream, so you are getting all the gut-friendly good stuff.

Ghee. Ghee is clarified butter, which means that the milk solids have been removed from the butter. Ghee has a very distinct nutty flavor and therefore you may not love it in every dish. While it is good to use at higher temperatures, it cannot be substituted all the time for butter in baking since the moisture contents are different. I love using ghee for cooking scrambled eggs, making Kitchari (page 98) or combined with olive oil to roast potatoes.

Virgin Coconut Oil. Coconut oil is a saturated fat from a vegetable source; it is metabolized by the body as energy as opposed to being stored as fat. Coconut oil has antibacterial and antiviral compounds and an immune-boosting fatty acid called lauric acid. Since it is saturated, it is solid at room temperature and needs to be melted prior to using it to get it into liquid form. Coconut oil is a fantastic substitute for butter in many baked goods, and can be used for savory applications as well. Refer to the roasted vegetable chart

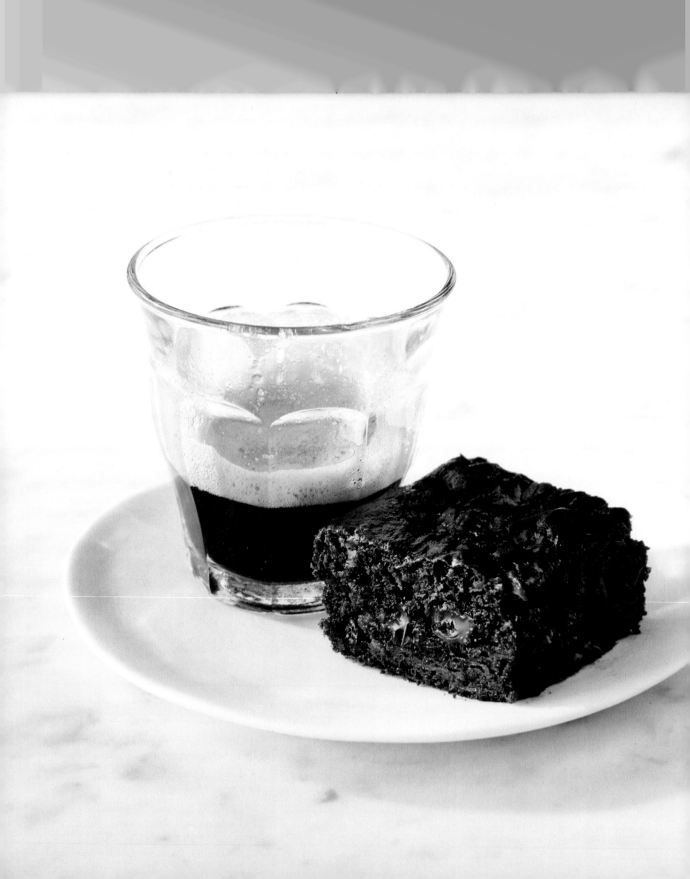

on pages 104–105 to see what vegetables are compatible (flavor-wise) with coconut oil.

Extra-Virgin Olive Oil. Olive oil is made up of mostly heart-healthy monounsaturated fats and is full of antioxidants and anti-inflammatory compounds. I like extra-virgin olive oil, which is produced by cold-pressing and without the use of chemical solvents. High heat is also avoided since it can damage the healthy fatty acids and nutrients in the oil.

Extra-Virgin Avocado Oil. Vitamin E–rich avocado oil can be found unrefined and is mostly monounsaturated. It can be used to sauté or roast vegetables or cook eggs, or really anyplace where olive oil is used.

Toasted Sesame Oil. Pressed from sesame seeds, this oil is great for using in stir-fries and other Asian-influenced dishes. The flavor is strong, so I tend to use it in small amounts or combine it with another more neutral oil, such as olive or avocado.

TIPS: Make sure that your sesame oil is labeled as "unrefined" and look for toasted to ensure a deeper, richer flavor. (Untoasted sesame oil doesn't have much flavor).

You can store sesame oil in your pantry, or refrigerator if you don't use it often.

THESE ARE UNREFINED FATS/OILS I USE ONLY RAW (AND STORE IN THE REFRIGERATOR):

Flaxseed oil. Flaxseed oil is a polyunsaturated fat that should only be used raw because it is sensitive to oxidation if heated. Flax oil is nutty in flavor and adds a healthy dose of fat; drizzle it on oatmeal, toast, or salad or use it in place of some olive oil in vinaigrettes.

Hemp seed oil. Derived from hemp seeds, this oil is rich in omega 3 and omega 6 fatty acids, protein, and essential amino acids. Like flaxseed oil,

hemp seed oil is not to be used for cooking and is highly perishable. You can drizzle it over savory oatmeal or use as a finishing oil over salad.

VINEGARS

Best-Quality Aged Balsamic Vinegar. Not only is balsamic vinegar thick and sweet, it is rich in antioxidants and several essential minerals. Unlike regular balsamic vinegar, thick aged balsamic vinegar is great for finishing dishes. You can drizzle it over veggies, burrata, and even fruit desserts; using aged white balsamic provides rich flavor without adding color to your dish.

Unpasteurized Cider Vinegar. Cider vinegar promotes digestion, good immune health, and helps flush toxins out of the body. It is super important to buy raw and unpasteurized cider vinegar so as to benefit from the live enzymes and probiotics that aid in digestion. I love to use it in salad dressings especially.

Unseasoned Rice Vinegar. This is a lighter and mildly sweeter vinegar used in Asian cuisines. It comes seasoned with salt and sugar or unseasoned, so be sure to look for the bottle labeled as "rice vinegar" rather than that labeled as "seasoned." I love it mixed with cider vinegar in my Everyday Salad Dressing (page 255).

White Wine Vinegar. White wine vinegar is less acidic and pungent than red wine vinegar. It's great to use in salad dressings.

SWEETENERS

I prefer to use sweeteners that have been minimally processed and are less destructive to our body's delicate mineral balance. Many of these can be subbed in for white sugar, which promotes inflammation, is addictive, and has zero nutritive value.

That said, concentrated sweeteners are not health food and should be enjoyed in moderation. A healthy approach to using sweeteners is to try to use natural, unrefined products that still maintain their nutrients and do not cause as severe a spike in blood sugar as processed white sugar or high-fructose corn syrup, and, most important, to use less overall. These natural sweeteners will add amazing sweetness and complexity to your recipes. Store all of them in the pantry, except for maple syrup, which should be stored in the refrigerator after being opened.

Please do not resort to chemical-laden artificial substitutes, thinking you are doing a good thing by avoiding sugar. Artificial sweeteners are even more inflammatory than regular sugar and have been shown to not aid in weight loss.

Brown Rice Syrup. Rice syrup is sometimes referred to as rice malt and is essentially brown rice boiled down until it becomes maltose, so it does have a ricelike aftertaste. It has a sticky quality to it that makes it a great replacement for corn syrup and has a nice subtle sweetness to it.

Substitution: one to one for corn syrup

Coconut Palm Sugar. Coconut sugar, or palm sugar as it is sometimes called, is the dried sap from a coconut palm tree. It has an appearance similar to that of brown sugar yet is drier, has a more distinct flavor, and is a little bit richer than brown sugar—it is almost smoky.

Substitution: one to one for sugar if the recipe can handle a sugar with a dark color and smoky flavor

Dried Dates. Dates are one of my favorite sweeteners because they have not been altered in any way. Because dates are a whole food, all of the fiber, enzymes, and nutrients are still intact, and your body will be able to absorb the sugar content much more efficiently. Dates have a caramel-like taste and texture to them when made into a paste and can add more depth to your food than white sugar.

Substitution: For quick bread and muffin recipes, soak 1 cup of pitted dates in ½ cup of warm water for at least 10 minutes and puree both together until a paste is formed. Substitute for ½ cup of the sweetener in the recipe and decrease the fat by 25 percent.

Maple Syrup and Maple Sugar. Maple syrup should be bought in pure form so as to avoid selecting products that are essentially just maple-flavored corn syrup. Pure maple syrup is the sap of the maple tree and goes through minimal processing before being bottled, so the trace minerals and nutrients are still intact. Maple syrup is categorized by "grade" and contrary to popular belief, one grade does not mean a higher quality over another. Rather, Grade A represents an earlier press in the season, and therefore a lighter maple taste. Grade B maple syrup will have a deeper, more intense maple flavor. I prefer Grade A when using maple syrup to act as white sugar replacement, and I use Grade B when I want to impart an actual maple flavor, such as on pancakes or for a barbecue sauce.

Substitution: In baked goods, for every 1 cup of white sugar substitute ¾ cup of maple syrup and reduce the liquid in the recipe by 3 tablespoons. Keep in mind that maple syrup is less sweet than sugar, so the resulting product will be less sweet than the original recipe. Maple syrup and honey can be substituted in recipes one to one. Maple sugar is much less sweet than sugar and can be substituted one to one for any dry sugar, but the result will be a little less sweet.

Muscovado Sugar. An unrefined brown sugar derived from sugarcane juice, muscovado sugar has a more molasses-y flavor than standard brown sugar.

Substitution: one to one with brown sugar, and one to one with white sugar if the recipe can handle a dark color and more molasses-y flavor.

Raw Honey (not pasteurized). Raw honey is a natural, versatile liquid sweetener that contains trace vitamins and minerals. It is great not only to use as a finishing drizzle to sweeten such things as yogurt and smoothie bowls, but can be used in baking and salad dressings as well. Because honey is made from flowers, it can have a floral undertone that can be a bit overpowering. Try and find a neutral honey that you enjoy the taste of.

Substitution: Substitute one to one with maple syrup; for every 1 cup of sugar, substitute ½ to ⅔ cup of honey and reduce the liquid by 25 percent. In addition, check your baked goods early to avoid overbrowning.

WHOLE GRAINS

Whole grains have not been refined, which means they have not been stripped of fiber, protein, and fatty acids that slow down the process of converting the carbohydrate into sugar; they do not spike blood sugar levels the way refined grains can. There is a whole world of tasty, hearty grains that provide fiber, protein, vitamins, and minerals, and in my opinion, have a more delicious flavor, to boot!

Be aware of how your body responds to certain grains, especially ones containing gluten, such as wheat, barley, and farro. Also be aware of whether you are overexposing yourself to any one particular grain, and seek more variety, which offers new and different nutrients to your diet!

Once you have made the leap to whole grains, you may want to consider getting into the habit of soaking them for any length of time before cooking, but for at least an hour. Soaking grains helps them to become more digestible. A bonus is a slight reduction in cooking time once they've been soaked. See page 128 for how to soak grains.

GLUTEN-FREE GRAINS:
Buckwheat
Millet
Oats (look for specially packaged GF varieties)
Quinoa (there are different colors, which have different phytonutrients)
Arborio rice, for risotto
Brown basmati rice
Long-grain brown rice
Short-grain brown rice
Sushi rice
Wild rice (technically a grass and not a rice)
White basmati rice

GLUTEN-CONTAINING GRAINS:
Barley
Farro
Freekeh
Spelt
Wheat berries

PASTA

This is a processed food and one we eat occasionally. Because I try to limit our gluten intake, I have experimented successfully with a few good gluten-free pastas. My two favorites are a brown rice pasta by Tinkyada and a quinoa and brown rice pasta by Trader Joe's. Otherwise I keep whole wheat, spelt, and durum wheat pastas handy, as well. I have recently experimented successfully with bean-based pastas and I love the added protein and fiber they provide. Try the black bean pasta by Trader Joe's or the chickpea pasta by Banza.

Soba Noodles. These are thin Japanese noodles traditionally made with buckwheat flour. They are great for noodle soups and salads. I use either 100 percent buckwheat by Eden or the wheat-buckwheat blend.

LEGUMES

Legumes are rich in protein, iron, and fiber, and are low in fat. Like whole grains, legumes should be soaked before cooking to help make them more digestible and reduce the cooking time. To help tenderize beans and reduce gas, you can add a piece of kombu (a sea vegetable, available at most health stores) to the pot. Seek out beans from a source that has a high turnover. Old beans take much longer to cook and are generally more challenging to work with.

Even though I prefer beans and other legumes made from scratch, it is helpful to have canned beans in the pantry for last-minute cooking. I love the Eden brand because it uses kombu in the cooking process and restricts the use of BPA in its cans. Or seek out cooked beans in glass jars. The beans I use regularly are pinto, cannellini or great northern, black, kidney, and chickpeas.

Lentils. Lentils are an extremely versatile legume that can be used in place of ground meat in some recipes. They are an excellent source of plant-based protein, and are high in iron and folate, two extremely important nutrients. Lentils cook more quickly than dried beans and therefore do not need to be soaked before using (although it will make them more digestible), but do need a good rinse and sorting.

BAKING ESSENTIALS

Baking soda
Aluminum-free non-GMO baking powder
100 percent pure vanilla extract (check to make sure there's no added sugar or corn syrup)
Organic, dark chocolate 70 percent cacao or higher
Pure almond extract

NUTS AND SEEDS

Nuts and seeds contain so many nutrients that are supportive of brain function, heart health, the immune system, and battling diabetes. All nuts and seeds have health benefits, but almonds are high in vitamin E and magnesium, Brazil nuts are rich in selenium and walnuts and flaxseeds are loaded with omega-3 fatty acids. As with other whole foods, try to buy organic nuts and seeds. (Refrigerate the ones you don't use frequently.)

Almonds
Walnuts
Pecans
Pine nuts
Brazil nuts
Pumpkin seeds (pepitas)
Sesame seeds
Sunflower seeds
Gomasio (sesame seed and sea salt condiment; I love the variety with seaweed by Eden)
(For hemp seeds, chia seeds, and flaxseeds, see Superfoods.)

CONDIMENTS AND OTHER BASIC INGREDIENTS

Sea salt (try Celtic gray sea salt, which contains trace minerals and no additives.)
Herbamare organic herbal seasoning
Dried herbs and spices (especially turmeric, cumin, cinnamon, oregano, smoked paprika, coriander, and curry powder)
Glass-jarred tomatoes
Tomato paste in a glass jar
Anchovy paste
Canned or jarred wild tuna and salmon
Arrowroot powder
Unsulfured, unsweetened dried fruit
Culinary coconut milk
Unsweetened shredded coconut
White wine (I keep a 4-pack of mini glass bottles for risottos and sauces)

SUPERFOODS

The label "superfood" implies a nutrient-dense, whole-food source of concentrated antioxidants, protein, essential fats, minerals, and vitamins. The following are the ones you'll find in this book's recipes. If you are ready to elevate your healthy eating to the next level, try adding a new superfood to your routine! Most of the time, it is easiest to add the powders to smoothies and the seeds and berries to porridges, or as a topping for parfaits and smoothie bowls. Keep them visible front and center inside your pantry or fridge if you want to remember to use them more often. If you're not ready to add bee pollen to your oatmeal, no big deal! These are just really nutrient-dense foods that are fun to try.

Bee Pollen. After bees collect pollen, it is brought back to the hive and mixed with the bees' digestive enzymes, resulting in pellets of bee pollen. Bee pollen is approximately 40 percent protein and is considered one of nature's most completely nourishing foods. It contains nearly all the nutrients required by humans! About half of its protein is in the form of free amino acids that are ready to be used directly by the body. Many of bee pollen's health-supportive claims have been challenged, but I truly feel that I have more energy when I eat bee pollen. Bee pollen tastes slightly citrusy, slightly bitter, with a touch of a honey flavor. Add it to smoothies, oatmeal, and parfaits. Bee pollen should be stored in the refrigerator. Those highly allergic to bee stings should avoid bee pollen.

Chia Seeds. Chia seeds are naturally rich in omega-3 fatty acids, which are super anti-inflammatory, as well as chock-full of fiber and calcium. The seeds have no taste at all, which makes them very easy to use. When chia seeds come into contact with liquid, they become very gelatinous and thick. They make an awesome "pudding" when mixed with almond milk and can help thicken your morning smoothie. The key is knowing just the right ratio of chia to liquid, so your pudding or smoothie doesn't get too thick or too thin, and giving the chia seeds a little time to work their magic. You can also add them to muffin or quick bread batter for a little extra crunch or sprinkle on salads or in dips, such as hummus.

Dried Mulberries. Mulberries are similar in flavor and chewiness to a dried fig. They are an excellent source of iron, calcium, vitamin C, protein, and fiber. And, the major bonus, they contain resveratrol, which is also known as the antiaging nutrient. These are perfect for sprucing up your morning oatmeal and granola; you can also add them to smoothies or baked goods.

Flaxseeds. Flaxseeds contain loads of fiber and the highest concentration of plant-based omega-3 fatty acids. The body cannot digest whole flaxseeds, so grinding them is a must. For maximum freshness, I buy the seeds whole, as opposed to preground, and grind a small amount at a time at home in a coffee grinder.

Try stirring a few tablespoons into pancake or muffin batter, warm porridge, or smoothies or smoothie bowls for an extra boost of fiber, protein, and good fats.

TIP: 1 tablespoon of flax meal mixed with 3 tablespoons of warm water is a fantastic substitute for 1 egg in baking. Allow the mixture to sit on the countertop for 10 to 15 minutes before adding to batter.

Goji Berries. Not only do these dried berries have a unique tart flavor, they are loaded with antioxidants and actually have the highest concentration of protein of any fruit! Believe it or not, this superfood also boasts fifteen times the amount of iron than what spinach has. They are delicious paired with coconut, cacao nibs, and walnuts and can top everything from multigrain porridge to açai bowls to homemade trail mix. Try substituting them for dried fruit in muffin recipes.

Hemp Seeds. Also known as hemp hearts, these seeds come from a variety of the cannabis plant, and are considered to be one of nature's perfect foods. Hemp seeds are packed with a type of protein that is a lot more easily digestible by our bodies than animal proteins. They also carry all nine of the essential amino acids needed for optimum health, and the rarely found gamma-linoleic acid (GLA), a powerful anti-inflammatory omega-6 fatty acid. Hemp seeds are also high in vitamin E, fiber, zinc, and iron. Hemp seeds have a pleasant, slightly nutty flavor with a smooth texture that allows them to be blended easily. Their light flavor is hard to detect when added to cookies, granolas, smoothies, and so on. Hemp milk is also a popular alternative to dairy milk.

Lucuma Powder. Lucuma is a Peruvian fruit that actually looks similar to an avocado, but is bright yellow on the inside. This supernutritious fruit contains iron, zinc, calcium, protein, and fiber, just to name a few of the benefits. The flavor is pretty unique and similar to that of maple, caramel, and custard. This sweetener is not only unrefined and low-glycemic but actually has lots of health benefits! Try adding lucuma powder to smoothies, hot chocolate, yogurt, oatmeal, or puddings.

Maca Root Powder. Maca, a root vegetable grown in the Peruvian Andes, is well known for its ability to help enhance strength and endurance. Maca contains calcium, magnesium, and potassium, and some claim it boosts fertility, balances hormones, and gives a natural energy boost.

I think maca tastes like a smoky peanut butter and jelly sandwich; some people think maca tastes a little like butterscotch. I pair it in smoothies with peanut, almond, or cashew butter. Besides using it in smoothies, I also add it to my Peanut Larabars (recipe on my blog).

Raw Cacao Nibs. Raw cacao can be an acquired taste, for sure. It has a crunchy texture and bitter chocolate flavor that is great added to porridges, puddings, raw desserts (e.g., Bliss Balls, pages 76–77) and smoothie bowls. You can even use the nibs as you would chocolate chips, in cookies and baked goods. And when paired with unrefined sweeteners such as maple syrup or dates, cacao is the perfect substitute for sugar-laden chocolate in sweets.

REFRIGERATOR

Organic, Free-Range Eggs. Eggs are an inexpensive source of high-quality protein. But interpreting all the labels on eggs can be discouraging. Such terms as *free-range* and *cage-free* don't really mean much in relation to the nutrition of the egg or how the chickens are treated.

The two words you should look for are:

Organic. This means the chickens have been fed non-GMO organic feed and have not been given antibiotics.

Pastured. This means that chickens live outdoors and eat bugs, worms, grass, and other foods natural to a chicken's diet.

I suggest you buy pastured eggs from the farmers' market, but if that's not an option, choose eggs labeled "organic and pastured."

Miso Paste. This savory paste is made from fermented soybeans, sometimes with the addition of grains such as rice or barley, or even beans such as chickpeas. Unpasteurized and naturally fermented miso contains live, beneficial enzymes. The darker the miso, the longer it has aged and the stronger the flavor. There are many kinds, but I find the light or white to

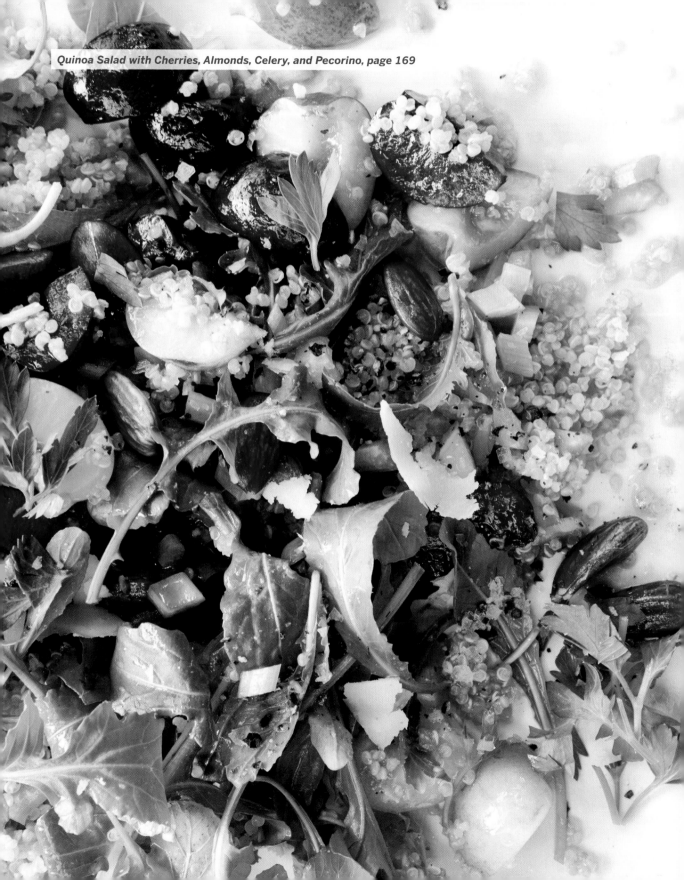

Quinoa Salad with Cherries, Almonds, Celery, and Pecorino, page 169

be the most versatile. Always buy organic or at least non-GMO, since soybeans are a genetically modified crop.

Shoyu (naturally fermented soy sauce) and Wheat-Free Tamari. These traditionally brewed options are better for you than commercial, flash-pasteurized soy sauces. Again, choose organic, non-GMO brands.

Nut Butters. Look for pure, organic nut butter without added oils or sweeteners and packed in glass jars.
Peanut butter
Raw almond butter
Cashew butter

Mustard. Whole-grain and Dijon.

FREEZER
Organic peas
Organic berries and bananas, for smoothies
Edamame
Homemade chicken and vegetable stocks

TIPS: How to freeze stock and other liquids
    You can freeze in glass (my preference) as long as the sides of the container are straight (if using jars, wide-mouth only), in BPA-free plastic containers, or in resealable bags.
    Since liquids expand when frozen, the key is to fill your container three-quarters full or within 2 inches from the top of the container so the liquid has room to expand. For a quart-size container, that means you pour in only 3 to 3½ cups of liquid.
    Next, place your container of stock in the freezer without the lid. This is a key step! Allow the stock to freeze solid and then cover with the lid. If you secure the lid on the jar before freezing, the stock may expand more than you have allowed for and that's how glass or thin plastics crack.
    I don't recommend freezing in containers larger than a quart; I haven't always had success with half-gallon glass containers.
    To freeze in a resealable bag, open up the bag in a medium-size pot or bowl and then pour in the stock (remember to fill only three-quarters full). The pot will allow you to have two hands free. Seal and freeze flat.

A PRIMER ON ANIMAL PRODUCTS

Animal products can be a part of a healthful diet. But most animal foods create inflammation in the body, which is the basis for most chronic disease. Meat consumption also has a serious negative impact on the environment—more than planes, trains, and automobiles combined.

I suggest limiting animal products to a few ounces at a time, a few times per week.

While red meat, poultry, and seafood are high in protein and contain vitamin B12 (which is not available from plant sources), not all animal products are high quality or are equally nutritious. With all the labels and confusing marketing terms, it's no wonder consumers have a hard time making the healthiest choice. Here's what you need to know. First, some terms:

Natural. "Natural" only implies that the product has been minimally processed with no artificial ingredients. This word really means very little with respect to ethics, health, organics, or sustainability.

Organic. The organic label is associated only with the food the animal ate and the lack of hormones, drugs, genetically modified feed, animal by-products, and antibiotics. The animals could have eaten grains, but they were certified organic. "Organic" does not mean the animals were treated ethically, however. I still recommend buying organic poultry and meats over nonorganic as much as possible.

NOW, SOME SPECIFICS ON TYPES OF ANIMAL PRODUCTS.

Poultry. According to the USDA, "free-range" means the poultry has had access to the outdoors. Unfortunately, what this translates to is that the birds for a very limited time each day are permitted to exit the barn through a small opening and graze outside *if* they choose to.

Pastured, on the other hand, implies animals (namely chickens and pigs) that have been raised in open fields and woods, foraging for food (primarily seeds and insects, with the occasional small rodent or reptile if they can get them), and going back into a henhouse (in the case of chickens) at night to roost, nest, and lay eggs.

Beef. Cows are biologically designed to graze on grass, not grains. Meat from cows that have been raised exclusively on grass contains a health-supportive fatty acid called conjugative linoleic acid (CLA), and more omega-3 fatty acids and less saturated fat than do grain-fed cows. It's like comparing a vegetable-eating, fit person to a fast food–eating couch potato. Which sounds like a healthier creature to you?

"Grass-fed" is technically supposed to mean that the cows have had a partial grass diet and access to pasture year-round. There is no third-party verification of this, however, and the cows can be fed grains before they go to slaughter. You want to look for a label of "100 percent grass-fed" or "grass-finished."

FISH AND SEAFOOD

I personally favor fish and seafood over meat and poultry, but there are concerns about sustainability, mercury, nuclear radiation from Japan, industrial chemicals, and pesticides in our waters. So, it's best to limit your fish consumption; I eat only a few ounces once or twice each week, and I only buy wild-caught fish that have lived in an environment natural to the fish. Wild fish have higher concentrations of anti-inflammatory omega-3 fatty acids, which are critical for brain and heart health.

Seafoodwatch.org, published by the Monterey Bay Aquarium, is a great resource for helping you make choices that lower your risk and maximize the potential health benefits of eating fish.

DAIRY

Human beings weren't designed to regularly digest milk and it is certainly not essential for good health. If you can tolerate dairy, I recommend enjoying it in small quantities with these tips in mind for better digestibility and nutrition:

Try sheep or goat dairy. The fat composition of sheep and goat milk is closer to human's than cow milk and easier to digest. For this reason, I tend to use more grated pecorino (sheep's milk) rather than Parmesan (cow's milk.)

Choose cultured dairy, such as yogurt or kefir, which contain health-supportive good bacteria for gut health.

Consume raw dairy over pasteurized. Raw contains beneficial bacteria and is more digestible.

Opt for full-fat instead of low-fat or nonfat. Studies have shown that people who eat full-fat dairy are more satisfied, snack less, and weigh less than people who eat low-fat dairy. Also, without the presence of fat, our body cannot absorb the important fat-soluble vitamins A, D, E, and K.

What to Buy Organic

With respect to food, there are many reasons to choose organic as often as possible, from your health to the health of the workers who pick the crops and the health of the planet.

Unfortunately, organic goods usually come with a higher price tag, so most people need to make choices as to what are the more important items to buy organic. Here's my own organic buying guide to help you get the most (or fewest pesticides) for your dollar.

Butter. Many toxins, including pesticides, are fat-soluble and tend to concentrate in the fat of animals and humans. Since butter is 100 percent fat, it is not surprising that nonorganic butter can contain up to twenty times as many pesticides as nonorganic vegetables do.

Meat and Poultry. According to Elson Haas in his book *Staying Healthy with Nutrition*, [conventionally raised] meat is among the most contaminated products in our food supply. The animals are raised under inhumane and unsanitary feedlot conditions and result in very unhealthy animals treated with antibiotics, steroids, and hormones. Organic meat is free of these things; in addition, organic meat indicates animals that have been fed pesticide-free food. To locate organic beef or poultry in your area, visit organicconsumers.org or your local farmers' market.

Dairy Products. In general, I'm not a big fan of pasteurized milk, but I realize not everyone has access to or is comfortable with the idea of raw dairy, so if you do choose to consume dairy, please buy organic and preferably nonhomogenized. Conventional milk can contain high levels of antibiotics and hormones, as well as pesticides. Many pediatricians are concerned that these hormones could initiate early puberty, given how much milk kids drink on a daily basis.

Produce—The "Dirty Dozen." According to the Environmental Working Group (EWG), the top ten conventionally grown fruits and veggies with the highest pesticide load are:

Apples
Peaches
Nectarines
Strawberries
Grapes
Celery
Spinach
Sweet bell peppers
Cucumbers
Cherry tomatoes
Snap peas
Potatoes

Just buying the organic versions of these fruits and vegetables will reduce your exposure by up to 90 percent.

Corn, Soybeans, Canola. Along with cotton, these are the largest genetically modified crops in America. A genetically modified organism, or GMO, is a food that has been spliced with the genes of another organism, such as a tomato with a fish gene. There is plenty of controversy as to whether GMO foods are safe, especially since their effects haven't been studied over a long period of time. My gut tells me to stick with foods that are natural, whose DNA hasn't been tinkered with, so I try to avoid GMO foods like the plague. Corn, soybeans, and canola labeled "organic" is supposed to mean that they are not only grown without pesticides, but have also *not* been genetically modified.

New on the GMO scene are alfalfa, papaya, sugar beets, tomatoes, and zucchini. So, if you are trying to avoid GMOs, you must look for certified organic versions of these foods, too.

Peanut Products. Peanuts have a tendency to grow a toxic mold called aflatoxin, so they are very heavily sprayed. According to the Pesticide Action Network, peanuts rank among the top ten foods contaminated with persistent organic pollutants. The good news is that you can find organic, GMO-free peanut products, including peanut butter, pretty easily.

Baby Food. Babies and children eat more for their body weight than adults do and their body can't process as many toxins as an adult body can. Their immune and nervous systems are more vulnerable, so I wouldn't think twice about buying organic baby food. You can easily make your own organic baby food or choose from many high-quality brands.

Foods That You Consume Regularly. This is important for minimizing your overall exposure to chemicals. For example, if you consume olive oil, oats, rice, and eggs most days of the week, then those would be good to buy organic.

The Clean 15. It's not all gloom and doom. The Environmental Working Group has also published a list of "The Clean 15," which are lower-pesticide foods and therefore okay to buy conventionally grown.

Avocados
Pineapple
Cabbage
Sweet peas
Onions
Asparagus
Mangoes
Papayas
Kiwis
Eggplant
Grapefruit
Cantaloupe
Cauliflower
Sweet potatoes
Mushrooms

12 EASY WAYS TO GET HEALTHIER

The best way to make changes that last a lifetime is to start small. Here are a few easy ways you can be healthier every day.

Start your day with a mug of warm water with the juice of half a lemon.
Meditate for 5 minutes (or more!).
Drink 2 quarts of water.
Move! Do some form of exercise (a walk, jumping jacks, dancing) even if it's just 20 minutes.
Eat a vegetable at every meal.
Chew your food more than you normally do—aim for 30 chews per bite.
Cut some vegetables and store in the refrigerator for snacking during the week.
Start taking a high-quality probiotic.
Throw away your bottled salad dressings and make one from scratch with an unrefined oil.
Do a digital detox 2 hours before bedtime.
Go to sleep by 10:00 p.m.
Feel gratitude.

Common Substitutions

It's crucial to make informed choices when it comes to our well-being. The decision to buy organic may cost a bit more, but you are making an investment in your health, that of your family, and the environment.

Interacting with hundreds of students regularly has helped me understand the challenges that allergies and dietary intolerances impose on the home cook when planning a meal that needs to accommodate the whole family. The recipe codes on page 28 are provided at the top of each recipe to help you quickly know whether that recipe fits your needs. That said, whenever possible, for the recipes in this book I have provided substitutions for several common allergens, such as gluten and dairy, and for dietary preferences, such as vegetarian or vegan.

I have been asked for a substitution for literally every single ingredient I have ever used from the most common allergens, including gluten, dairy, soy, nuts, and eggs, to seemingly innocuous foods, such as olive oil and peaches. I am very aware that there are many people who need to know basic substitutions due to intolerances, but it's good to know these swaps in the event you are out of something.

Butter. Butter does add a unique flavor to recipes and helps to promote browning. But if you are dairy-free, you can use unrefined virgin coconut oil or vegan organic butter, such as Earth Balance, in any recipe. Keep in mind that coconut oil may impart a slight coconut flavor to the recipe.

Earth Balance contains some salt, so you may consider reducing the salt slightly in the recipe.

Buttermilk. I do like using buttermilk occasionally since it provides acidity that helps keep such things as pancakes and muffins tender, and can lend creaminess and tang to some salad dressings.

1 cup of buttermilk
Swap: ½ cup of plain, unsweetened whole yogurt (dairy or nondairy) + ½ cup of milk (dairy or nondairy)

or 1 cup of plain, unsweetened kefir

or place 1 tablespoon of cider vinegar in a 1-cup measuring cup and add dairy or nondairy milk to make 1 cup

Egg. Eggs that are used as a binder in baked goods or to add leavening can go with these substitutes:

1 egg
Swap: 1 flax or chia egg: 1 tablespoon of flax meal or ground chia seeds + 3 tablespoons of warm water

In a small bowl, combine the chia seeds or flax meal with the water and stir. Let the mixture sit and stir it occasionally for about 10 minutes, or until the mixture has the consistency of a raw egg white.

Or swap: aquafaba (a.k.a. liquid from cooked white beans or chickpeas—the thicker, the better)

Use 3 tablespoons of liquid for each whole egg,

2 tablespoons for each egg white, and 1 tablespoon for each egg yolk.

In the case of actual eggs in a frittata or a scramble, there are substitutes for that, too:

For every 2 eggs, sub 7 ounces of extra-firm tofu, preferably organic and sprouted

+ 1 tablespoon of nutritional yeast + ¼ teaspoon of ground turmeric

For 1 egg in custard or in the cheesecake recipe, swap ¼ cup of silken tofu, pureed.

Flour. Flours, such as wheat or spelt, are used in baking, for pancakes and waffles, or for coating meats, just to name a few examples. If you have a gluten-free flour blend that you find consistently works one for one in place of gluten flours, it should work in the recipes in this book.

1 cup of gluten flour, such as wheat

To make a recipe gluten-free, I recommend substituting 1 cup of King Arthur Gluten-Free Multi-Purpose Flour for the original flour. I also recommend adding xanthan gum. Xanthan gum mimics the elasticity of gluten and will help provide structure to your batter. Refer to the package instructions for how much xanthan gum to add per cup of flour because it varies according to what you are making. You do not need to add xanthan gum to gluten-free pancake or waffle batter, or if the flour is being used to thicken a pie or for dredging meat.

If you are wheat-intolerant, but not gluten-free, you can substitute spelt flour one for one for wheat flour. The only exception is pancake batter, which can take about ⅞ cup of spelt flour for 1 cup of wheat flour.

If a recipe calls for oat flour, you may use a gluten-free oat flour.

You cannot substitute a nut flour or coconut flour for a grain flour.

Honey. Honey is not vegan nor should it be given to babies under the age of twelve months because it can cause a rare type of botulism (food poisoning). Maple syrup may be substituted in equal amounts in any recipe in this book.

Milk. Nut or seed milks can be substituted for dairy milk in any recipe in this book. You may also substitute half culinary coconut milk and half nut milk for dairy milk. See specific substitution suggestions for buttermilk.

Nuts. If you have a nut allergy and a recipe contains nuts, you have a couple of options. With respect to any recipe in the Salad or Vegetable chapter, you can either omit the nuts altogether or substitute seeds such as pumpkin or sesame seeds, or crunchy chickpeas. For pesto recipes, replace nuts one for one with sunflower seeds.

If you are allergic to a specific nut, feel free to substitute another nut in its place.

Almond extract may be omitted in every recipe.

Red Pepper Flakes, Cayenne, Hot Sauce, Sriracha, or Fresh Chiles. If you cannot tolerate any heat or spiciness, just omit any of the above, or reduce the amount. They are not equal in terms of heat level, so you cannot substitute them one for one with each other.

Shoyu/Soy Sauce. Gluten-free tamari can be substituted one for one for shoyu if you are trying to avoid wheat. If you are trying to avoid soy, you can substitute coconut aminos one for one.

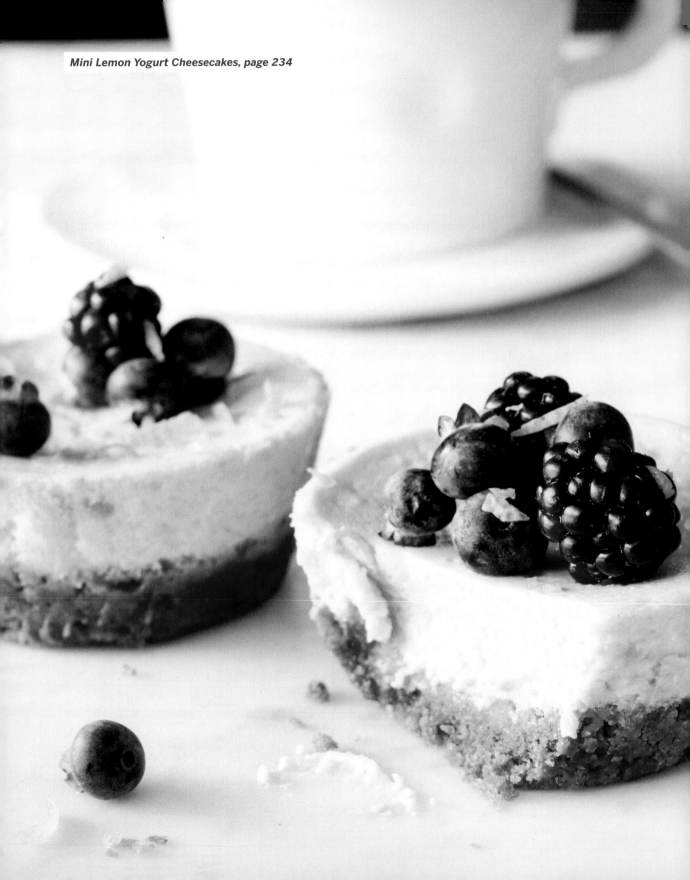

Mini Lemon Yogurt Cheesecakes, page 234

How to Create a Balanced Meal

Imagine a dinner plate. Now, place nonstarchy vegetables, such as Crispy Stovetop Brussels Sprouts (page 106) on half of the plate. On one quarter of the plate, add whole grains or a starchy vegetable, such as Herbed Mixed-Grain Pilaf (page 149). On the remaining quarter of the plate, add lean animal protein or a vegetarian protein, such as legumes. This is just one way to create a balanced meal, but the exercise here is to emphasize plant foods, especially nonstarchy vegetables, which will provide you with the most nutrition for the fewest calories.

In addition, consider how the flavors of everything will complement one another as well as the complexity of the recipes; you don't need to overcomplicate anything by making more than one time-consuming dish at once!

CREATING A WEEKLY MEAL PLAN

I have been making a weekly dinner plan on Sunday mornings for at least twenty years and honestly, given my schedule, it is the only way dinner happens. Knowing on Sunday what you are cooking for the week allows you to go through each day without the "dinner cloud" over your head. You know, the one that is always nagging, "What are you going to make for dinner tonight?" "Should you start defrosting that chicken?" "Hurry and run to the market before after-school pickup!" That is all way too stressful.

After I started posting my weekly dinner plan on my blog and offering it in my classes, I was flooded with feedback from people who said it changed their lives. They were cooking more and stressing less; they were saving money because they approached grocery shopping with a list and only bought what would be used. Their families were thrilled! That's the idea.

Here's how to do it:

Set up the calendar: Check your calendar for the week and look to see who is home for dinner each night and how busy you are each day. For example, if my husband and I are out and the kids are home, I will choose one of the kids' favorite dinners that I don't mind missing out on. You might see that you're busy in the late afternoon and need a slow cooker meal that night or something that can be prepared ahead, such as a casserole that can be easily popped in the oven. Write down the days on which you would like to cook at home and whether you're accommodating more or less than the normal crew.

Check the current inventory: Make a note of anything in the refrigerator and freezer that needs to get used up so that it doesn't go to waste. These items should be incorporated into the week's meals.

Create your own cookbook: I love having all my favorite recipes in one place; that way I can scan the repertoire quickly and make decisions as to what goes on the meal plan. You can photocopy your go-to recipes from cookbooks or print them from blogs and file them in a binder by category (e.g., meatless mains, soups, etc.). I use Pinterest to save recipes that I would like to make or that inspire me.

Be democratic: Ask your family for suggestions for meals. (Or don't!)

Be strategic: The most perishable items should be placed on the meal plan earlier in the week. For example, fresh fish doesn't last more than a day in the refrigerator. So, fresh fish should go on the menu on the day you go shopping. You can double a recipe so you have leftovers for lunch or dinner the next day. You can also use leftovers in a different way. Making chili on Tuesday? Wednesday's baked potatoes can be topped with the remaining chili.

Find balance: If you cook six nights a week, maybe try to prepare two or three vegetarian meals, one or two fish, two poultry, and one or no beef. Look for where you can incorporate leafy green vegetables and cruciferous vegetables into several meals. It's also good to try to provide a wide variety of different whole grains and starches.

Learn what is in season: Planning your meals around what is in season has its benefits, namely more flavorful, more nutritious food; lower cost due to greater supply; and following the cycle of eating as nature intended, by consuming a diverse set of nutrients appropriate to the season. Here are some seasonal basics:

Spring: artichokes, asparagus, avocados, beets, chard, cherries, leeks, mangoes, peas, radishes, spinach, strawberries

Summer: bell peppers, berries, cucumbers, eggplant, figs, grapes, green beans, melons, stone fruit, sweet corn, tomatoes, zucchini

Fall: apples, fennel, pears, persimmons, pomegranate, sweet potatoes, winter squashes

Winter: broccoli, Brussels sprouts, cauliflower, citrus, kale, rutabaga, turnips

Year-round: cabbage, carrots, celery and celery root, lettuces, mushrooms, onions, potatoes

RECIPE CODES

Vegan: Contains no products derived from an animal, including honey or bee pollen

Vegetarian: Contains no meat, poultry, game, fish, or shellfish; may contain animal-derived dairy or eggs.

GF (gluten-free): Contains no wheat, spelt, rye, barley, Kamut, or farro. If oats or other grains that may be contaminated with gluten are required, those ingredients will be clearly noted.

DF (dairy-free): Contains no products derived from the milk of an animal.

Vegan adaptable: Ingredients may be substituted or omitted to create a vegan recipe. In vegan-adaptable recipes, the nonvegan ingredients will be clearly noted.

Vegetarian adaptable: Ingredients may be substituted or omitted to create a vegetarian recipe. In vegetarian-adaptable recipes, the nonvegetarian ingredients will be clearly noted in parentheses.

GF adaptable: Ingredients may be substituted or omitted to create a recipe free from gluten. In GF-adaptable recipes, the ingredients that contain gluten will be clearly noted in parentheses.

DF adaptable: Ingredients may be substituted or omitted to create a recipe free from dairy. In DF-adaptable recipes, the ingredients that contain dairy will be clearly noted in parentheses.

Tips for Prepping in Advance

When it comes to prepping recipes for your week in advance, you really have to do what works for you. A basic rule of thumb regarding produce: It slowly loses its nutritional value beginning the moment that it is harvested. So, the fresher, the better. If you have the flexibility, the longer you wait to prep fresh produce, the better. The following is a guide to which vegetables and foods can be prepped in advance and which are best to do as you go.

Vegetables. Whether you are cooking a vegetable on its own or to be mixed with other ingredients (e.g., a stir-fry or soup), you can prep it in advance. By "prep," I mean wash, dry, peel (if appropriate), and cut up. To prevent drying out in the refrigerator, put a damp paper towel on top of the cut vegetables and store in an airtight container.

You can also blanch vegetables 1 to 2 days in advance and store in the refrigerator. Blanching is to boil in salted water until just tender and then to shock in ice water to stop the cooking process. Drain, pat dry, and refrigerate.

Vegetables to be added to a dish cooked, such as in a frittata or casserole, can be sautéed or roasted the day before and stored in the refrigerator. Same goes for a stand-alone vegetable, such as spaghetti squash.

Asparagus and Green Beans: Can be washed, trimmed, and stored in an airtight container or a resealable bag for 2 to 3 days.

Avocado (technically a fruit, but I've included it here with veggies): Can be peeled, pitted, sliced or cubed 2 to 3 hours in advance. Arrange in one layer on a plate and cover tightly with plastic wrap, adhering the wrap to the avocado to prevent any exposure to air.

Carrots: Carrots can be peeled in advance (if roasting them whole) or peeled and chopped, shredded, or grated up to 3 to 4 days in advance. Store in a sealed bag or container with an airtight lid in the refrigerator.

Bell Peppers: Can be washed, cored, and seeded 2 to 3 days in advance. Store whole or sliced/chopped in a sealed bag or container with an airtight lid in the refrigerator.

Broccoli and Cauliflower: Can be washed and cut into florets 2 to 3 days in advance. Store in a sealed bag or container with an airtight lid in the refrigerator.

Brussels Sprouts: Brussels sprouts can dry out, so you can slice these as you go. But prepping the day ahead is fine, especially if you're going to cook them versus use them raw.

Cabbage: Can be washed and chopped, sliced, or shredded 1 to 2 days in advance. Store in a sealed bag or container with an airtight lid in the refrigerator.

Celery: Celery can be washed and chopped 3 to 4 days in advance. Store in a sealed bag or container with an airtight lid in the refrigerator.

Eggplant: Can brown when exposed to air, so it's good to peel/cut/cube/slice as you go.

Fennel: Can be washed, then thinly sliced or chopped 2 to 3 days in advance. Store in a sealed bag or container with an airtight lid in the refrigerator.

Garlic: Can be peeled and whole cloves stored in a glass jar or resealable bag until ready to use. Stays good for 7 to 10 days. Fresh minced garlic can lose its flavor/potency when prepared too far in advance, so chop as you go to preserve the flavor. You can also find frozen, minced garlic in markets. These are fine as long as there are no preservatives added.

Ginger: Can be peeled in advance and stored in the freezer. No need to defrost before grating.

Onions: Chop or slice 1 to 2 days in advance, but keep in a tightly sealed glass container or a double-bagged resealable bag (if you don't double the bags, your refrigerator will likely smell like onions and infuse the foods surrounding it).

Potatoes: Peel or pare and chop up to a day in advance. Store in a bowl of cold water in the refrigerator.

Sweet Potatoes: Peel and chop 3 to 4 days in advance. Store in a sealed bag or container with an airtight lid in the refrigerator.

Winter Squash: Peel, seed, and chop 3 to 4 days in advance. Store in a sealed bag or container with an airtight lid in the refrigerator.

Zucchini: Wash and chop, slice, or shred 2 to 3 days in advance. Store in a sealed bag or container with an airtight lid in the refrigerator.

Greens: Heartier greens such as collard greens, kale, Swiss chard, and beet greens can be washed and sliced or chopped 2 to 3 days in advance.

More tender greens such as butter, romaine, red leaf, or green leaf lettuce can be washed 2 to 3 days in advance. Allow to dry for a few hours on a clean towel on your countertop or upright in a dish drainer in the sink. Store in a clean bag in the crisper drawer. Tear or cut for salads just before serving to prevent oxidation.

Herbs. Cilantro, parsley, dill, thyme, rosemary, and mint: Trim the stems, wash, dry, and store in a glass jar with an inch of water at the bottom, and cover with a plastic bag. After 1 week, change the water. If using within a few days, washed herbs can be put in a resealable plastic bag and stored in the fridge. These herbs can be chopped a few hours in advance, if necessary, but will give you the best results if you cut as you go, and even better if you tear by hand. They can oxidize and lose flavor.

Basil, Sage, and Chives: Wash these herbs as you need (they will brown or wilt if done too far in advance) and chop as you go.

Fruits. Certain fruits will never get eaten in my house unless I have done the work in advance (hello, pomegranates!). But many fruits are susceptible to oxidation and should be prepped as needed.

Apples: If slicing a few hours in advance, store in cold water to prevent oxidation.

Berries: Strawberries are the only berry you should wash or prep (hull, slice, or dice) in advance, and perhaps only 1 day ahead. Blackberries, raspberries, and blueberries are all best to wash as needed; otherwise they can become soggy or moldy.

Citrus: Can be peeled and segmented 3 to 4 days in advance. Store in an airtight container in the refrigerator.

Grapes: Can be washed and stored 4 to 5 days in the refrigerator in an open container.

Melons (Cantaloupe, Honeydew, Watermelon), Mangoes, and Pineapple: These can all be cut 3 to 4 days in advance and kept in an airtight container in the refrigerator.

Pomegranate seeds: Can be stored 4 to 5 days in the refrigerator in an airtight container.

Stone Fruits (Peaches, Plums, Nectarines) and Pears: Best to wash and prep these as needed.

Grains and Legumes. Quinoa, farro, rice, barley, millet, beans, and lentils can be cooked 3 to 4 days advance and stored in the refrigerator. You can also prepare these 2 to 3 months in advance and store them in the freezer. If preparing any of these from scratch, you can always make extra and freeze. (See pages 130, 131 for how to cook basic quinoa and brown rice, and page 129 for how to cook beans from scratch.) Defrost in the refrigerator or countertop and reheat on the stove with a little water when ready to consume.

Salad Dressings. Salad dressings can be made up to a week in advance and stored in the refrigerator or in a cool, dark place in the kitchen. Dairy-based dressing should be refrigerated and will only last for a couple of days. If refrigerated, dressings made with olive oil will solidify. So, leave them on the counter for an hour to come to room temperature, and shake to re-emulsify. See page 255 for the best vinaigrette that goes with any salad.

Stock. Chicken and vegetable stock can be made in advance and kept in the refrigerator for 3 to 4 days, or frozen for up to 3 months (see page 20 for how to freeze). Defrost in the fridge overnight or on your countertop for a few hours. See the Basics section for homemade stock recipes.

Cheese. Most cheeses can be shredded or sliced up to 5 days in advance.

Poached or Roasted Chicken. Precooked chicken is convenient to have on hand for casseroles, salads, soups, quesadillas, and enchiladas. Cooked chicken can be stored for up to 2 days in the refrigerator in an airtight container.

Dry Mixes. If you want to bake a cake or make pancakes, for example, you can mix all the dry ingredients ahead and store in an airtight container at room temperature for a month (or two!).

Hard-Boiled Eggs. Cook and shock in cold water (to stop the cooking process) and refrigerate for either 2 days peeled or up to a week

10 EASY SWAPS TO MAKE TODAY

If you are motivated and committed to getting healthy, why not give your pantry an overhaul? Remove chemical-laden foods and expired items and replace them with higher-quality, health-promoting ones. Or take the slow, but steady approach and make one new swap or try one new food each week.

Out: processed table salt
In: moderate amounts of mineral-rich, unrefined sea salts—Celtic, Himalayan, or Maldon.

Out: refined vegetables oils such as corn, canola, and soybean
In: unrefined, cold-pressed olive oil, avocado oil, coconut oil, and ghee (clarified butter)

Out: acid-forming, nonnutritive white sugar
In: limited quantities of pure maple or brown rice syrups, coconut sugar, stevia, and raw honey

Out: excess gluten, especially refined flours made from wheat, spelt, rye, and barley
In: brown rice, quinoa, millet, legumes, and sweet potatoes

Out: refined, nutrient-stripped white flour
In: fiber-rich whole wheat pastry flour or whole spelt flour

Out: mass-produced, factory-farmed animal meat
In: healthier animals raised in their natural environment

Out: imitation vanilla extract with corn syrup solids
In: pure vanilla extract

Out: processed, GMO cornstarch
In: arrowroot powder

Out: artificial food coloring
In: natural or homemade food colors

unpeeled (see page 248 for how to cook hard-boiled eggs).

Casseroles. Anything that is to be assembled and then baked can usually be made up to the point of baking and refrigerated, covered, 8 to 12 hours in advance (or even the night before). Examples include baked ziti, mac and cheese, gratins, rice bake, and millet casserole.

Marinades. Make the day before you need them and store in the refrigerator. Marinate meats or fish according to the recipe.

A NOTE ABOUT CONTAINERS

As much as possible, use glass for storage in the pantry, refrigerator, and the freezer. Plastic is something to be avoided if you have a choice. Toxins such as BPA, BPS, and phthalates, leach from plastic containers into our food and have been shown to disrupt the endocrine system, wreak havoc with our hormones, and are even linked with certain cancers. Remember that children have a lower body weight and toxins disproportionately affect their body. It is virtually impossible to avoid plastic, but you still have many opportunities to make a better choice. I removed all plastic from my kitchen in favor of glass and stainless steel.

My favorite containers for storing food in the refrigerator and freezer are by Glasslock because they are easy to clean, don't leach, keep things airtight and stack well. I recommend the square and rectangular shapes over round since they use space more efficiently. You can find these containers at many supermarkets, Bed Bath and Beyond, the Container Store, and Amazon.

I use Neat-os reusable canvas bags for storing clean produce in the refrigerator.

In the pantry, I keep all my nuts, seeds, coconut flakes, and dried fruit in hermetic glass storage jars. All of our reusable water bottles are glass or stainless steel. For little ones, there are silicone options.

For those of you looking for dishes that are not breakable, you can try enameled tin or at least look for BPA-free plastic, but never reheat food in plastic.

CLEANING UP AS YOU GO

The only part about cooking that I don't love is doing the dishes. It's not so fun to sit down to a meal with piles of dirty bowls and pots in the background. My grandmother taught me to clean up as I go and that was excellent advice. While you're cooking, keep a bowl of warm soapy water in the sink to use as you move through a recipe. When you have a minute, wash whatever you just used; it makes cleanup at the end much less painful. Try to use the least toxic products you can find.

You must wash your dishes with hot water for them to get very clean. Washing in hot water also helps the dishes dry more quickly in the dish drainer. Wear rubber gloves when washing dishes so that you can use the hottest water possible without being uncomfortable.

The dishwasher is also very efficient at cleaning a lot of dishes for less water than when you hand-wash.

If your stainless-steel pots and pans start to lose their luster, you can use a little Bar Keepers Friend or Bon Ami powder to shine them back up.

Lastly, keep baking soda on hand for burnt-on messes. Sprinkle a few tablespoons of baking soda on your pot or pan and add an inch or two of water. Put the pan over the heat and bring the water to a boil. Scrape the pan with a wooden turner or a plastic scraper while the baking soda helps lift the burnt bits off the surface.

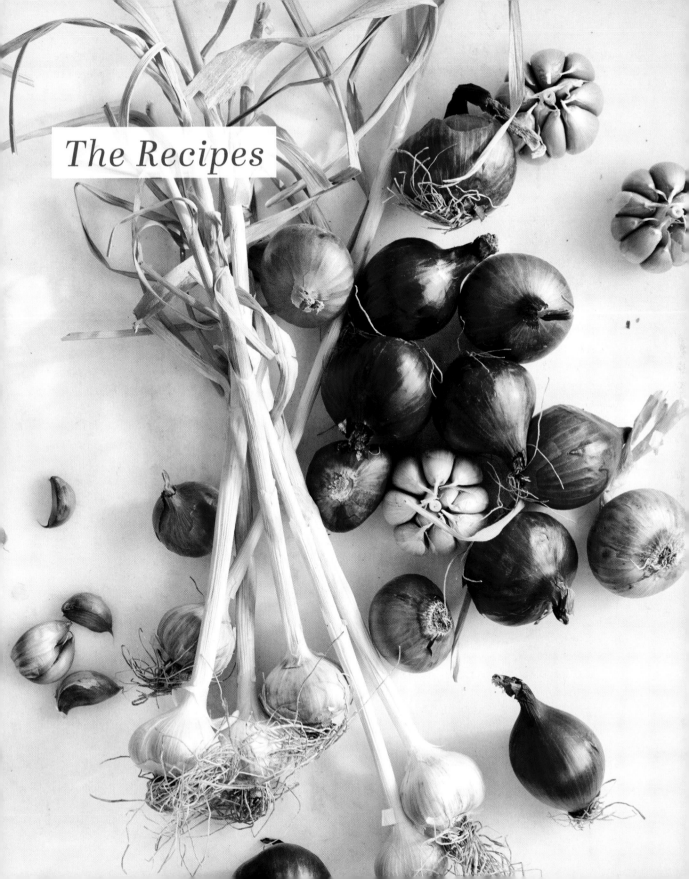

The Recipes

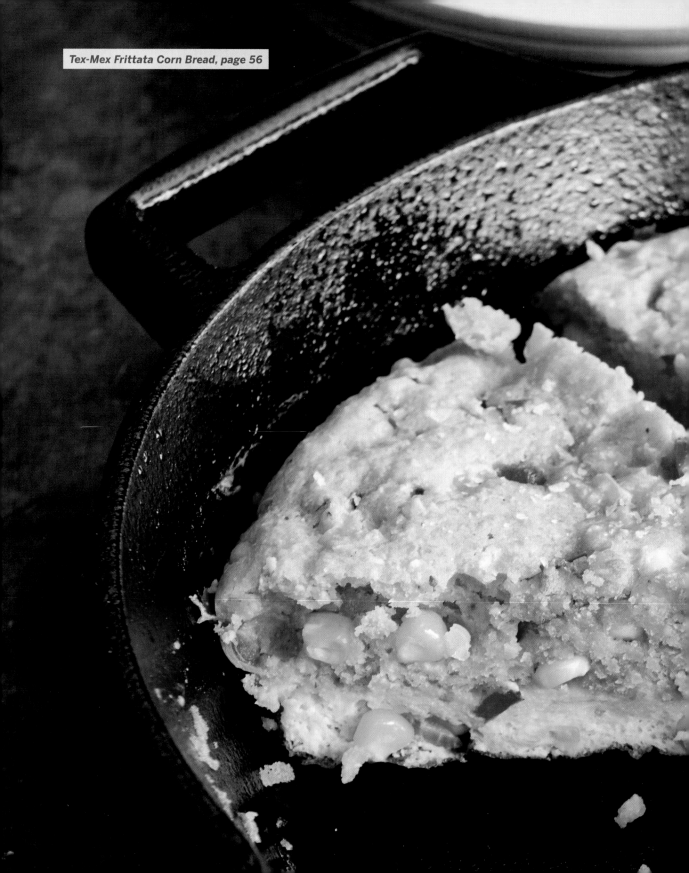

Tex-Mex Frittata Corn Bread, page 56

BETTER BREAKFASTS

Every morning is an opportunity for a fresh start. I believe that breakfast sets the tone for the rest of the day. My kids know they're not leaving the house without a proper breakfast, one that contains protein, good fats, and complex carbohydrates—and is filling and satisfying. Children especially need to eat breakfast in the morning to help stimulate their brain, provide blood sugar stability (for energy, mood, and focus), and supply their cells with enough fuel to make it through to their next meal.

Even though most of these recipes are more traditional, breakfast doesn't have to be. One of my favorite things to eat in the morning during the cooler months is soup. Furthermore, there's nothing wrong with last night's leftovers or a sandwich with protein or a quesadilla for breakfast.

But for many people, the struggle with eating a good breakfast is not in finding the recipes; it's finding the time to make them! Remember when I said being organized is the key to eating healthfully? That is especially true for breakfast. Make a breakfast plan for yourself at the beginning of the week or come up with a repeating schedule of oatmeal on Monday, eggs and toast on Tuesday, yogurt and granola on Wednesday, pancakes on Thursday, and so on, leaving the weekends for experimenting with new and more time-consuming recipes. There are several recipes here that can be made the night before, or that can be frozen and defrosted overnight. No time to cook? Look at the page of my go-to quick breakfasts.

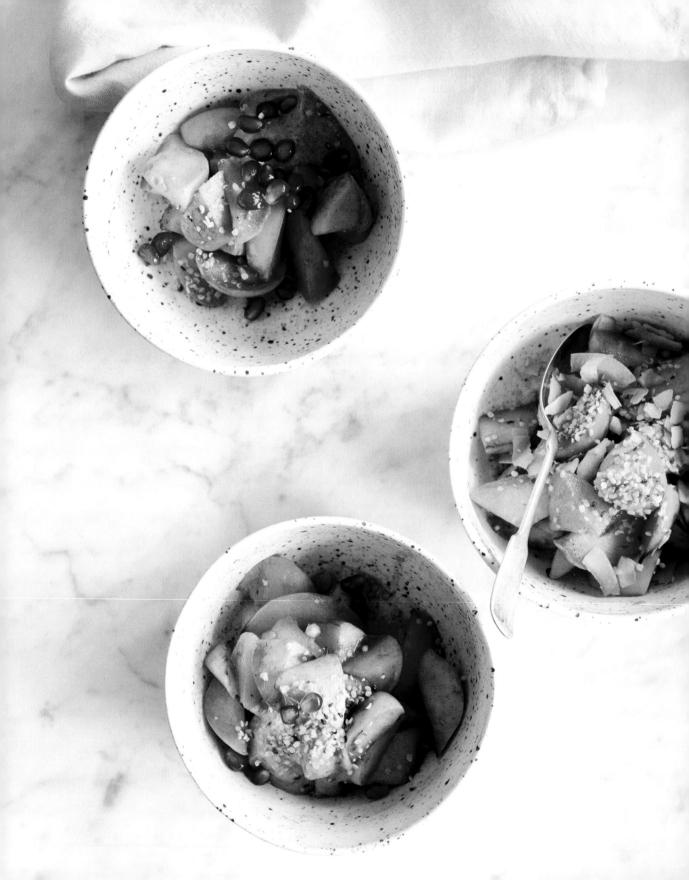

Sautéed Apple Power Bowl

SERVES 2 · GF, VEGAN ADAPTABLE, DF ADAPTABLE

You'll be surprised how satisfying a bowl of warm, cinnamon-laced apple chunks can be. I originally came up with this after my son asked me to make him "the inside of an apple pie." Once I added some protein and good fats, it became one of our favorite breakfasts. Note: Although this recipe serves two, it can easily be increased to serve more.

1. Warm the coconut oil in a 9- or 10-inch skillet over medium heat. Add the apple chunks to the skillet and sauté until lightly golden brown on all sides, 5 to 6 minutes.
2. Add the juice, cinnamon, and a pinch of salt and increase the heat to high so that the juice simmers, stirring the apples occasionally. Cook until the juice is almost all evaporated, 4 to 5 minutes. The apples should be tender, but not falling apart. Remove from the heat.
3. Serve with your favorite protein and crunchy add-ins. My favorites are a drizzle of almond butter, pomegranate seeds, hemp seeds, and toasted coconut flakes.

TIPS: There are so many varieties of apples to choose from. Tart apples include Granny Smith and Pippin, sweet include Fuji and Golden Delicious, and my favorites are the tart-sweet varieties, such as Pink Lady and Honeycrisp. Since apple is a heavily sprayed fruit, try to buy organic whenever possible.

The antioxidants in apples are concentrated in the peel, which also contains a compound that helps suppress breast cancer cells.

2 teaspoons unrefined virgin coconut oil

2 apples, any variety, unpeeled, cored and chopped into 1-inch pieces

½ cup unsweetened apple juice or water

½ teaspoon ground cinnamon

Pinch of sea salt

Add some protein: a drizzle of nut or seed butter, or a dollop of Greek yogurt (not vegan/DF)

Add something crunchy: chopped nuts, seeds, toasted coconut, pomegranate seeds, GF/DF granola (for homemade, see page 40)

Smoothie Bowls

SERVES 2 TO 3 · GF, DF, VEGAN ADAPTABLE

While smoothie bowls are everywhere these days, I prefer to make them at home; I have control over bulking up the smoothie without adding an excess of sweet stuff and I'll save money, too. The key is to make the consistency of the smoothie base thick enough that your toppings won't sink. My bowls all revolve around frozen, ripe bananas, which make the creamiest smoothies. If you can't tolerate bananas, frozen figs and frozen pears are pretty good substitutes. If you don't have frozen fruit, you can use fresh, but the smoothie will be thinner. Although I have provided recipes here, I never make a smoothie or a smoothie bowl the same way twice! Feel free to start with these measurements and adapt to create your own favorites.

Banana-Berry Smoothie Bowl

3 ripe bananas, peeled and cut into 1-inch pieces, frozen (about 2 cups), or 1½ ripe bananas, frozen + 4 frozen figs

1 cup frozen strawberries or blueberries

⅔ to ¾ cup unsweetened almond milk (page 257) or DF milk of choice, or coconut water

½ teaspoon pure vanilla extract (optional)

Optional filler to add fiber and cut down on the sweetness: ½ cup or more of one of the following: sprouted tofu (any kind), cold or frozen steamed cauliflower, frozen green peas, fresh or frozen mild greens such as spinach or chard, cold certified-GF oatmeal, cold pumpkin puree or cooked sweet potato, cooked white beans, avocado

Optional toppings: bee pollen (not vegan), hemp seeds, raw cacao nibs, toasted coconut, chopped walnuts or almonds, fresh berries, GF/DF granola (for homemade, see page 40)

1. Place the bananas and strawberries in a food processor or high-powered blender. Add the almond milk and vanilla and filler of choice, if using. Process until smooth and creamy. I find that the food processor needs a little more liquid and a few more seconds to achieve the desired consistency, which is anywhere between a thick smoothie and soft-serve ice cream.

2. Pour the smoothie into bowls and serve immediately with your desired toppings, if using.
3. You can also store the smoothie bowl in the freezer for another time, but you'll need to allow it to sit on the countertop to soften up for a few minutes before eating.

Chocolate Smoothie Bowl

4 frozen bananas (about 2⅔ cups banana chunks)

2 tablespoons raw cacao powder

6 tablespoons to ½ cup unsweetened almond milk (page 257) or DF milk of choice, or coconut water

½ teaspoon pure vanilla extract

Optional filler to add fiber and cut down on the sweetness: ½ cup or more of one of the following: sprouted tofu (any kind), cold or frozen steamed cauliflower, frozen green peas, fresh or frozen mild greens such as spinach or chard, cold certified-GF oatmeal, cold pumpkin puree or cooked sweet potato, cooked white beans, avocado

My favorite healthy toppings: bee pollen (not vegan), hemp seeds, raw cacao nibs, toasted coconut, chopped walnuts or almonds, fresh berries, GF/DF granola (for homemade, see page 40)

I also like stirring chopped cherries into the smoothie base.

Mint Chip Smoothie Bowl

2 cups baby spinach leaves or other baby greens

1 small avocado, peeled and pitted (about ²/₃ cup diced)

3 frozen bananas

½ teaspoon pure vanilla extract

⅛ teaspoon peppermint extract

½ cup unsweetened almond milk (page 257) or DF milk of choice, or coconut water

Sometimes I like to add ½ teaspoon chlorella or 2 teaspoons matcha powder to this one.

Optional filler to add bulk and cut down on the sweetness: ½ cup or more of one of the following: sprouted tofu (any kind), cold or frozen steamed cauliflower, frozen green peas, cold certified-GF oatmeal, cold pumpkin puree or cooked sweet potato, cooked white beans

Top with raw cacao nibs, DF mini dark chocolate chips, or shaved DF dark chocolate.

Mocha Smoothie Bowl

4 frozen bananas (about 2²/₃ cups banana chunks)

2 tablespoons raw cacao powder

6 tablespoons to ½ cup unsweetened almond milk (page 257) or DF milk of choice, or coconut water

½ teaspoon pure vanilla extract

2 teaspoons instant coffee powder or replace half the almond milk with cold brewed coffee

Optional filler to add fiber and cut down on the sweetness: ½ cup or more of one of the following: sprouted tofu (any kind), cold or frozen steamed cauliflower, frozen green peas, fresh or frozen mild greens such as spinach or chard, cold certified-GF oatmeal, cold pumpkin puree or cooked sweet potato, cooked white beans, avocado

My favorite healthy toppings: bee pollen (not vegan), hemp seeds, raw cacao nibs, toasted coconut, chopped walnuts or almonds, fresh berries, GF/DF granola (for homemade, see page 40)

Peanut Butter Smoothie Bowl

4 frozen bananas about (2²/₃ cups banana chunks)

6 tablespoons to ½ cup unsweetened almond milk (page 257) or DF milk of choice, or coconut water

½ teaspoon pure vanilla extract

4 to 6 tablespoons unsweetened, unsalted peanut butter

Pinch of sea salt

You can also add 2 tablespoons of raw cacao powder to this to make a chocolate version.

Optional filler to add bulk and cut down on the sweetness: ½ cup or more of one of the following: sprouted tofu (any kind), cold or frozen steamed cauliflower, frozen green peas, fresh or frozen mild greens such as spinach or chard, cold oatmeal, cold pumpkin puree or cooked sweet potato, cooked white beans, avocado

My favorite healthy toppings: bee pollen (not vegan), hemp seeds, raw cacao nibs, toasted coconut, chopped walnuts or almonds, fresh berries, GF/DF granola (for homemade, see page 40)

TIPS: If you're using a Vitamix or another high-powered blender, you can cut bananas into larger pieces and use the smaller quantity of liquid.

How to freeze fresh fruit: Bananas should be very spotty and ripe. Peel them and cut them into chunks, smaller if your blender is weak. For other fruit, wash, dry, and remove stems, pits, and anything else you wouldn't eat. Cut into bite-size pieces.

Arrange the pieces in one layer on a plate or whatever can fit into your freezer. Freeze until firm, then place all the pieces into a container or resealable bag.

Grain-Free Superseed Granola

MAKES ABOUT 8 CUPS · VEGAN, GF, DF

2 cups raw pecans, walnuts, or a combo, roughly chopped

1 cup unsweetened flaked coconut

1 cup raw pumpkin seeds (pepitas)

¾ cup raw hulled sunflower seeds

¼ cup hemp seeds

¼ cup sesame seeds

1¼ teaspoons ground cinnamon

½ teaspoon flaky sea salt, such as Maldon (or sub fine-grain sea salt)

¼ cup unrefined virgin coconut oil, melted

¼ cup pure Grade A maple syrup

¼ cup muscovado sugar, coconut sugar, or light brown sugar

1 teaspoon pure vanilla extract

¼ teaspoon pure almond extract

I created this grain-free recipe for my daughter and it instantly became my family's preferred granola recipe—and a favorite in my cooking classes. It is remarkable how light and crispy this mixture is, and the combo of sweet and salty is completely addictive. You can use a mix of nuts; I prefer pecans as they are a little sweeter than walnuts. This recipe doesn't contain dried fruit, but feel free to customize to your likes; if you do add dried fruit, just do so after the granola has finished baking.

1. Preheat the oven to 350°F. Line a rimmed baking sheet with unbleached parchment paper.

2. Pulse 1 cup of the nuts in a blender or a food processor until very finely chopped. Transfer to a large bowl with the remaining cup of roughly chopped nuts and the coconut flakes, seeds, cinnamon, and salt and stir to combine.

3. In a small bowl, whisk together the melted coconut oil, maple syrup, sugar, vanilla, and almond extract until well blended. It is really important to mix the oil and syrup so that everything is emulsified, otherwise the syrup may burn. Add the syrup mixture to the nut mixture and stir to coat well.

4. Transfer to the prepared baking sheet and spread out evenly. Bake for 20 to 30 minutes (ovens vary), stirring occasionally, until golden brown. The mixture will not be crunchy at this point, but will become so out of the oven. Allow to cool and transfer the granola to an airtight container. Store at room temperature for up to 1 week or freeze for up to 3 months.

ASK PAMELA: How do I measure and melt coconut oil? *You can measure coconut oil by packing it into a dry measuring cup and then scooping it out to melt it. You don't need to remeasure the melted coconut oil, since it will be same amount. You can melt the oil in a small pot or metal measuring cup over low heat or place the oil in a heatproof bowl in the oven for a few minutes while it is preheating. You can also use a microwave.*

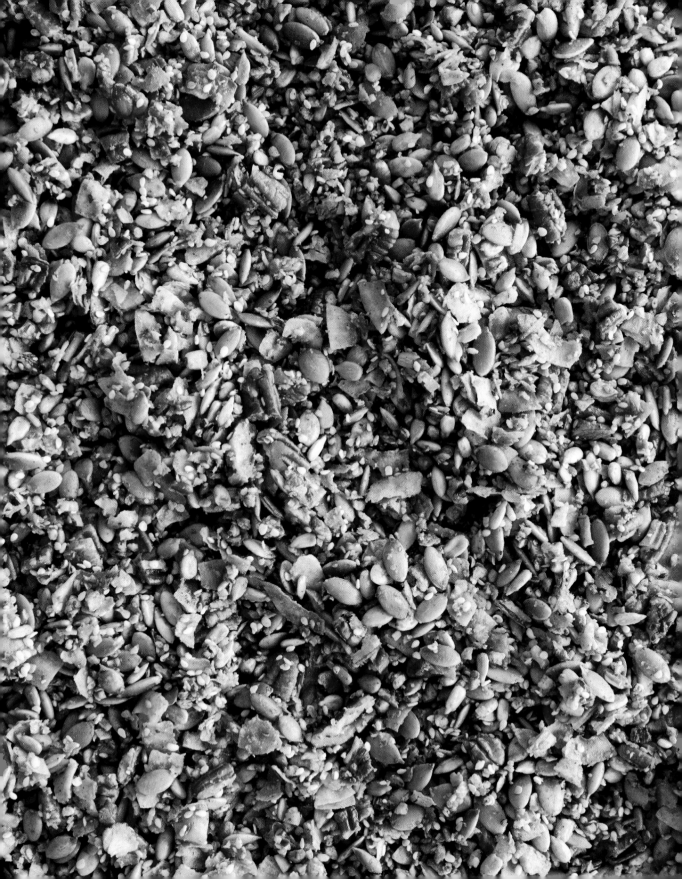

Savory Steel-Cut Oats

SERVES 4 · VEGAN ADAPTABLE, GF ADAPTABLE, DF ADAPTABLE

1 cup certified-GF steel-cut oats

Sea salt

2 tablespoons unrefined, cold-pressed extra-virgin olive oil, plus more for drizzling

3 garlic cloves, thinly sliced

Pinch of crushed red pepper flakes

1 big bunch kale, stems stripped and discarded, leaves coarsely chopped

½ pound shiitake mushrooms, stems discarded, caps wiped clean with a damp paper towel and sliced

Freshly ground black pepper

Flax, hemp, or avocado oil, for drizzling (optional)

⅓ cup chopped walnuts, or another nut or seed, toasted or raw

Gomasio, for sprinkling on top

It may seem strange to eat oats with vegetables but I promise, savory oats are incredibly delicious and even more satisfying than the typical sweetened version. Anything you would combine with risotto or polenta would be great with oatmeal, which is a perfect blank canvas for any number of toppings. I've listed my favorite versions here, but since oats are so bland, the sky's the limit. Make sure to include protein and some healthy fats for a well-balanced breakfast—or lunch or dinner! If you want to make the oats easier to digest, soak them overnight and drain (see instructions on page 128).

1. Place the oats, 4 cups of water (use 3¾ cups of water if the oats were soaked and drained), and a pinch of salt in a medium-size saucepan and bring to a boil over high heat. Lower the heat and simmer oats uncovered until tender, about 40 minutes. (Soaked oats only take 30 minutes.)
2. In a large skillet, heat the olive oil over medium heat. Add the garlic and a pinch of red pepper flakes. Sauté until fragrant, 30–60 seconds.
3. Add the vegetables and a pinch of salt and black pepper, and sauté until tender, about 6 to 8 minutes.
4. Portion the oats into four bowls and top with the vegetable mixture. Add an extra drizzle of olive oil or a different oil, such as flax, hemp, or avocado. Top with the walnuts and sprinkle with gomasio.

Other variations I love:

- Sauté 4 cups of chopped cabbage and 4 sliced scallions in 2 teaspoons of sesame oil and 2 teaspoons of olive oil, drizzle with 4 teaspoons of shoyu (sub tamari for GF), add to the oats, sprinkle with gomasio or sesame seeds, and top with a fried or poached egg (omit for vegan).

- Sauté two small shredded zucchini or ½ bunch of asparagus, chopped, in 1 tablespoon of olive oil and a pinch of salt, add to the oats, and top with 1 to 2 ounces of goat cheese (omit for vegan/DF) and ⅓ cup of toasted, salted pistachios.

- Sauté four sliced garlic cloves, a pinch of red pepper flakes, and ½ pound of halved cherry tomatoes with a pinch of salt in 1 tablespoon of olive oil until they release their juices, about 5 minutes, then add to oats and top with a handful of thinly sliced fresh basil and grated pecorino or Parmesan (omit for vegan/DF).
- Finish the cooked oats with ⅓ to ½ cup of coconut milk (page 255); stir in ½ cup of toasted, unsweetened dried coconut; ⅓ cup of toasted, chopped cashews; ⅓ cup of sliced scallions; and sriracha to taste.

Overnight Oat, Chia, and Buckwheat Porridge SERVES 2 TO 3 · GF, DF, VEGAN ADAPTABLE

This recipe is a combination of my three favorite overnight porridges—muesli, raw buckwheat, and overnight chia and oats, all of which save me on busy weekday mornings. Stir the ingredients together the night before and refrigerate for an instant breakfast the next day. Soaking the grains and nuts in this way also neutralizes the hard-to-digest phytic acid present in all of them, making this a very digestible dish. I like to eat this porridge as is, but my kids top it with sliced bananas or berries.

¼ cup raw buckwheat groats

¾ cup certified-GF old-fashioned rolled oats

2 tablespoons chia seeds

2 cups unsweetened almond milk (page 257) or DF milk of choice

½ teaspoon orange zest

¼ cup freshly squeezed orange juice

¼ teaspoon pure vanilla extract

2 tablespoons unsulfured raisins

2 tablespoons chopped hazelnuts or walnuts, or pumpkin seeds

Pinch of sea salt

½ teaspoon ground cinnamon

Optional sweetener: raw honey (not vegan), pure maple syrup, or a few drops of stevia

1. Place all the ingredients, except the sweetener, in a glass container and stir to combine. Cover and refrigerate overnight or for at least 6 hours.

2. Remove from the refrigerator and stir to mix everything well. Eat cold or at room temperature, or heat gently in a saucepan, if desired. Taste for sweetness and add your choice of sweetener, if desired. This porridge lasts for up to 3 days in the refrigerator.

TIP: Buckwheat is considered a pseudo-cereal, which means it's not technically a grain. It is naturally gluten-free and very high in fiber, as well as in amino acids. Buckwheat can be helpful in regulating blood pressure.

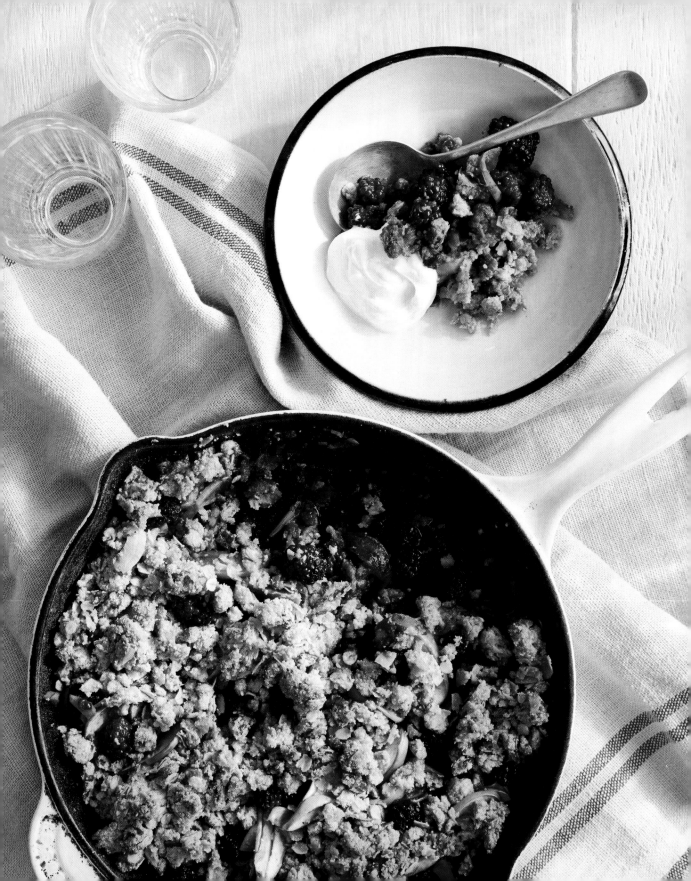

Apple-Blackberry Breakfast Crisp

SERVES 6 · GF, VEGAN ADAPTABLE, DF ADAPTABLE

I love making fruit crisps for dessert, especially when I have friends over. I am always tempted to sneak some for breakfast the next morning, but dessert isn't the best way to start the day—so I developed this low-sugar, high-protein crisp that's suitable for brunch or breakfast. And guess what? Most of my students think this is plenty sweet and could work for dessert as well. You can definitely adapt the fruit according to what's in season.

1. Preheat the oven to 375°F.

2. Prepare the filling: Combine the apples, blackberries, orange juice, and arrowroot in a bowl and pour everything into a 9- or 10-inch pie plate or cast-iron skillet and spread evenly.

3. Prepare the topping: Combine all the topping ingredients in a bowl and mix with your hands until no longer dry, forming small "nuggets" of topping. Alternatively, use an electric mixer to combine everything. Using your hands, arrange the crisp topping on the filling and place the baking dish or skillet on a rimmed baking sheet. Bake for 40 to 50 minutes, or until the fruit is soft and bubbling and the topping is golden brown. If the topping is getting too golden before the fruit is soft, tent with aluminum foil. Serve warm with yogurt, if desired.

TIP: The crisp topping can be made up to 3 days ahead and kept refrigerated. Remove from refrigerator and break up into pieces and arrange directly on top of fruit. The topping can also be frozen for up to 3 months.

ASK PAMELA: Can I make my own almond meal in a blender and substitute that for almond meal in any recipe? *Not exactly. You won't be able to duplicate the fine texture of almond meal or almond flour, and you'll probably turn it into almond butter trying!*

FILLING:

1 pound apples, peeled only if desired, cored and sliced thinly (4 to 5 small apples)

12 ounces fresh or frozen and defrosted blackberries

Juice of ½ orange (about 3 tablespoons)

1 tablespoon arrowroot powder

TOPPING:

1¼ cups almond meal or almond flour

¾ cup certified-GF old-fashioned rolled oats

⅔ cup raw pecans, chopped

6 tablespoons unsweetened coconut flakes

5 tablespoons pure Grade A maple syrup

½ teaspoon sea salt

1 teaspoon ground cinnamon

Pinch of ground nutmeg

½ cup unrefined virgin coconut oil, at room temperature, or 8 tablespoons (1 stick) unsalted butter (not vegan/DF)

Greek yogurt for serving (optional; omit for vegan/DF, or look for coconut or almond milk yogurt as a vegan/DF alternative)

Hash Brown Waffles

MAKES 2 WAFFLES · GF, VEGETARIAN ADAPTABLE, DF ADAPTABLE

2 large eggs, beaten (see page 24 for substitutions)

2 tablespoons unsalted butter or ghee, melted (not DF), or unrefined extra-virgin olive oil, plus more for greasing the waffle iron

½ teaspoon sea salt

A few grinds of freshly ground black pepper

⅛ teaspoon paprika

1 pound Yukon Gold potatoes, unpeeled

Add-ins, up to 2 tablespoons of each:

Minced onion

Finely diced bell pepper

Shredded Cheddar or Monterey Jack cheese (omit for DF)

Chopped chives or herbs

Cayenne pepper (use no more than a pinch)

Cooked, diced bacon (omit for vegetarian)

I have put many unlikely foods in a waffle iron, but this is my family's favorite. If you've ever struggled with achieving really crispy hash brown potatoes, a waffle iron will get the job done. This is a great basic recipe, but the optional add-ins make these waffles extra-special. What's great about waffles is that you can customize each one. Hash brown waffles also make a terrific dinner with eggs, crispy chicken, or a fresh green salad on top.

1. Preheat a waffle iron to high heat. Preheat your oven to 300°F.
2. In a medium-size bowl, mix together the eggs, melted butter, salt, pepper, and paprika.
3. Grate the potatoes in a food processor fitted with a shredding disk or with a box grater. Squeeze any excess moisture out of the potatoes with a nut milk bag or a clean kitchen towel. Add the potatoes to the egg mixture as well as any additional desired add-ins.
4. Brush the preheated waffle iron with butter, ghee, or oil. Spread half the batter on the waffle iron and close. Remove the waffle when it is golden brown and crispy on the outside and tender on the inside. The amount of time will vary from machine to machine.
5. Keep the waffles warm in a 300°F oven on a cooling rack set on a rimmed baking sheet.

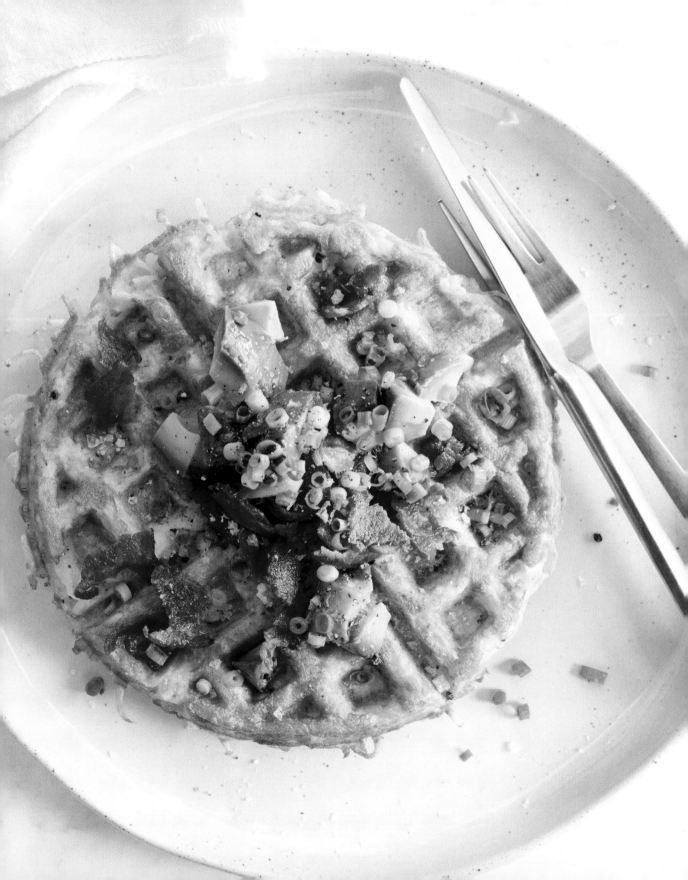

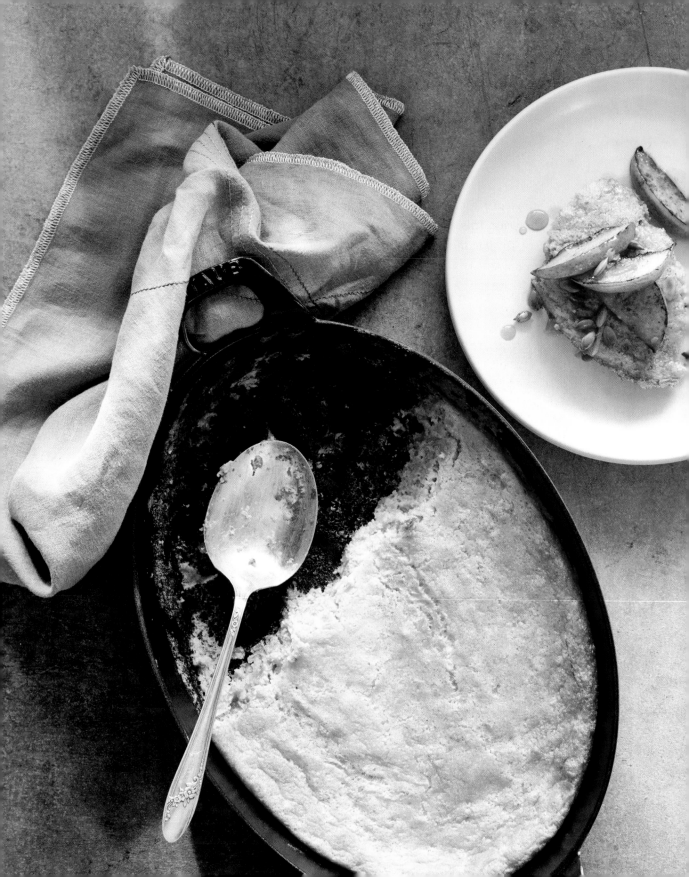

Pumpkin Oatmeal Soufflé

SERVES 4 · VEGETARIAN, GF, DF ADAPTABLE

I originally saw a recipe for an oatmeal soufflé in Food & Wine *magazine and instantly knew it would be delicious and a welcome change from baked oatmeal. Oatmeal soufflé is not like a bowl of oatmeal; it's light, fluffy, and creamy on the inside, with a dry exterior. This version is like a pumpkin pie meets fluffy oatmeal. Try it with sautéed apples or pears for a warm and delicious breakfast.*

1. Preheat the oven to 350°F and generously grease a 9- to 10-inch skillet or baking dish.

2. In a large saucepan, combine the oats, milk, pumpkin puree, maple syrup, pumpkin pie spice, and salt and bring to a simmer. Cook over medium heat, stirring occasionally, until thickened to a soft porridge consistency, about 15 minutes. Remove from the heat and allow to cool slightly, about 5 minutes.

3. Working quickly, stir the egg yolks into the oatmeal until well blended.

4. In a large bowl or using an electric mixer, whisk the egg whites at medium speed until medium-stiff peaks form, 2 to 3 minutes. Using a spatula, gently fold the whites into the oatmeal until just combined. You don't want to see big clumps of white, but you don't want to deflate all the egg whites, either.

5. Pour the mixture into the prepared skillet or baking dish and bake for 30 to 40 minutes, until golden and puffed. If using a nondairy milk, the soufflé will not get as golden, but it will still be delicious. Serve warm with your desired accompaniments, although I have eaten this cold the next day and it is quite good!

Note: If you are out of pumpkin pie spice, mix together 1 teaspoon of ground cinnamon, 1/2 teaspoon of ground ginger, 1/4 teaspoon of ground cloves, and 1/4 teaspoon of ground nutmeg

TIP: Pumpkin is rich in carotenoids, a powerful class of phytonutrients and antioxidants that give the gourd its orange color. Carotenoids, including beta-carotene, support the health of your eyes and skin and boost the immune system.

Unrefined coconut oil or unsalted butter (not DF), for pan

1 cup certified GF old-fashioned rolled oats

2½ cups whole milk (not DF), unsweetened almond milk (page 257), or coconut milk (or a combination of any of these)

½ cup pure pumpkin puree (not pumpkin pie filling)

3 tablespoons pure Grade A maple syrup

2 teaspoons pumpkin pie spice (see headnote)

¼ teaspoon sea salt

3 large eggs, separated

Apple compote, fresh fruit, and/ or maple syrup, for serving (optional)

Banana-Walnut French Toast Casserole

SERVES 4 TO 6 · VEGETARIAN, GF ADAPTABLE, DF ADAPTABLE

Unrefined coconut oil or unsalted butter (not DF), for pan

5 large eggs

1¼ cups unsweetened almond milk (page 257) or milk of choice

2 teaspoons pure vanilla extract

1 teaspoon ground cinnamon

⅛ teaspoon ground nutmeg

¼ teaspoon sea salt

6 slices sprouted bread (certified-GF, if necessary) (thawed if frozen), cut into 1-inch pieces (about 5 cups)

2 large ripe bananas, sliced into ½-inch slices

STREUSEL (OPTIONAL):

3 tablespoons certified-GF oat flour

¼ cup certified-GF old-fashioned rolled oats

⅓ cup raw walnuts, chopped

2 tablespoons maple sugar, muscovado or brown sugar

2 tablespoons pure Grade A or B maple syrup

Pinch of sea salt

3 tablespoons unrefined coconut oil or unsalted butter (not DF)

Accompaniments: pure maple syrup, Greek yogurt (not DF) or DF yogurt of choice

This version of the classic breakfast is very easy to make and allows me to get a few more protein-rich eggs into our breakfast. I'll use whatever bread I have on hand, from sprouted sliced bread to hamburger buns to the ends that no one wants—they will all work here (cinnamon raisin is especially delicious). Most of the time I make the casserole without the streusel on weekday mornings and save the added sweet crunchy topping for the weekends. Even though there is no added sugar, the bananas provide enough sweetness that you can enjoy this without adding maple syrup.

1. Prep the night before you plan to serve this dish: Grease an 8- or 9-inch square glass baking dish with a little coconut oil or unsalted butter.
2. In a large bowl, beat together the eggs, almond milk, vanilla, cinnamon, nutmeg, and salt. Add the bread cubes, pressing on the bread to make sure it soaks up half of the egg mixture. Gently stir in the bananas. Pour into the prepared baking dish.
3. Cover and refrigerate the dish overnight.
4. Make the streusel, if using: Combine all the streusel ingredients until moistened. Cover and refrigerate overnight.
5. The next morning, preheat the oven to 350°F.
6. Crumble the streusel into small clumps on top of the bread mixture and bake, uncovered, for 40 to 45 minutes, or until set. Serve warm with desired accompaniments.

Note: To double this, use a 9 x 13-inch baking dish and bake for closer to 55 to 60 minutes.

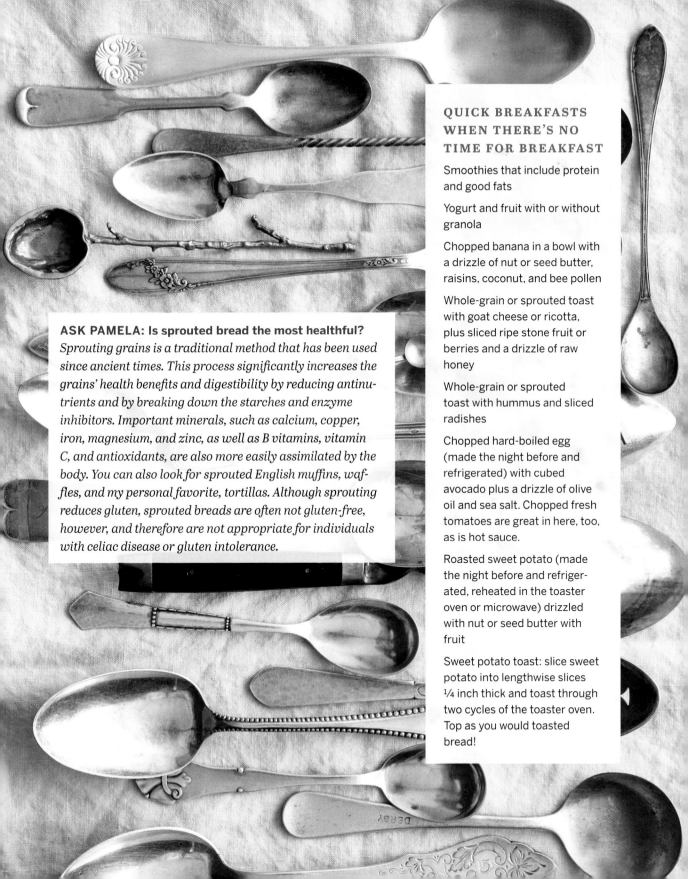

ASK PAMELA: Is sprouted bread the most healthful?
Sprouting grains is a traditional method that has been used since ancient times. This process significantly increases the grains' health benefits and digestibility by reducing antinutrients and by breaking down the starches and enzyme inhibitors. Important minerals, such as calcium, copper, iron, magnesium, and zinc, as well as B vitamins, vitamin C, and antioxidants, are also more easily assimilated by the body. You can also look for sprouted English muffins, waffles, and my personal favorite, tortillas. Although sprouting reduces gluten, sprouted breads are often not gluten-free, however, and therefore are not appropriate for individuals with celiac disease or gluten intolerance.

QUICK BREAKFASTS WHEN THERE'S NO TIME FOR BREAKFAST

Smoothies that include protein and good fats

Yogurt and fruit with or without granola

Chopped banana in a bowl with a drizzle of nut or seed butter, raisins, coconut, and bee pollen

Whole-grain or sprouted toast with goat cheese or ricotta, plus sliced ripe stone fruit or berries and a drizzle of raw honey

Whole-grain or sprouted toast with hummus and sliced radishes

Chopped hard-boiled egg (made the night before and refrigerated) with cubed avocado plus a drizzle of olive oil and sea salt. Chopped fresh tomatoes are great in here, too, as is hot sauce.

Roasted sweet potato (made the night before and refrigerated, reheated in the toaster oven or microwave) drizzled with nut or seed butter with fruit

Sweet potato toast: slice sweet potato into lengthwise slices ¼ inch thick and toast through two cycles of the toaster oven. Top as you would toasted bread!

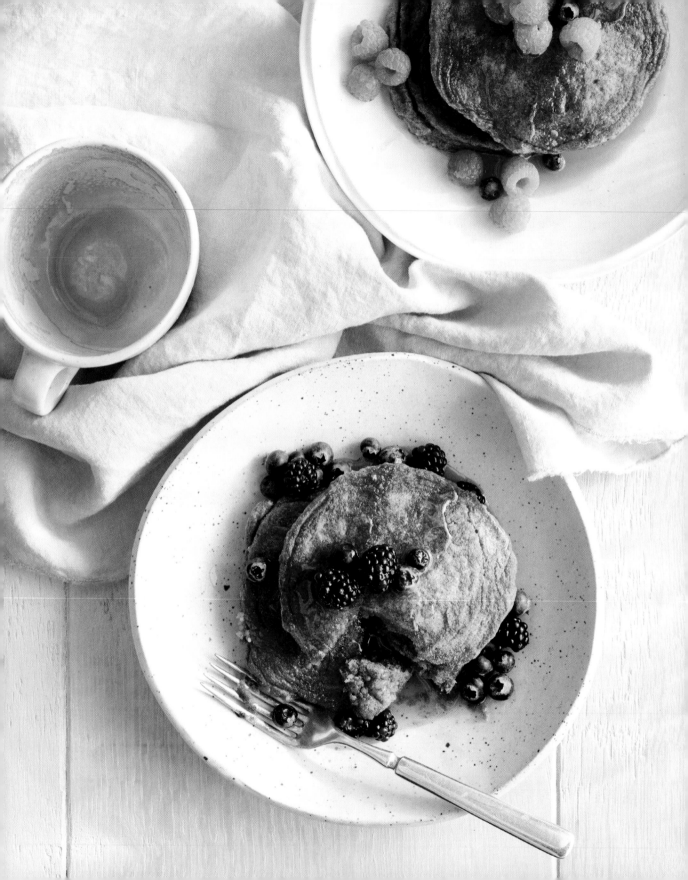

Hearty Multigrain Pancakes with Flax

SERVES 4 TO 5 · VEGETARIAN, GF ADAPTABLE, DF ADAPTABLE

We make pancakes in our house twice a week. I love that the batter can be prepared the night before so my kids can make their own pancakes if I have to leave for work early in the morning. These are my heartiest pancakes yet, with lots of protein, fiber, and good fats to keep everyone's blood sugar stable through the morning. My favorite part? Adding the cooked grains to the batter before flipping so the bottoms of the pancakes develop a lovely crunchy texture. Note that you can use one premixed multigrain flour or any combination of whole wheat pastry, whole spelt, buckwheat, millet, sorghum, or certified-GF oat flour; the latter four grains are gluten-free. For a refresher on these flours, see pages 9–11.

1. Preheat a griddle to 375°F or heat a heavy-bottomed skillet over medium heat.

2. In a medium-size bowl or in a blender, combine the buttermilk, eggs, vanilla, maple syrup, and melted butter until well blended.

3. In a large bowl, combine the flours, flax meal, hemp seeds, baking powder, baking soda, salt, cinnamon, and nutmeg.

4. Pour the wet mixture into the dry ingredients and stir until just combined.

5. Brush the griddle with coconut oil and spoon about ¼ cup of batter onto the griddle. Once the pancakes have set around the edges, about 1 minute, sprinkle 1 to 2 tablespoons of cooked grains evenly on the surface of each pancake. When bubbles start to form on the surface of the pancake and the edges become slightly dry, flip it over and cook for another couple of minutes, or until done. Maintain the heat at 375°F or medium-low and repeat with the remainder of the batter.

TIP: Flaxseeds cannot be digested in whole form; however, I don't recommend preground flax meal. Because flaxseeds are high in fragile omega-3 fats that can go rancid quickly when exposed to light, heat, and air, it is much better to grind flaxseeds fresh at home. I use a coffee grinder to do this. Any flax meal you do not use can be stored in the refrigerator for up to 2 weeks.

- 1½ cups buttermilk (not DF) (see page 24 for substitutions, including DF)
- 2 large eggs (see page 24 for substitutions)
- 1½ teaspoons pure vanilla extract
- 1 tablespoon pure Grade A or B maple syrup, or honey
- 3 tablespoons unsalted butter (not DF), melted or unrefined virgin coconut oil, melted
- 1½ cups mixed-grain flours (see headnote)
- ¼ cup flax meal, freshly ground (ground from about 2½ tablespoons of whole flaxseeds)
- 2 tablespoons hemp seeds
- 1 teaspoon aluminum-free baking powder
- 1 teaspoon baking soda
- ¾ teaspoon sea salt
- ½ teaspoon ground cinnamon
- Pinch of ground nutmeg
- 1 cup cooked grains (e.g., brown rice, quinoa, millet, farro [omit last for GF])
- Unrefined virgin coconut oil, melted, for brushing the griddle

Apple-Dipped Pancakes

SERVES 4 TO 5 · VEGETARIAN, GF ADAPTABLE, DF ADAPTABLE

2 large or 3 medium-size apples, cored and sliced crosswise into ¼-inch slices

1⅔ cups whole spelt flour (see headnote for GF substitutions)

1 teaspoon aluminum-free baking powder

1 teaspoon baking soda

1 teaspoon sea salt

½ teaspoon ground cinnamon

Pinch of ground nutmeg

2 cups buttermilk (not DF) (see page 24 for substitutions, including DF)

2 large eggs (see page 24 for substitutions)

1 teaspoon pure vanilla extract

1 tablespoon pure Grade A or B maple syrup

4 tablespoons unsalted butter (not DF), melted, or unrefined virgin coconut oil

Unrefined virgin coconut oil, melted, for brushing the griddle

These pancakes taste like an apple fritter, only much more nutritious! And your kitchen will smell heavenly when you make them. The key is slicing the apples to just the right thickness—too thick and they won't become tender; too thin and they can break easily when dipped into the batter. Try eating these without syrup—they're perfectly sweet without it. Gluten-free: Substitute half buckwheat flour and half brown rice flour for the spelt flour. Or you can use certified-GF oat flour, too, such as part oat flour, part buckwheat flour, and part brown rice flour.

1. Preheat a griddle to 375°F or over medium heat.
2. Combine the flour, baking powder, baking soda, salt, cinnamon, and nutmeg in a large mixing bowl.
3. In a medium-size bowl or 4- to 6-cup measuring cup, whisk together the buttermilk, eggs, vanilla, maple syrup, and melted butter until well blended. (A blender can do this easily, too.)
4. Pour the wet mixture into the dry ingredients and stir until just combined.
5. Brush the griddle with a little coconut oil.
6. Dip the apple slices one at a time into the batter and turn to coat. I do this with my fingers, but you can use a toothpick or a wooden skewer, if you prefer.
7. Cook the dipped apple slices as you would regular pancakes, flipping once the bottoms are golden and the edges are dry. Cook until the second side is golden brown and the pancake is cooked through.

Grain-Free Banana Muffins

MAKES 9 MUFFINS · VEGETARIAN, GF, DF

Whole-grain, fiber-rich muffins and quick breads are a staple in my house. They are easy to pull together and freeze beautifully. But standard wheat flour muffins don't have the protein I desire for a hearty breakfast. So, I turn more often to nut-based batters to start the day. These muffins became a fast favorite with my students and their families. As opposed to grain-based muffins, these stay fresh for up to a week in the refrigerator.

1. Preheat the oven to 350°F. Line a muffin tin with nine unbleached parchment liners.

2. Place all the ingredients, except the optional add-ins and optional toppings, in a food processor and blend until completely smooth and well combined.

3. Stir in your choice of optional add-ins. Pour the batter evenly into the prepared muffin cups. You will be filling the cups almost up to the top. Sprinkle the tops with your choice of optional toppings. Bake for 30 to 40 minutes, or until just set and a toothpick inserted into the center of a muffin comes out clean or with dry crumbs.

- Espresso-chip muffins: Add 1 tablespoon of instant espresso powder and an additional ⅛ teaspoon of salt. Omit the nutmeg. Stir ⅓ cup of DF chocolate chips into the mixture.

- Blueberry: Stir ⅓ cup of fresh blueberries into the mixture.

- Peanut butter: Sub an equal amount of unsalted, unsweetened peanut butter for the almond butter.

TIP: To make these nut- and peanut-free, you can substitute an equal amount of unsweetened, unsalted sunflower seed butter. But, there's a compound in sunflower seeds that will react to the baking soda and turn the muffins bright green. They are completely edible, but the color may be shocking if you're not expecting it.

1 cup creamy, unsweetened, unsalted almond butter, raw or roasted (see below for nut-free tip)

¼ cup pure Grade A maple syrup

¼ teaspoon sea salt

1 teaspoon baking soda

1 teaspoon ground cinnamon

Pinch of ground nutmeg

2 large eggs

1 teaspoon pure vanilla extract

1 cup very ripe mashed bananas (2 to 3 bananas)

Optional add-ins: ¾ cup chopped walnuts or pecans, raisins, fresh cranberries or blueberries, diced fresh banana, DF chocolate chips or raw cacao nibs

Optional toppings: shredded coconut, pumpkin seeds, sliced banana, pecans

Tex-Mex Frittata Corn Bread

SERVES 6 TO 8 · VEGETARIAN, GF ADAPTABLE, DF ADAPTABLE

FRITTATA AND VEGETABLES:

1 tablespoon ghee (not DF) or unrefined extra-virgin olive oil

1 small red onion, diced

1 red bell pepper, seeded and diced

1/2 jalapeño pepper, seeded and minced (optional)

1/2 cup fresh or frozen and defrosted organic corn kernels

6 large eggs

1/2 teaspoon sea salt

Freshly ground black pepper

CORN BREAD:

1/2 cup whole wheat pastry flour or whole spelt flour (not GF) or King Arthur Gluten-Free Multi-Purpose Flour + 1/2 teaspoon of xanthan gum

1/2 cup yellow cornmeal, preferably stone-ground

1 teaspoon aluminum-free baking powder

1/4 teaspoon baking soda

1/4 teaspoon fine-grain sea salt

1/2 cup buttermilk (not DF) (see page 24 for DF substitutions)

4 tablespoons unsalted butter (not DF), melted or unrefined virgin coconut oil, melted, or unrefined extra-virgin olive oil

1 large egg (see page 24 for substitutions)

2 tablespoons honey or pure Grade A maple syrup

It's so easy to overeat corn bread and forget about consuming something more nutritious. A warm wedge of this frittata corn bread gives you the best of both worlds. Don't reverse the layers. This only works with the egg on the bottom. But change up the veggies and use whatever is in season, if you like.

1. Prepare the frittata and vegetables: Preheat the oven to 375°F. In a 9- or 10-inch cast-iron skillet, warm the ghee or olive oil over medium heat and sauté the onion, bell pepper, jalapeño, if using, and corn until the onion is tender and translucent, 5 to 6 minutes. Set aside half of the vegetable mixture in a bowl (just eyeball it) and keep the other half in the skillet.

2. In a medium-size mixing bowl, beat together the eggs, sea salt, and a few grinds of black pepper. Pour the egg mixture into the skillet and combine well with the vegetables that are in the pan.

3. Bake until the egg mixture is slightly set but still slightly undercooked, about 8 minutes.

4. Meanwhile, prepare the corn bread: In a medium-size bowl, whisk together the flour, cornmeal, baking powder, baking soda, and salt. In a separate medium-size bowl or a blender, combine the buttermilk, melted butter, egg, and honey until well blended. Pour the wet ingredients into the dry ingredients and stir until just combined. Gently fold the reserved sautéed vegetables into the batter.

5. Pour the corn bread mixture on top of the partially cooked frittata, distributing evenly. Carefully (the pan may still be hot) put the skillet back into the oven and bake until the corn bread layer is cooked through and springs back when you press lightly in the center, about 15 minutes. This tastes best warm out of the oven, but leftovers reheat well in a toaster oven the next day.

TIPS: If you like a more tender, less grainy corn bread, increase the flour by 1/4 cup and decrease the cornmeal by 1/4 cup.

If your skillet isn't cast iron or otherwise ovenproof, you can sauté the vegetables in a skillet and then bake the frittata in a greased pie plate.

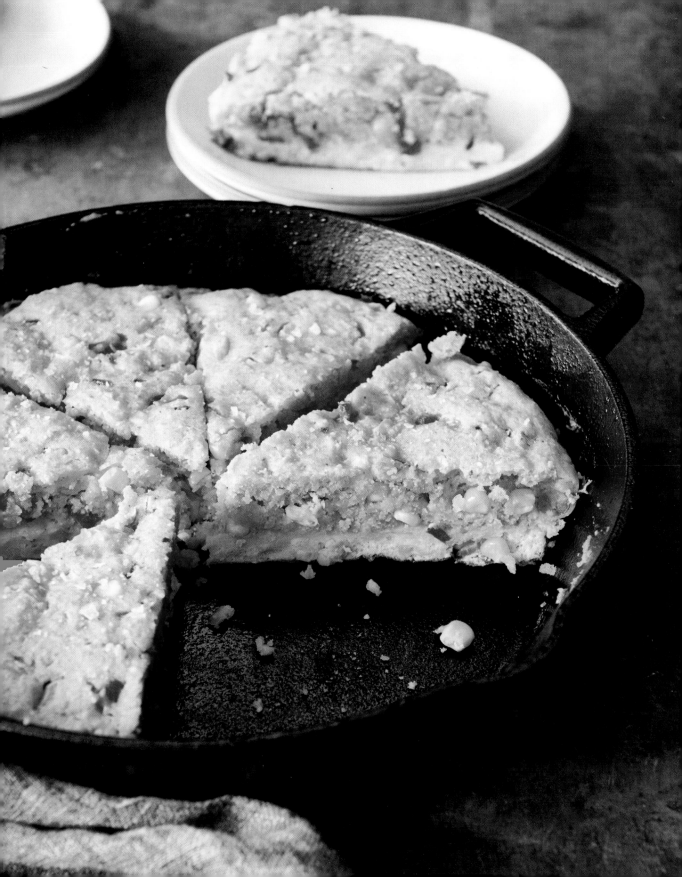

Migas (Egg and Corn Tortilla Scramble)

SERVES 2 · VEGETARIAN, GF, DF ADAPTABLE

1 tablespoon ghee (not DF) or unrefined avocado oil

Heaping ⅓ cup fresh pico de gallo
(salsa)

2 scallions, sliced (optional)

2 small GF corn tortillas, preferably
sprouted, cut into 2-inch pieces

Pinch of sea salt

A few grinds of black pepper

4 large eggs, beaten (see Ask
Pamela for an all-whites version)

1 small avocado, peeled, pitted, and
sliced

Fresh cilantro leaves

Hot sauce (optional)

I arrived to teach a class at a student's home one morning and she was scrambling an intoxicating mixture of eggs, corn tortillas, onions, and tomatoes. And she made it in minutes! I found out that this is a popular Mexican dish called migas, which is usually made by frying tortillas until crispy before adding the other ingredients. Let's just say I made this dish a bit healthier without sacrificing flavor. My family loves it; we always eat this scramble with fresh cilantro, avocado and lots of hot sauce.

1. Warm a medium-size (8-inch) cast-iron or nonstick skillet over medium heat. Melt the ghee and add the pico de gallo and scallions, if using. (Caution: The salsa will splatter a little.) Sauté for a few minutes, until the scallions have softened.
2. Add the corn tortilla pieces and sauté until softened, 3 to 4 minutes. Season with salt and pepper.
3. Pour in the beaten eggs and cook, stirring occasionally (use a wooden turner or a silicone spatula), until the eggs are cooked but not dry, about 1 minute. These eggs will be a little wet because of the salsa.
4. Serve the migas with sliced avocado, fresh cilantro, and hot sauce, if desired.

ASK PAMELA: If I wanted to substitute all egg whites, how many should I use? *You can use two egg whites for every whole egg. I don't advise eating only the whites though, since the yolks contain wonderful fats and vitamins necessary for brain health. Egg yolks do contain cholesterol, but the myth that dietary cholesterol leads to elevated blood cholesterol has been debunked.*

Cauliflower and Roasted Red Pepper Frittata

SERVES 6 TO 8 · VEGETARIAN, GF, DF, VEGAN ADAPTABLE

One of my favorite frittatas is the Spanish tortilla española, which is a dense mixture of eggs and fried potatoes. This much lighter version replaces the greasy potatoes with nutritious cauliflower, one of my favorite vegetables. To make this egg-free and vegan, puree in a food processor 15 to 16 ounces of firm or extra-firm tofu in place of the eggs and combine with the other ingredients. Bake for the same amount of time.

1. Preheat the oven to 375°F. Lightly grease a 9- or 10-inch pie plate with olive oil.

2. In a large, ovenproof skillet, heat the 2 tablespoons of olive oil. Add the cauliflower and onion and season with the salt and black pepper to taste. Cook over moderate heat, stirring occasionally, until the vegetables are tender and the onion is translucent, about 10 minutes. It is very important that the cauliflower be tender.

3. Add the garlic and sauté until fragrant, about 1 minute. Remove from the heat.

4. Beat the eggs in a large bowl and stir in the cauliflower mixture, red peppers, and smoked paprika.

5. Pour into the prepared pie plate and bake for 40 to 45 minutes, or until the center is set and the edges are golden brown.

6. Alternatively, bake in a larger, ovenproof skillet for less time for a thinner frittata. Or cook gently over medium-low heat, covered, until slightly set on the bottom, 15 to 20 minutes, then transfer the skillet to the oven and broil until the top is slightly puffed and golden, 3 to 5 minutes. Let rest for a few minutes before serving.

TIP: Cauliflower is one of the most versatile vegetables as well as one of the most nutritious. A member of the cruciferous family, which also includes broccoli, bok choy, Brussels sprouts, cabbage, and kale, cauliflower is loaded with anti-inflammatory and anticancer compounds as well as a host of vitamins and minerals. Cauliflower supports brain and heart health and is very effective in detoxifying the body.

2 tablespoons unrefined, cold-pressed, extra-virgin olive oil, plus more for pan

3 cups small cauliflower florets, thinly sliced

1 small onion, halved and thinly sliced

1 teaspoon sea salt

Freshly ground black pepper

2 garlic cloves, finely chopped

8 large eggs (see the headnote for a vegan version and Ask Pamela on page 58 for an all-whites version)

1 cup roasted red peppers, sliced (see page 251 for how to roast peppers)

1 teaspoon smoked paprika, or more to taste

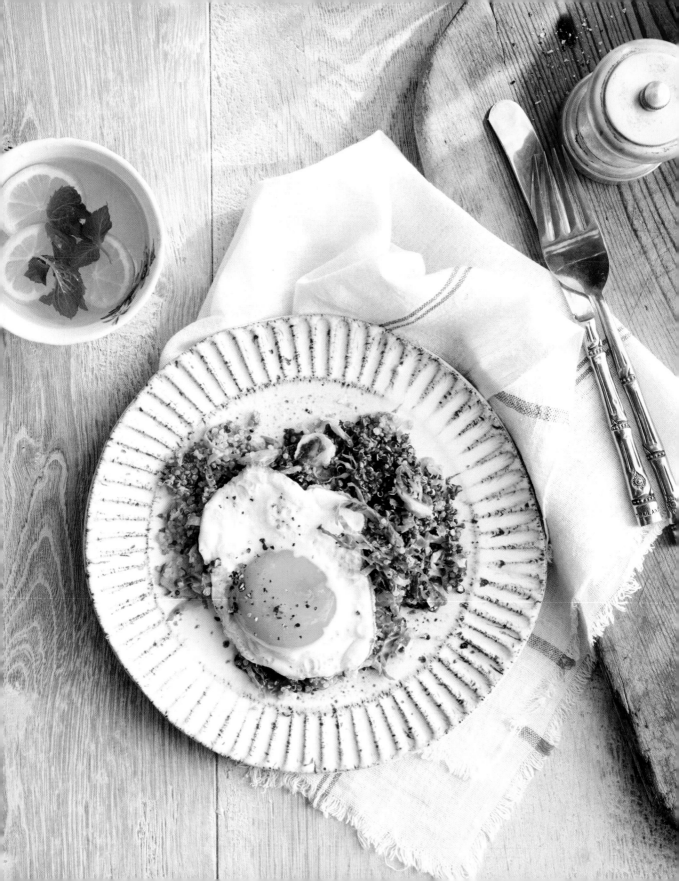

Brussels Sprout and Quinoa Hash with Fried Eggs

SERVES 2 · VEGETARIAN, GF, DF ADAPTABLE

My kids often give me puzzled looks for some of the combinations I come up with to use up leftovers. One morning I sautéed leftover Brussels sprout hash in a skillet with leftover quinoa and I wondered to myself, why have I not done this before? It was so delicious and checked off all the important boxes for me: good fats, protein, complex carbohydrates, and fiber. Although you do need already cooked quinoa to make this, the rest of the prep is really fast, making this very doable for a weekday morning or a really quick dinner.

1. Heat 2 tablespoons of the ghee in a medium-size skillet over medium heat. Add the Brussels sprouts and sauté until tender but still slightly crisp, 4 to 5 minutes.

2. Add the quinoa, salt, and pepper to taste and cook until the quinoa is warmed through. Stir in the sriracha. Taste for seasoning. Set aside.

3. In a medium skillet, heat the remaining 2 tablespoons of ghee. Crack one egg into a small bowl, then slide into the skillet. Repeat with the remaining egg. Cook until the whites are set and you achieve desired doneness on the yolks, about 4 minutes for soft, runny yolks.

4. Divide the sprout mixture between two bowls and top each with a fried egg.

ASK PAMELA: Should I crack my eggs one at a time in a separate bowl before adding them to the rest of the recipe's ingredients? *Yes, I advise cracking eggs in a separate bowl in case you get a bad egg.*

How do I know if I have a bad egg? *You'll know!!! Without getting too graphic, let's just say there is no mistaking a bad egg.*

What about a red dot on the egg yolk or white? *A red dot is nothing to worry about. A red dot on the yolk is likely from a burst capillary in the hen's ovary or yolk sac. A red dot in the white of the egg is probably either a brown blood spot or a tiny bit of tissue sloughed off from the oviduct wall. Both are harmless.*

4 tablespoons ghee (not DF), unrefined extra-virgin olive oil, unrefined avocado oil, or unrefined virgin coconut oil

½ pound Brussels sprouts (about 2 cups), halved and thinly sliced, ends discarded

½ cup cooked quinoa, millet, or brown rice

2 big pinches of sea salt

Freshly ground black pepper

½ teaspoon sriracha, or more to taste

½ teaspoon sea salt

2 large eggs

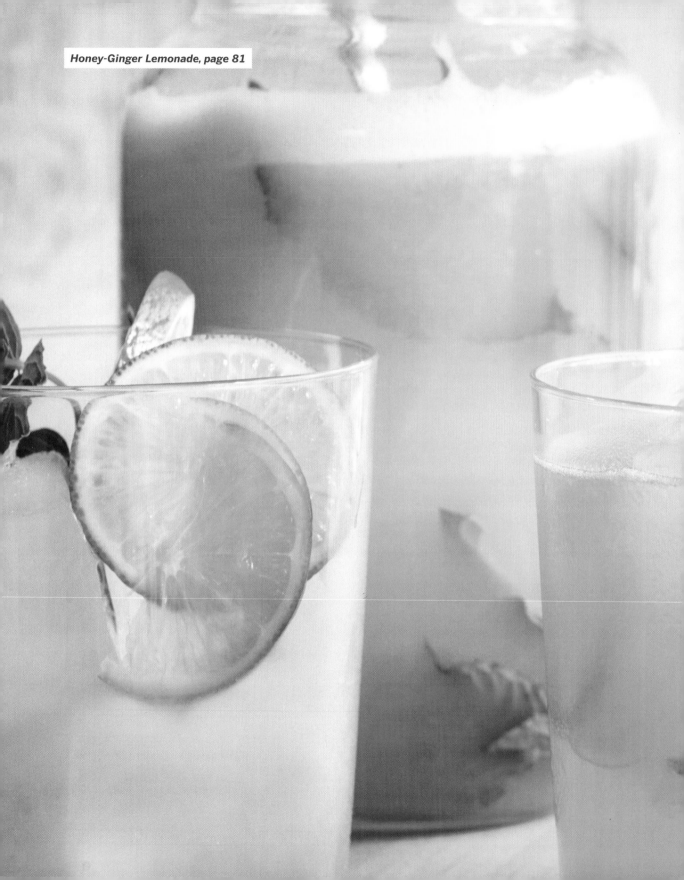

Honey-Ginger Lemonade, page 81

SNACKS AND DRINKS

It is easy to succumb to packaged convenience snacks when hunger strikes and there's nothing nutritious in sight. But junk food will set off a blood sugar spike and crash, and then you'll be craving more foods with false energy. Instead of feeling energized and satisfied, you'll be feeling cranky and tired. Here's the deal—the best snacks don't come from a vending machine; they are ones made with high-quality protein, good fat, and/or complex carbohydrates. These nutrients provide nourishment, satiate hunger, and combat cravings.

To avoid the quick-fix options, it's a good idea to always have a stash of whole food–based alternatives. These snack recipes are easy and very adaptable for a variety of flavors. Many of them can be made ahead and stored at room temperature or frozen.

Of course, a snack doesn't have to be a traditional "snacky" food. Great snacks to tide you over until the next meal can be a small cup of soup, half a sandwich, raw vegetables and hummus, a hard-boiled egg, or even a small salad.

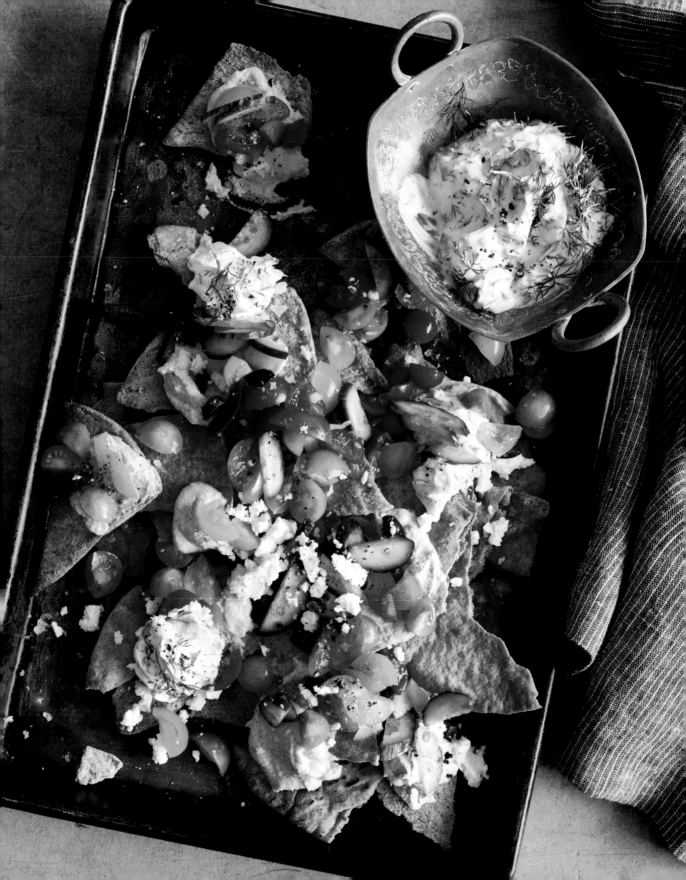

Greek Nachos

SERVES 8 · VEGETARIAN

Nothing says "fun food" like nachos, but who says it has to be the typical tortilla chips with fake cheese? These Greek nachos are loaded with fresh veggies and healthful dips, such as hummus and tzatziki. These can just as easily be set out for snack time as they can for dinnertime. If you don't want to make your own hummus and tzatziki, there are plenty of great, clean ones you can find in your local supermarket. Just read your ingredients and look for no added preservatives.

1. Arrange half of the pita chips on a platter.
2. Scatter half of the cucumber, tomatoes, feta, and olives on top. Make sure every chip has something on it.
3. Dollop half of the hummus and tzatziki all over the pita and vegetables or use a squeeze bottle.
4. Layer the remaining pita chips on top and repeat with the remaining toppings.

TIP: DIY pita chips: Preheat the oven to 350°F. Line two baking sheets with parchment paper.

Split the pita into two separate disks. Brush each pita round on both sides with olive oil. Sprinkle with a pinch of sea salt. Bake until crisp, 15 to 20 minutes.

6 ounces whole-grain pita chips (10 to 12 cups) or whole pitas, split, toasted, and broken into chip-size pieces

1 to 2 cucumbers, diced, large seeds removed

1½ pints cherry tomatoes, diced

8 ounces feta cheese, preferably goat or sheep, crumbled

1 cup pitted kalamata olives, diced

½ pint tzatziki

½ pint hummus

Pizza Muffins

MAKES 12 MUFFINS · VEGETARIAN, GF ADAPTABLE

2 cups whole wheat pastry flour, white whole wheat flour, or whole spelt flour (not GF), or King Arthur Gluten-Free Multi-Purpose Flour + 1½ teaspoons xanthan gum

1 tablespoon aluminum-free baking powder

½ teaspoon baking soda

1 teaspoon sea salt

2 teaspoons dried oregano

2 large eggs

2 tablespoons unrefined cold-pressed extra-virgin olive oil

¾ cup buttermilk (see page 24 for substitutions)

1¼ cups marinara sauce (see page 253 for a recipe)

1 tablespoon pure Grade A or B maple syrup

½ cup shredded mozzarella cheese

½ cup grated pecorino cheese, plus more for topping

Sometimes I'll make soup or a salad for lunch or dinner and my kids are looking for an extra something to go with it. These pizza muffins have all the flavor of pizza, but are made with wholesome ingredients, including whole-grain flour and fresh tomato sauce, as well as minimal amounts of cheese. The best part is that they are portable and perfect for lunchboxes or picnics.

1. Preheat the oven to 350°F. Line a 12-cup muffin pan with unbleached parchment liners or reusable silicone liners.
2. Whisk together the flour, baking powder, baking soda, salt, and oregano in a medium-size bowl to combine.
3. In a large bowl beat the eggs and add the olive oil, buttermilk, marinara sauce, and maple syrup, and stir. Add the cheeses and stir to combine. Slowly stir in the dry mixture until just combined. Do not overbeat.
4. Using a large ice-cream scoop fill each muffin cup. Top each with 1 teaspoon of sauce and sprinkle with pecorino cheese.
5. Bake for 20 to 22 minutes, or until a toothpick inserted into the center of a muffin comes out clean. Allow to cool for 10 minutes in the pan and then transfer to a wire rack to completely cool.

Note: You can top each muffin like a pizza with your favorite toppings, such as nitrate-free pepperoni, sautéed spinach, chopped fresh basil, or chopped olives. Or you can stir these toppings into the batter before baking.

ASK PAMELA: How do I freeze and defrost muffins? *Allow the muffins to cool completely before wrapping and freezing. If you will use them within 2 weeks, place them in glass containers or freezer bags. If you'd like them to last up to 3 months without freezer burn, wrap each one individually in aluminum foil and place them in a resealable freezer bag. Don't forget to label what is in the bag and the date!*

Thaw frozen muffins at room temperature for about an hour.

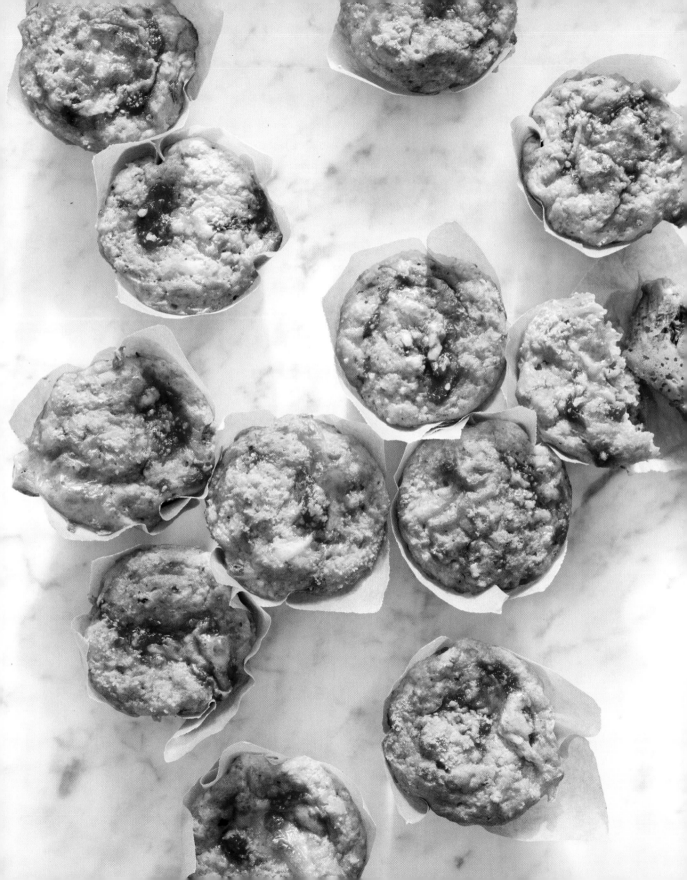

Chocolate-Zucchini Bread with Apple and Carrot

MAKES 1 (8½ X 4½-INCH) LOAF · VEGETARIAN, GF ADAPTABLE

¼ cup unrefined cold-pressed olive oil or melted coconut oil

¼ cup plain, unsweetened whole Greek yogurt

½ cup pure Grade A or B maple syrup

2 large eggs

1 teaspoon pure vanilla extract

1½ cups whole spelt flour, whole wheat pastry flour, or white whole wheat flour (not GF) (or ¾ cup flour + ¾ cup almond pulp from making almond milk; see page 257) or King Arthur Gluten-Free Multi-Purpose Flour + 1½ teaspoons xanthan gum

¼ cup unsweetened cocoa powder or raw cacao powder

1 teaspoon baking soda

½ teaspoon aluminum-free baking powder

½ teaspoon sea salt

1½ teaspoons ground cinnamon

Pinch of ground nutmeg

¾ cup shredded, unpeeled zucchini (about 1 small)

¾ cup shredded, unpeeled apple (about 1 small)

¾ cup shredded carrot

½ cup chopped walnuts or pecans (optional)

When your zucchini are abundant and you're trying to get creative with them, here's a lovely recipe for an after-camp snack or to take to the beach. This is zucchini bread to the next level: laced with carrot and apple, it is exceptionally moist and very lightly sweetened. It tastes amazing warm from the oven and sometimes we'll break off hunks and smear them with a little almond butter. Bake a few loaves before school starts and freeze them for those later months when you need a quick after-school treat.

1. Preheat the oven to 350°F. Lightly grease an 8½ x 4½-inch loaf pan, or if aluminum, grease it and line it with parchment paper.

2. In a blender, process the oil, yogurt, maple syrup, eggs, and vanilla until combined.

3. In a mixing bowl, whisk together the flour, cocoa powder, baking soda, baking powder, salt, cinnamon, and nutmeg. Stir the wet ingredients into the dry. Fold in the zucchini, apple, carrot, and nuts. Pour into the prepared pan.

4. Bake for 50 to 60 minutes, or until a tester inserted in the center comes out clean. Allow to cool slightly, about 10 minutes. Remove from the pan and allow to cool completely.

TIPS: Use your food processor with the shredding disk to quickly and easily shred the zucchini, apple, and carrot.

You can also make these in a standard muffin tin and bake for 20 to 25 minutes. This will yield 12 muffins.

These freeze well; just tightly wrap them and store them in the freezer.

Black Bean Cookie Dough Bites

MAKES ABOUT 16 · VEGAN, GF, DF

I am an unapologetic chocoholic and I am not above sneaking a pinch of cookie dough if it's staring me in the face. This recipe for Black Bean Cookie Dough Bites is not to be believed. My kids all went crazy for them and thought I had gone temporarily insane when I was prancing around the house pushing raw chocolate cookie dough one day. It is hard not to get excited about a treat that is full of antioxidants, protein, fiber, and healthy fats. Just don't eat the whole bowl in one sitting, okay? (And yes, you read that right: black bean cookie dough. Read on!)

1. Combine all the ingredients, except the chocolate chips, in a food processor. Process until completely smooth.

2. Stir in the chocolate chips or cherries. Shape into balls and refrigerate on a baking sheet or a plate until firm. Store in the refrigerator in a covered container for up to 1 week.

1½ cups cooked black beans, or 1 (15-ounce) can, drained and rinsed

½ cup packed pitted dates (about 4 Medjool dates)

¼ cup pure Grade A maple syrup

3 tablespoons coconut butter

3 tablespoons unsweetened, creamy almond butter or raw cashew butter

4 tablespoons certified-GF oat flour or 3 tablespoons coconut flour

⅓ cup raw cacao powder or unsweetened cocoa powder

1 teaspoon pure vanilla extract

½ teaspoon sea salt

¼ cup DF mini chocolate chips or small diced, dried unsulfured cherries

Stovetop Popcorn 3 Ways

SERVES 6

POPCORN:

2 tablespoons unrefined virgin coconut oil

½ cup good-quality popcorn, such as Eden Organic

Don't even think about buying microwave popcorn. The chemicals, preservatives, and toxic packaging are all things to be avoided. You can easily make the most delicious popcorn on your stovetop just as quickly as in your microwave. My kids love snacking on popcorn after school or bringing it to sports games, but I'll also set it out when I have friends over to play cards or watch a movie. I included a basic technique here, as well as my three favorite flavored popcorn recipes—one sweet and two savory. The truffle one is definitely for grown-ups!

1. Heat the oil in a heavy-bottomed 3-quart pot over medium heat. (I use one that is 8 inches in diameter and 5 inches deep.) Add three kernels of popcorn to the pot and cover with a lid. When the kernels pop (this usually takes 2½ to 3 minutes), add the rest of the popcorn in an even layer and partially cover with the lid. Leave it open by about ½ inch to allow steam to escape but not wide enough to let the popcorn pop right out.

2. Shake the pot every now and then. If you can't shake it with the lid ajar, cover the pot, shake and open the lid again when you return the pot to the heat.

3. Once the popping reduces to several seconds between each pop, take the pot off the heat and remove the lid.

Truffle–Parmesan Popcorn

VEGETARIAN, GF, VEGAN ADAPTABLE, DF ADAPTABLE

10 to 12 cups stovetop popcorn

1 teaspoon unrefined, cold-pressed extra-virgin olive oil

3 teaspoons truffle oil

½ cup grated Parmesan cheese (not vegan or DF), or ¼ cup nutritional yeast

1 teaspoon garlic powder

Sea salt

1. Pour the popcorn into a large bowl and add the olive oil and truffle oil. Toss so it the oil is evenly distributed over the popcorn.
2. Sprinkle with the Parmesan and garlic powder. Toss to combine and add a sprinkle of sea salt, if desired.

Maple–Almond Butter Popcorn

VEGAN, GF, DF

10 to 12 cups stovetop popcorn

3 tablespoons pure Grade A or B maple syrup

2 tablespoons creamy, unsalted and unsweetened almond butter (or nut or seed butter of your choice)

1 teaspoon pure vanilla extract

¼ teaspoon sea salt, plus more to taste

⅛ teaspoon ground cinnamon

¾ cup toasted almonds, chopped

1. Preheat the oven to 350°F. Line a baking sheet with parchment and set aside.
2. Pour the maple syrup into a small pot and bring to a boil over medium heat. Remove from the heat.
3. Add the almond butter, vanilla, salt, and cinnamon to the maple syrup and whisk until combined.

4. Pour the popcorn into a large bowl along with the chopped almonds and then drizzle with the maple mixture. Toss so that it is evenly distributed over the popcorn.
5. Spread the popcorn in an even layer on the prepared baking sheet and bake for about 5 minutes. After 5 minutes, rotate the baking sheet and bake for another 2 minutes.
6. Remove the popcorn from the oven and let it cool until the popcorn becomes crunchy.

Nori–Sesame Popcorn

VEGAN, GF, DF

10 to 12 cups stovetop popcorn

1¼ teaspoons unrefined toasted sesame oil

1¼ teaspoons unrefined extra-virgin olive oil

1 (0.17-ounce) package roasted, salted seaweed snacks

1 tablespoon toasted sesame seeds

½ teaspoon sea salt

or 1½ tablespoons gomasio in place of the sesame seeds and salt

1. Pour the popcorn into a large bowl and add the sesame oil and olive oil. Toss so the oil is evenly distributed over the popcorn.
2. Crumble the seaweed snacks with your hands into the bowl and then add the toasted sesame seeds and salt. Toss to combine.

TIP: Toast sesame seeds in a dry skillet over medium heat for 3 to 5 minutes, or until slightly browned. Stir occasionally.

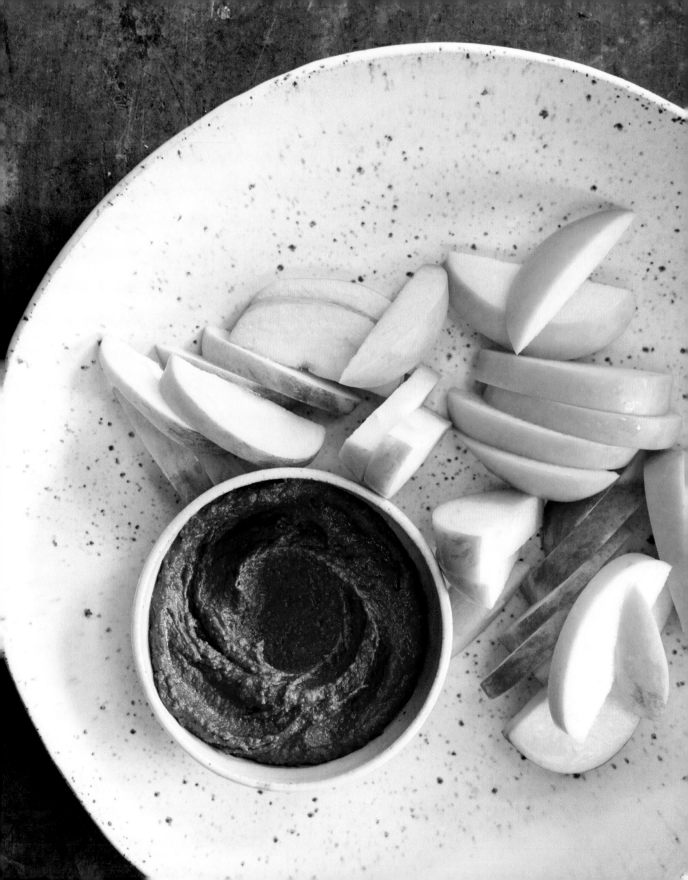

Chocolate Hummus

MAKES ABOUT 2 CUPS · VEGAN, GF, DF

I know what you're thinking. Chocolate, yes. Hummus, yes. Chocolate hummus, not so sure. Stay with me. Hummus, which is made from chickpeas, tahini, garlic, and lemon juice, is, hands-down, my favorite dip. But I didn't exactly throw chocolate into the pool, too. Instead, this is a blend of chickpeas, raw cacao, and some high-quality sweeteners that transforms into an insanely delicious chocolate dip. It's creamy, chocolaty, and the perfect snack, since it's high in protein, fiber, and good fats. I love an extra pinch of flaky salt on mine because chocolate and salt are BFFs! Serve with apple slices, celery sticks, or your favorite GF/DF crackers.

1. Place all the ingredients, except the water, in a food processor or high-speed blender. Process until smooth.
2. With the motor running, add the warm water and process until combined.
3. Serve at room temperature or chilled. Store leftovers, covered, in the refrigerator for up to 4 days.

1½ cups cooked chickpeas, or 1 (15-ounce) can, drained and rinsed (or sub white beans)

2 Medjool dates, pitted

⅓ cup unsweetened, unsalted, raw or roasted almond butter

¼ cup pure Grade A maple syrup

¼ cup raw cacao powder or unsweetened cocoa powder

½ teaspoon sea salt

½ teaspoon pure vanilla extract

¼ cup warm water

Nut Butter–Stuffed Dates

MAKES 4 · VEGAN, GF, DF

4 medium-size dates, pitted and
  split open slightly

4 teaspoons nut or seed butter, or
  8 shelled nuts*

4 teaspoons raw cacao nibs or DF
  dark chocolate chips

Pinch of sea salt or flaky sea salt, if
  your nut butter is unsalted

*Pecans, walnuts, and almonds would
be great here. Almond butter, peanut
butter, cashew butter, and sunflower
butter would work as well.*

When I am dying for something sweet and I don't want to give into my son's stash of Halloween candy hidden underneath his bathroom sink behind the extra towels, I split open a soft, sticky date and stuff it with creamy nut butter, crunchy cacao nibs, and a pinch of flaky salt. A stuffed date is a quick fix that leaves me both satisfied and feeling somewhat virtuous.

1. Stuff each date with nut butter (or two shelled nuts) and chocolate chips. Top with a pinch of salt, if desired, and enjoy.

ASK PAMELA: Should I store dates in the refrigerator? *If you are not going to eat your dates within a week or if they are particularly sticky, yes, you'll want to store them in the refrigerator. If you need to dice dates for a salad or porridge, for example, they'll actually be easier to cut cold.*

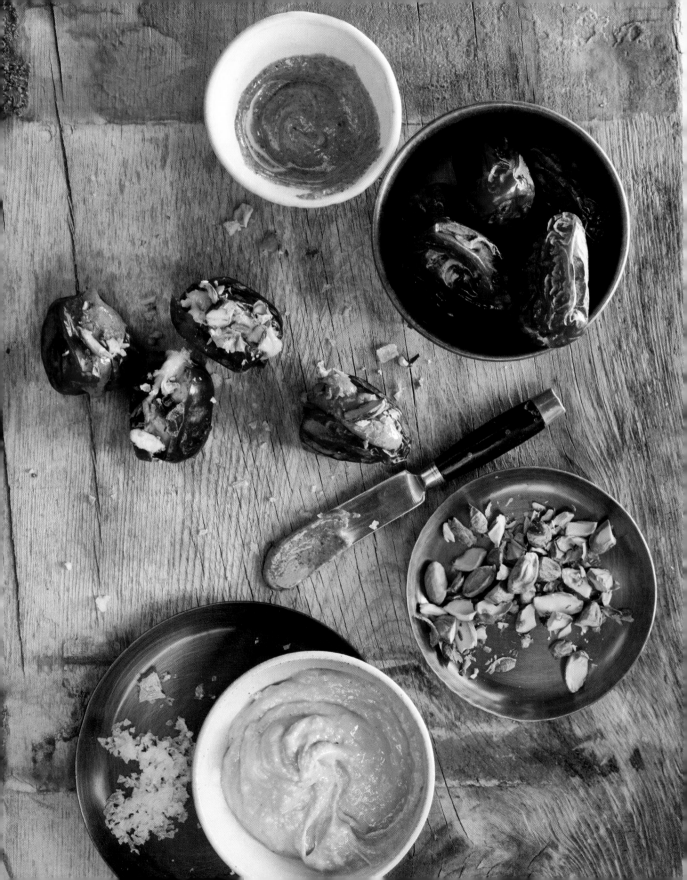

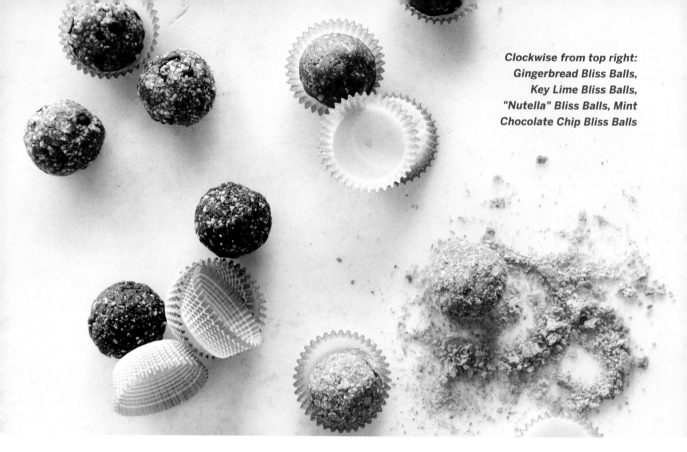

Clockwise from top right:
Gingerbread Bliss Balls,
Key Lime Bliss Balls,
"Nutella" Bliss Balls, Mint
Chocolate Chip Bliss Balls

Bliss Balls

MAKES 12 · VEGAN, DF, GF/GF ADAPTABLE

We had some good laughs on the set when we were shooting these Bliss Balls photos. But at the end of the day, literally and figuratively, everyone wanted to know when it was Bliss Ball o'clock. These energy balls not only taste amazing, but are an incredibly natural way to satisfy a sweet craving and give you a boost of energy. Bliss Balls are dead simple to make and I love having them on hand in the fridge for a quick afternoon snack or lunchbox treat. They also make a fabulous hostess or holiday gift. The following are a few of my favorite flavors, but once you get the basic formula, start playing around with different ingredients to create your own Bliss Balls!

"Nutella" Bliss Balls

1½ cups raw hazelnuts

1½ cups Medjool dates, pitted (about 12 dates)

¼ cup raw cacao powder

½ teaspoon pure vanilla extract

¼ teaspoon sea salt

1. Toast the hazelnuts: Preheat the oven to 350°F. Pour the nuts onto a pie plate and toast for 10 to 15 minutes, or until skins blister. Remove from the oven and allow to cool; rub the nuts in kitchen towel to remove the skins.

2. Place all the ingredients in a food processor

and blend until the nuts are finely chopped and you have a well-combined mass that is moist enough to roll into balls. Depending on your food processor, this could take a couple of minutes.

3. Roll the mixture, using your hands, to form 1½- to 2-inch balls.

4. These can be eaten immediately, or refrigerate to firm them for a few hours. Store them in the fridge in a covered container for up to 7 days.

Mint Chocolate Chip Bliss Balls

1⅛ cups raw almonds

1⅛ cups pitted Medjool dates (about 9 dates)

¼ teaspoon pure vanilla extract

⅜ teaspoon peppermint extract

1 tablespoon lucuma powder

1 tablespoon coconut butter

¼ teaspoon sea salt

3 tablespoons DF mini chocolate chips or raw cacao nibs

1. Place all the ingredients, except the chocolate chips, in a food processor and blend until the nuts are finely chopped and you have a well-combined mass that is moist enough to roll into balls. Depending on your food processor, this could take a couple of minutes.

2. Stir in the chocolate chips, using your hands or a spatula. Roll the mixture, using your hands, to form 1½- to 2-inch balls.

3. These can be eaten immediately or refrigerate to firm them for a few hours. Store them in the fridge for up to 7 days.

Gingerbread Bliss Balls

1 cup Medjool dates, pitted (about 8 dates)

¾ cup raw walnuts

¾ cup raw pecans

½ cup certified-GF old-fashioned rolled oats

1 teaspoon ground ginger

¾ teaspoon ground cinnamon

⅜ teaspoon ground cloves (this adds a little kick, so feel free to use a little less, if desired)

¼ teaspoon pure vanilla extract

¼ teaspoon sea salt

1. Place all the ingredients in a food processor and blend until the nuts are finely chopped and you have a well-combined mass that is moist enough to roll into balls. Depending on your food processor, this could take a couple of minutes.

2. Roll the mixture, using your hands, to form 1½- to 2-inch balls.

3. These can be eaten immediately or refrigerate to firm them for a few hours. Store them in the fridge for up to 7 days.

Key Lime Bliss Balls

1½ cups raw cashews

1½ cups Medjool dates, pitted (about 12 dates)

1½ tablespoons coconut butter

1½ teaspoons lime zest

¼ teaspoon pure vanilla extract

¼ teaspoon sea salt

2 to 3 DF graham crackers (look for certified-GF crackers for GF Bliss Balls), crushed into small pieces, using your hands (not completely into crumbs) (optional)

1. Place all the ingredients, except the graham crackers, in a food processor and blend until the nuts are finely chopped and you have a well-combined mass that is moist enough to roll into balls. Depending on your food processor, this could take a couple of minutes.

2. Roll the mixture, using your hands, to form 1½- to 2-inch balls. Roll the balls in the crushed graham crackers, pressing slightly so that they stick.

3. These can be eaten immediately or refrigerate to firm them for a few hours. Store them in the fridge for up to 7 days.

Crunchy Savory Chickpeas

MAKES 1½ CUPS · VEGAN, GF, DF

1½ cups cooked chickpeas, or 1 (15-ounce) can, drained and rinsed

1 tablespoon unrefined, virgin coconut oil

1 tablespoon pure Grade A or B maple syrup

⅛ teaspoon sea salt

⅛ teaspoon cayenne pepper

1 to 2 teaspoons fresh rosemary, finely chopped

Truly crisp-like-crackers chickpeas had eluded me for years until I realized the secret of roasting them in an oven and then allowing them to continue to dry out with the heat turned off. They are not only crunchy on Day 1, but forever and ever after that, too. These crunchy chickpeas remind me of my favorite bar nuts, which are a little salty, sweet, and spicy at the same time. However, these chickpeas are a delicious nut-free alternative. They're even great in place of nuts or croutons on a salad for extra crunch, on a vegan cheese board, or with predinner drinks.

1. Preheat the oven to 400°F. Line a baking sheet with unbleached parchment paper.

2. Pat the chickpeas as dry as possible with a paper towel. Remove whatever skins are loose. Place the chickpeas on the prepared baking sheet and roast for 20 minutes.

3. Remove from the oven and add the coconut oil, maple syrup, and salt. Toss to coat. Put back in the oven and roast for another 15 to 20 minutes, or until golden brown. If a few pop, that's okay.

4. Turn off the oven. Toss the chickpeas with the cayenne and rosemary. Return the pan to the oven and with the oven door closed and the heat off, allow the chickpeas to sit in the warm oven for another hour (check on them after 30 minutes), or until perfectly crunchy. You'll have to test one to be sure. It should be dry and airy. If they're still not crunchy, leave in the oven with the door closed and the heat off until they are crunchy through and through. Set aside to cool at room temperature. Once completely cool, the chickpeas can be stored at room temperature in a container for up to 1 week.

Strawberry-Watermelon Ice Pops

MAKES 6 (3-OUNCE) ICE POPS · VEGETARIAN, GF, DF

Don't be duped by ice pop boxes with beautiful pictures of real fruit on them. You would be shocked to learn how much sugar, high-fructose corn syrup, and artificial colors and flavors are added to these simple frozen treats. Fortunately, ice pops are incredibly easy to make and you can control the ingredients. These are a favorite in my house, but you can actually freeze any blend of fruit and juice or even your favorite smoothie in an ice pop mold.

1. Place all the ingredients in a blender and process until smooth; taste and add more honey, if desired.
2. Pour into ice pop molds and add sticks, leaving at least 3 inches out of the mixture. Freeze until solid, at least 2 hours. Running tepid water over the outside of the molds can help release the pops easily.

TIPS: Look for molds that are made from stainless steel or silicone, both of which do not leach toxins into your food. At the very least, seek out BPA-free plastic molds.

No ice pop molds? No problem: you can use small disposable cups instead.

2 cups whole hulled fresh or frozen strawberries

1½ cups fresh watermelon chunks

Juice of ½ lime (about 1 tablespoon)

1 tablespoon honey, plus more if desired

Pineapple Agua Fresca

MAKES 1 LARGE PITCHER · VEGETARIAN, GF, DF, VEGAN ADAPTABLE

1 whole pineapple, outside rind sliced off, core removed, and fruit cut into chunks (about 8 cups)

8 fresh mint leaves (optional)

3 tablespoons raw honey (not vegan) or granulated cane sugar, if you need it

Juice of ½ lime (about 1½ tablespoons) (don't skip this; it really perks up the flavor)

If you and soda are still hanging out together, even if it's just on the weekends, it's time to break up. Soda is one of the absolute worst things you can put into your precious body. It's highly inflammatory, full of sugar or high-fructose corn syrup, often with added colors, and if it's in a can, you're drinking some aluminum, too. Diet soda isn't any better for you. Say good-bye for good and get cozy with an agua fresca. Literally translated as "fresh water," an agua fresca is simply fresh fruit blended with water for a light, natural homemade fruit drink. I have made aguas frescas with every type of melon, as well as berries; this pineapple version is so tasty with a little mint. For a carbonated agua fresca, blend fruit with 2 cups of water and strain. Then add 2 cups of sparkling water.

1. Place half the fruit and 2 cups of water in a blender and puree until smooth. Taste for sweetness. If you think you will need to add sugar, add it in the next batch.

2. Strain the liquid through a fine-mesh sieve or cheesecloth into a pitcher or a large bowl. Discard any seeds that remain. Repeat with the remaining fruit and 2 cups of water, adding the mint leaves and sugar, if using them.

3. Blend until smooth. Strain. Stir in the lime juice.

4. Transfer to a pitcher and chill before serving. The flavor is better if it has a chance to sit.

TIPS: If you don't have fresh pineapple handy, frozen pineapple certainly works. Just defrost it first.

For a cocktail, add a splash of sparkling wine.

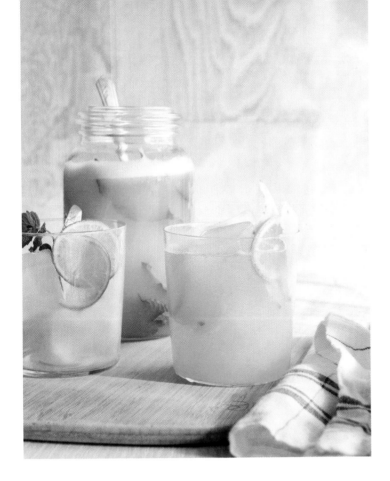

Honey-Ginger Lemonade

MAKES 8 CUPS · VEGETARIAN, GF, DF

One of my favorite flavor combinations is lemon and ginger. This is a healthier version of lemonade and my kids love it. I sweeten it with both raw honey and freshly squeezed orange juice instead of loads of refined sugar. I love the kick that ginger adds; if you're like me, feel free to add even more ginger!

1. Place 2 cups of the water and the honey and ginger in a blender and blend on high speed until emulsified. Strain the liquid through a fine-mesh sieve into a large bowl or pitcher.
2. Add the remaining 4 cups of water, lemon juice, orange juice, and ice to the pitcher and enjoy.

6 cups room-temperature water

½ cup honey, preferably raw, plus more to taste

⅓ cup peeled, sliced fresh ginger

1½ cups freshly squeezed lemon juice (9 to 11 lemons)

½ cup freshly squeezed orange juice

3 to 4 cups ice cubes

TIPS: If you don't like the flavor of honey or want to prepare this recipe as totally vegan, you can use ½ cup of superfine cane sugar instead, but honey is much more natural.

Raw honey is unrefined (except by bees) and contains many enzymes, vitamins, and phytonutrients, making it a higher-quality choice over refined sugar. Pasteurized honey, however, has lost all of its live enzymes and may have actually been chemically refined. Raw honey is still a concentrated sweetener and therefore should be consumed in moderation.

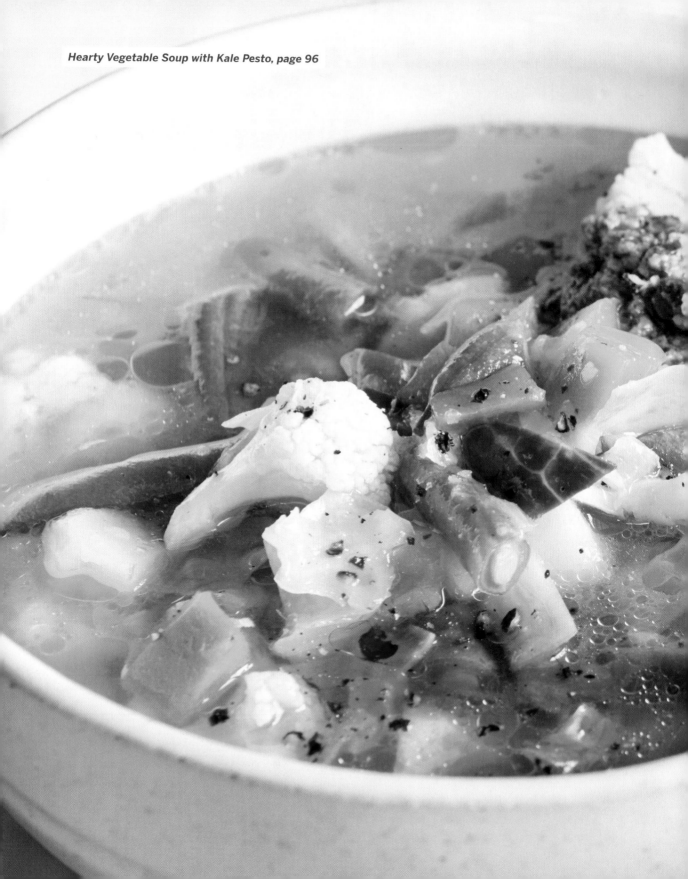

Hearty Vegetable Soup with Kale Pesto, page 96

SATISFYING SOUPS AND STEWS

There's nothing quite as comforting as a bowl of homemade soup. My whole family loves soup, and I often get requests from my students for more soup recipes. They are easy to make, nourishing, and often better the next day, making them the perfect lunchbox meal. Many can be frozen, which may encourage you to make a double batch for a rainy day or freeze individually for portable lunches.

I love the infinite potential of soups—brothy, creamy, chunky, spicy, light, hearty. Soup can be a starter to the meal or substantial enough to be an entrée. I find soups to be the perfect way to get in extra servings of vegetables and other wholesome foods.

I am a homemade stock-pusher, as I like to say in my classes. Yes, you can buy stock, but homemade stocks are a hundred, no, a thousand times more nutritious and better-tasting than store-bought (you'll find my homemade stocks and broths recipes in Basics, pages 248–250). The more brothy a soup is, such as my Italian Wedding Soup (page 90), the more the flavor of the stock will come through.

Soups are also very adaptable; as you start to cook more, you should also feel more confident adapting these and other soup recipes to different seasons or what you have on hand.

Keep in mind the salt measurements in these recipes are conservative since I don't know what kind of stock you'll be using. If you are using unsalted homemade stock, you'll definitely need to add more salt than what is listed.

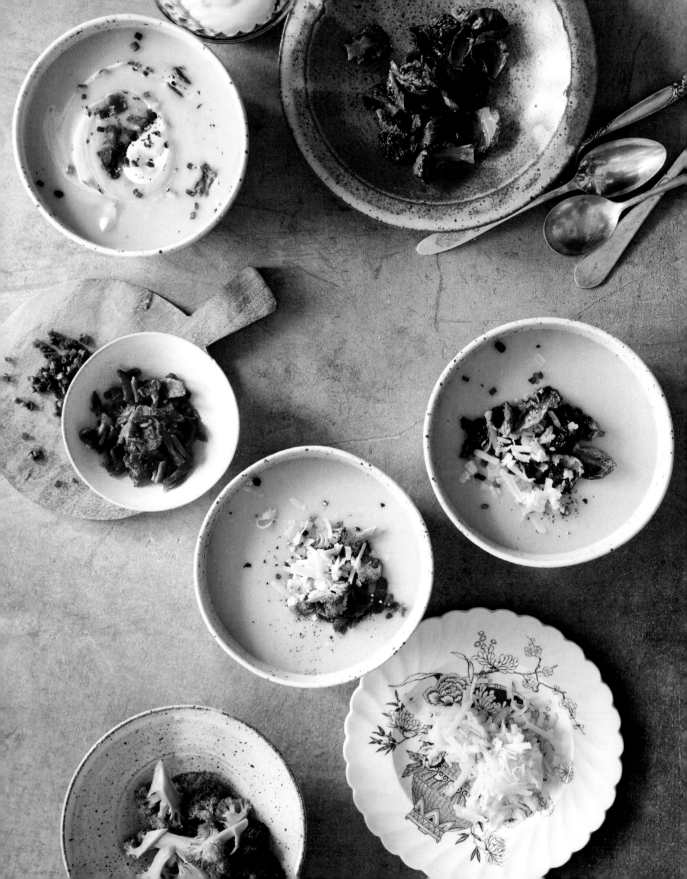

Loaded Baked Potato Soup

SERVES 6 · GF, VEGAN ADAPTABLE, VEGETARIAN ADAPTABLE, DF ADAPTABLE

Truth be told, there are no baked potatoes in this soup, but it really lends itself to loading it up with toppings, the way you would with a real baked potato. To keep this on the healthier side, try to choose more veggies and herbs and minimize the dairy. Speaking of healthier: This soup is so creamy you may be surprised to see cream nowhere in the ingredients. The secret? Cashews, which blend into a nice thick puree.

1. In a large pot, heat the butter until melted. Add the onions, celery, and garlic and sauté over medium heat until tender and translucent, about 6 minutes.

2. Add the chopped potatoes and toss to coat with the onion mixture. Add the cashews, mustard, salt, pepper, and stock. Bring to a boil and lower the heat to a simmer. Cook, covered, until the potatoes are tender, about 20 minutes.

3. Puree the soup with an immersion blender or in batches in a blender. Taste for seasoning. Serve immediately plain or with suggested toppings added on top or stirred in.

TIP: Bake turkey bacon on a parchment-lined baking sheet in a 375°F oven for 20 to 25 minutes, turning after 10 minutes. You can cook it longer or at a higher temperature if you like it crispier.

- Yukon Gold potatoes can be substituted for russet.

- You can also add carrot to give the soup a more golden color; add 1 medium-size carrot, diced, when you add the potatoes.

3 tablespoons unsalted butter or ghee (not vegan/DF), or unrefined avocado oil

2 medium-size onions, chopped

2 celery stalks, chopped

1 garlic clove, finely chopped

2 pounds russet potatoes, peeled, if desired, and chopped

½ cup raw cashews or cooked white beans

1 teaspoon Dijon mustard

2 to 3 teaspoons sea salt, plus more to taste

A few grinds of black pepper, plus more to taste

4 cups chicken stock (not vegan) or light-colored vegetable stock (for homemade, see pages 248–249)

Topping/add-in suggestions: chopped chives, shredded Cheddar cheese (omit for vegan/DF), sour cream or Greek yogurt (omit for vegan/DF), steamed or roasted broccoli florets, pesto (vegan/DF, if necessary), salsa and diced avocado, roasted Brussels sprout leaves, diced cooked turkey bacon (omit for vegan)

Mexican Vegetable Soup with Rice and Beans

SERVES 6 TO 8 · GF, DF, VEGAN ADAPTABLE

2 tablespoons unrefined, cold-pressed extra-virgin olive oil or avocado oil

1 medium-size onion, coarsely chopped

2 celery stalks, coarsely chopped

2 medium-size carrots, coarsely chopped

4 garlic cloves, thinly sliced

1 teaspoon ground cumin

1 teaspoon dried oregano

¼ teaspoon chipotle chile powder

1 pound fresh tomatoes, peeled, seeded and coarsely chopped, or 1 (18-ounce) jar, diced with juice

½ cup fresh cilantro leaves and tender stems, chopped

2 teaspoons sea salt

Freshly ground black pepper

6 cups chicken (not vegan) or vegetable stock (for homemade, see pages 248–249)

½ cup uncooked white or brown, long- or short-grain rice

4 small zucchini, cut into medium dice (about 4 cups)

1½ cups cooked pinto beans, or 1 (15-ounce) can, drained and rinsed

Handful of greens, such as spinach, baby kale, beet green leaves or Swiss chard, coarsely chopped (optional)

Optional toppings: crumbled Cotija cheese (omit for DF), julienned radish, avocado, GF/DF tortilla chips

One month I was testing soup recipes like crazy for my upcoming Mexican cooking class and nothing was hitting the mark. Finally I decided to follow the advice I give my students: when you have a recipe that you love, start tweaking the flavors to create something totally different. I turned to my Late Summer Minestrone recipe and adapted it with Mexican spices and toppings. The verdict—a winner! You can easily serve this soup as a full meal since it is really substantial and provides a complete protein with the beans and rice together. If you really need more, serve it with the Mexican Salad (page 166) or a simple quesadilla.

1. Heat the oil in a large, heavy-bottomed pot over medium-low heat and add the onion, celery, carrots, and garlic. Cook until the vegetables are tender and the onion translucent, about 10 minutes. Add the spices and sauté for 1 minute, or until fragrant.

2. Add the tomatoes with their juice, half of the cilantro, and ½ teaspoon of sea salt. Cook for 5 minutes more, until the tomatoes are fragrant.

3. Add the stock, rice, 1½ teaspoons of salt, and pepper to taste, and bring to a boil. Lower the heat so that the soup simmers. Cook for about 10 minutes for white rice, 30 minutes for brown.

4. Add the zucchini and beans and cook for another 10 to 15 minutes, until the rice is tender.

5. Add the chopped greens, if using, and stir until wilted. Serve with the remaining chopped cilantro and your desired toppings.

6. To freeze, follow the instructions on page 20 for freezing stock.

TIP: Soups with grains tend to thicken up as they sit at room temperature or in the refrigerator. To bring them back to a thinner consistency, warm them on the stove and then add extra stock or water.

Peruvian Chicken and Cilantro Soup with Quinoa

SERVES 6 TO 8 · GF, DF

There's a popular restaurant close to my house called El Pollo Inka that serves up traditional Peruvian food. My favorite item on the menu is Aquadito, a light and fresh brothy chicken soup infused with lots of cilantro. It normally contains rice, but this recipe uses quinoa, which happens to be native to Peru and Bolivia and is a natural fit here. Besides the flavor, what so many of my students love about this recipe is the ease of starting with water and making your own stock from the beginning.

1. Bring the chicken, quinoa, potatoes, celery, garlic, 1 teaspoon of the salt, and 8 cups of water to a boil in a soup pot over high heat. Skim off any impurities that rise to the surface. Lower the heat to medium and simmer, partially covered, until the chicken is tender, about 30 minutes.
2. Remove the soup from the heat. Remove the chicken and celery stalk.
3. Add the frozen mixed vegetables to the soup.
4. Process the cilantro and ½ cup of water in a blender. Stir into the soup mixture.
5. When the chicken is cool enough to handle, remove the meat from the bones and shred into bite-size pieces. Discard the skin, bones, and celery stalk or freeze and save for making stock.
6. Return the chicken meat to the soup and add 2 teaspoons of salt and pepper to taste. Bring to a simmer over medium heat and cook for 5 minutes. Sprinkle with lime juice to taste just before serving, if desired.
7. To freeze, follow the instructions on page 20 for freezing stock.

continued on page 89

- 2½ pounds bone-in, skin-on chicken pieces, or a whole small chicken, quartered
- 6 tablespoons quinoa, rinsed and drained
- 2 Yukon Gold potatoes or boiling potatoes, unpeeled or peeled and cut into bite-size pieces
- 1 celery stalk, halved crosswise
- 1 tablespoon chopped garlic
- 3 teaspoons sea salt
- 1 cup organic fresh or frozen, diced mixed vegetables (e.g., carrots, green beans, whole corn kernels, and/or peas)
- ½ bunch cilantro
- Freshly ground black pepper
- Freshly squeezed lime juice (optional)

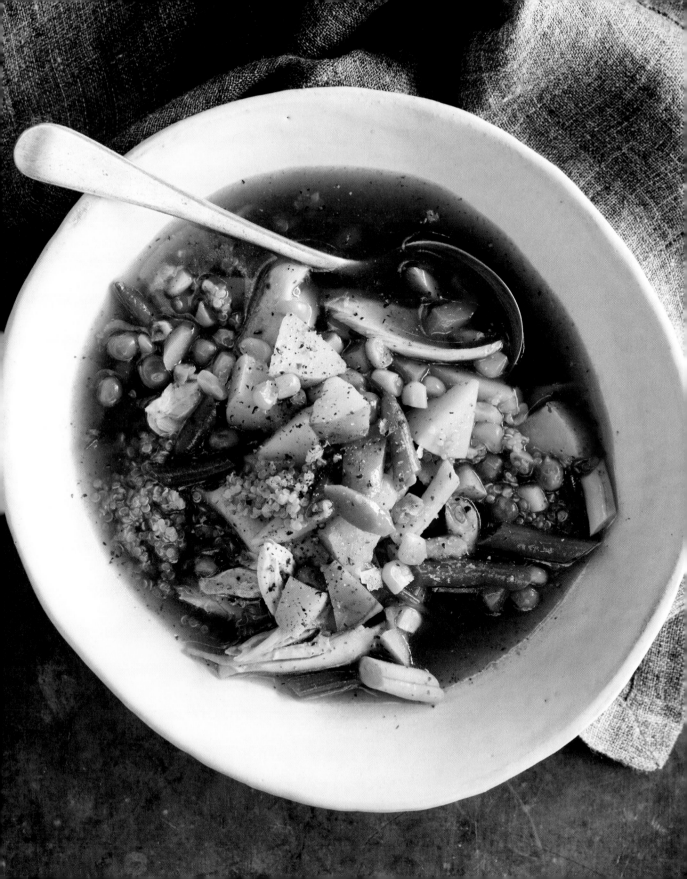

■ White rice or brown rice can be used in place of the quinoa. White rice will cook the same as quinoa. To make with brown rice, you should still take out chicken after 30 minutes. Allow brown rice to cook for another 15 before adding the shredded chicken back to the pot.

ASK PAMELA: Frozen vegetables seem like they wouldn't be nutritious. Are they okay to use? *No one seems to be discouraged by using frozen fruit, but frozen vegetables get a bad rap. I'm not sure why! Fresh is certainly best, but frozen vegetables are picked at their peak and frozen within hours of harvest, thereby locking in the nutrients. Once produce is picked, vitamins start to degrade immediately. By the time it has reached your plate, that fresh vegetable may have fewer nutrients than its frozen counterpart. So, frozen veggies are fine by me, and they are nice to have on hand for convenience. Unfortunately, the same does not hold true for canned vegetables!*

TIP: Cilantro is an amazing detoxifying and chelating herb, which means it can attach itself to heavy metals and pull them out of the body. Cilantro is also a polarizing food; people either love it or hate it. Most haters tell me cilantro tastes like soap or lotion to them. There are theories that disliking cilantro can be genetic. Sometimes you can leave it out of a recipe or substitute another herb, such as parsley. But if you really dislike cilantro, this soup recipe is probably not the one for you.

Italian Wedding Soup

SERVES 8 GF ADAPTABLE, DF ADAPTABLE

MEATBALLS:

1 large egg

¼ onion, finely grated

¼ cup (DF, if necessary) dried whole-grain bread crumbs or dried GF bread crumbs

½ cup (DF, if necessary) fresh whole-grain or GF bread crumbs (1 slice of bread, crusts removed, chopped roughly in a food processor)

⅓ cup grated pecorino or Parmesan cheese (omit for DF)

1 pound ground turkey, preferably dark meat

1 tablespoon finely chopped fresh flat-leaf parsley

1 garlic clove, finely chopped

¾ teaspoon sea salt

Freshly ground black pepper

SOUP:

2 tablespoons unrefined extra-virgin olive oil

1 medium-size yellow onion, diced

2 large carrots, diced

2 celery stalks, diced

10 cups chicken or turkey stock, preferably homemade (page 249)

1½ cups cooked cannellini beans, or 1 (15-ounce) can, drained and rinsed

Sea salt and freshly ground black pepper

8 ounces baby spinach, stems trimmed, or 1 head escarole, chopped

2 tablespoons freshly grated Parmesan or pecorino, plus more for garnish (omit for DF)

Wedding soup is an Italian-American creation and is often broth-based with meat or meatballs and leafy greens. My grandmother used to make this for us when we were little and I can remember my sisters fighting over the tiny meatballs. She used beef for the meatballs and pastina or orzo, but I use turkey as well as white beans, which are a nutritious whole food. Now my kids are the ones fighting over the meatballs!

1. To make the meatballs: Stir together the egg, onion, bread crumbs, and cheese in a bowl. Add the remaining meatball ingredients and combine well with your hands. Using a half-tablespoon or mini ice-cream scooper, scoop the meat mixture into your hands and form about 24 (1-inch-diameter) meatballs. Set aside on a plate or baking sheet. These can be made up to a day ahead, and kept covered and refrigerated.

3. To make the soup: Heat the olive oil in a large pot over medium heat. Add the onion, carrots, and celery and sauté until the onion is translucent.

4. Add the stock, beans, and 2 teaspoons of salt (or more, to taste, if your stock is unsalted). Bring to a boil and carefully add the meatballs (if using escarole, add this now). Lower the heat to a simmer and cook until the meatballs are cooked through, 8 to 10 minutes.

5. Stir in the spinach and grated cheese and cook until the spinach is just wilted. Taste for seasoning, adding pepper to taste. Serve immediately with additional grated cheese.

TIP: If you prefer to use the more traditional pastina or orzo, add already cooked pasta to the soup at the end with the spinach. Another option is cooked Arborio rice or green peas.

ASK PAMELA: What is the difference between dried and fresh bread crumbs? *Fresh bread crumbs are prepared at home with fresh bread that is processed in a blender or food processor until crumbs are made. Dried bread crumbs can be made at home or purchased. They are a dried, finer version. Panko crumbs are a coarse, dried bread crumb.*

Thai Coconut Chicken Soup

SERVES 4 TO 6 · GF, DF

Thai cuisine is one of my favorites. I love the emphasis on fresh ingredients, the balance of flavors, and the lightness of most of the dishes. Many of the herbs and spices used in Thai cooking have wonderful immune-boosting properties and healing benefits. This recipe is my version of the Thai soup tom ga kai; it may not be completely authentic, but it hits all the notes—sour, spicy, salty—and it will fix you up if you're under the weather. You can adjust many of the ingredients according to taste, especially the spiciness. You can also adjust the amount of chicken you use in this recipe according to what else you are making in the meal.

1. Heat the oil in large saucepan over medium heat. Stir in the onion and garlic and sauté until the onion is translucent.
2. Add the ginger, red pepper flakes, salt and lemongrass. Cook until fragrant, about 2 minutes.
3. Add the chicken to the pot and cook, stirring, until the chicken is white on the outside.
4. Stir in the coconut milk, stock, fish sauce, and lime juice and simmer until the chicken is thoroughly cooked and the flavors are well blended, about 10 minutes.
5. Add the bok choy, mushrooms, and cilantro and simmer for another 5 minutes. Taste for seasoning.
6. Remove the ginger and lemongrass stalk before serving.
7. To freeze, follow the instructions on page 20 for freezing stock.

TIPS: For more of a kick, try grating a teaspoon or two of fresh ginger into the soup instead of cutting it into chunks and removing it.

A little mint and/or basil is nice to add with the cilantro.

This soup traditionally contains coconut sugar, which is a higher-quality unrefined sugar. If you would like to balance the sour and spicy with some sweet, add about 2 teaspoons.

2 tablespoons unrefined virgin coconut oil

1 onion, chopped

2 garlic cloves, minced

1 (3-inch) piece fresh ginger, peeled and sliced into big chunks for easy removal

1/4 teaspoon crushed red pepper flakes (optional), or sriracha or red chile paste

1 teaspoon sea salt, plus more to taste

1 (6- to 8-inch) stalk lemongrass, white part only, split down the middle or smashed

1/2 to 1 pound boneless, skinless chicken breast, pounded and thinly sliced

1 (14-ounce) can culinary coconut milk or homemade (page 255)

4 cups homemade chicken stock or light vegetable stock (for homemade, see pages 248–249), or water

3 tablespoons Asian fish sauce

Juice of 1 lime

1 large baby bok choy, thinly sliced

A handful of mushrooms (any type), thinly sliced

1/4 cup fresh cilantro, chopped

Chipotle Turkey Chili with Sweet Potatoes

SERVES 6 TO 8 · GF, VEGAN ADAPTABLE, DF ADAPTABLE

2 tablespoons unrefined, cold-pressed extra-virgin olive oil

1 pound ground dark turkey meat (not vegan) or crumbled plain tempeh

1 medium-size onion, diced

1 jalapeño pepper, diced

4 garlic cloves, minced

1 tablespoon chili powder

2 teaspoons ground cumin

½ teaspoon chipotle chile powder

Pinch of ground cloves

2 teaspoons sea salt

Freshly ground black pepper

14 to 15 ounces diced tomatoes and their juice

3 cups cooked pinto beans, or 2 (15-ounce) cans, drained and rinsed (or use 1 can kidney beans and 1 can pinto)

2 small sweet potatoes (about 1 pound), peeled and shredded (about 4 cups)

Topping suggestions: diced avocado, fresh cilantro, Greek yogurt or sour cream (omit for DF), GF/DF tortilla chips

TIP: Believe it or not, chiles are actually loaded with antioxidants and antibacterial properties and can give a boost to your metabolism.

I absolutely love chili, especially when the weather is cool and there's a good football game on TV. I am definitely more partial to vegetable chilis and ones that are as much beans as they are meat, like this one. Sweet potatoes, which are one of my favorite foods and so incredibly nutrient-dense, add subtle body to this chili. Chipotles are technically smoked, dried jalapeño peppers; they have an intense smoky flavor—and can pack some heat. This recipe is about a 5 on a 1–10 heat scale. Adding avocado, or yogurt or sour cream (omit for DF), will definitely tone down the heat.

1. Heat the oil in a large pot over medium heat. Add the turkey meat and brown, breaking up the meat with a wooden spoon. When just cooked through, remove from the pan, using a slotted spoon, and set aside. If the pot looks dry, add more oil.

2. Add the onion, jalapeño, and garlic and sauté until the onion is tender and translucent, about 6 minutes.

3. Add the spices, salt, and pepper to taste and stir until fragrant, about 1 minute.

4. Add the tomatoes and their juice and cook for another minute or two.

5. Add the turkey meat back to the pot, along with the beans, sweet potatoes, and 2½ cups of water. Bring to a boil, lower the heat to a simmer, and cover. Cook until the sweet potatoes are tender and everything is nice and thick, about 1 hour.

6. Taste for salt and pepper. Serve with your desired toppings.

7. To freeze, follow the instructions on page 20 for freezing stock.

ASK PAMELA: How can I adjust a recipe that contains chiles if my family doesn't like spicy food? *Heat can easily be adjusted in a recipe. You can leave out such ingredients as cayenne or hot sauce. If a recipe calls for chipotle chile powder, you can substitute an equal amount of smoked paprika, which is ground, smoked, and dried bell pepper. Crushed red pepper flakes don't add that much heat in small quantities.*

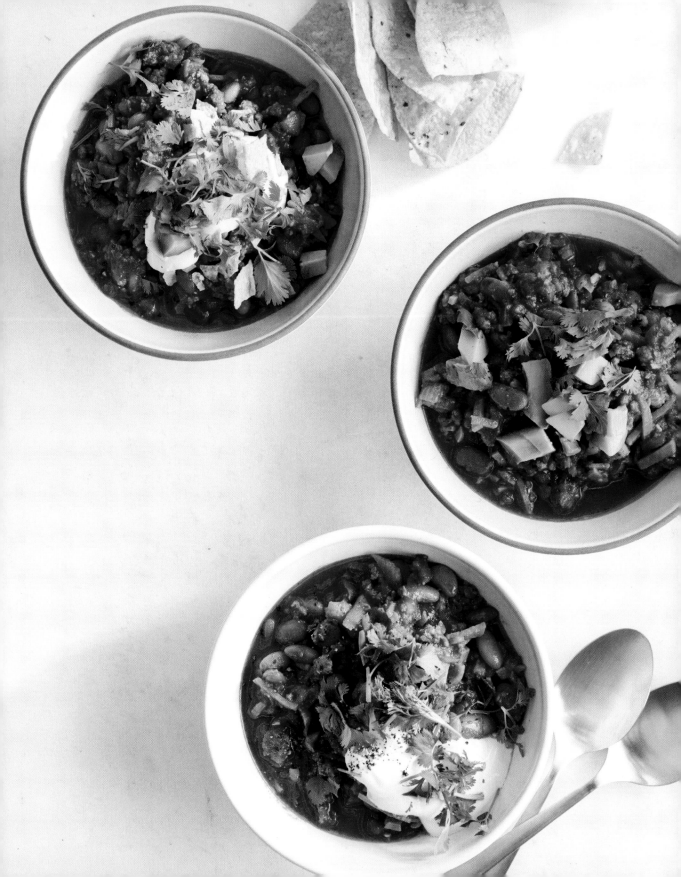

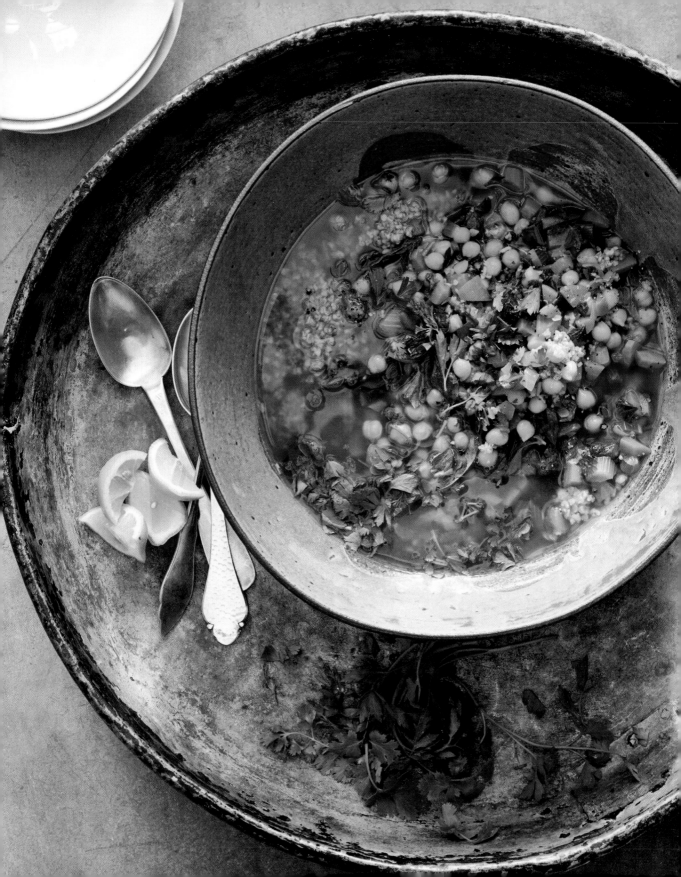

Middle Eastern Vegetable Soup with Freekeh

SERVES 6 · DF, VEGAN ADAPTABLE, GF ADAPTABLE

This soup is at once both comforting and hearty, but at the same time light and fresh. Turmeric, cinnamon, and cumin are a winning, earthy combination with incredible anti-inflammatory properties. Freekeh is a terrific ancient grain popular in the Mediterranean and Middle East. It is wheat that is harvested when it is still green, or young, and then roasted for a really unique and nutty flavor. Check the Resources for where to buy it (page 263). For a gluten-free option, you can always sub 2 cups of cooked millet or brown rice instead.

1. Bring 1½ cups of water to a boil in a small saucepan. Add the freekeh, lower the heat to a simmer and cook, covered, until the grains are tender, 30 to 35 minutes. Set aside.

2. In a large soup pot, heat the olive oil over medium heat. Sauté the onion, carrots, celery, and garlic until tender and translucent.

3. Add the spices, salt, and pepper to taste and cook for a minute, or until fragrant.

4. Add the chickpeas and stock and bring to a boil. Lower the heat to a simmer and cook, partially covered, until the vegetables are tender, 15 to 20 minutes. Add the cooked freekeh and turn off the heat.

5. Add the herbs and spinach and stir until just wilted. Stir in the lemon juice and taste for seasoning.

TIP: "⅓ cup fresh parsley leaves and tender stems, chopped" means you measure out ⅓ cup of herbs and then chop them. If the recipe was written "⅓ cup chopped fresh parsley leaves and tender stems," you would chop the herbs and then measure ⅓ cup.

¾ cup uncooked cracked freekeh (not GF)

2 tablespoons unrefined, cold-pressed extra-virgin olive oil

1 onion, diced

2 carrots, diced

2 celery stalks, diced

3 garlic cloves, finely chopped

1 teaspoon ground cumin

¼ teaspoon ground turmeric

Pinch of ground cinnamon

2 teaspoons sea salt, plus more to taste (double if using unsalted stock)

Freshly ground black pepper

1½ cups cooked chickpeas, or 1 (15-ounce) can, drained and rinsed

6 cups chicken (not vegan) or vegetable stock, preferably homemade (pages 248–249)

⅓ cup fresh parsley leaves and tender stems, chopped

⅓ cup fresh cilantro leaves and tender stems, chopped (omit if you want)

A few handfuls baby spinach leaves

Juice of 1 lemon (3 to 4 tablespoons), or give everyone his or her own lemon wedge

Hearty Vegetable Soup with Kale Pesto

SERVES 4 TO 6 · GF, DF, VEGAN ADAPTABLE, VEGETARIAN ADAPTABLE

3 tablespoons unrefined, cold-pressed extra-virgin olive oil

1 large onion, diced

2 celery stalks, diced

2 carrots, diced

4 garlic cloves, smashed and roughly chopped

2 cups red potatoes, chopped

4 cups green cabbage, chopped, or 3 cups cabbage plus 1 cup cauliflower

1 large Parmesan rind (optional, but it gives great flavor; omit for DF)

1 bay leaf

6 cups vegetable or chicken stock (not vegan), preferably homemade (pages 248–249)

2 teaspoons sea salt

Freshly ground black pepper

6 ounces green beans, trimmed and cut into bite-size pieces

½ cup Kale Pesto, or more as desired (recipe follows), or Basil-Parsley Pesto (page 252)

A basic vegetable soup recipe is easy to master and great to have in your back pocket for those times you need to clean out the crisper drawer (or the freezer—frozen veggies are fine here!). By no means do you need to follow this recipe exactly. I have used everything from turnips to fennel in this soup. If you are struggling with consuming enough vegetables, this soup can help. In addition, cooked vegetables are easier for many people to digest than raw. You certainly don't need to top this soup with pesto, but it does add a fantastic punch of flavor. If you can't have dairy, make the pesto without the cheese and it will still taste great here. This is definitely the time to use that homemade broth you have been saving!

1. Heat the oil in a soup pot over medium heat. Add the onion, celery, carrots, and garlic. Sauté until the onion is tender and translucent, about 6 minutes.

2. Add the potatoes and cabbage. Sauté for 1 minute.

3. Add the Parmesan rind, if using, bay leaf, stock, salt, and pepper to taste and increase the heat. Bring to a boil, lower the heat to a simmer, and cook, partially covered, until the potatoes are just tender, about 15 minutes.

4. Add the green beans and simmer until tender, about 5 minutes. Taste for seasoning.

5. Ladle the soup into bowls and dollop with a spoonful of kale pesto.

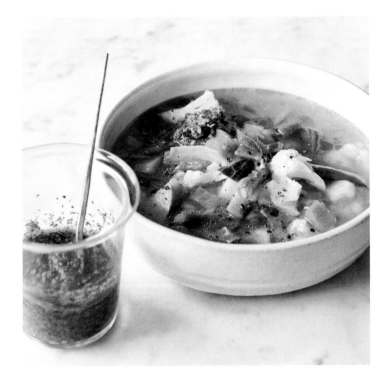

1/2 cup blanched almonds, walnuts, pine nuts, or a combination (or raw sunflower seeds for a nut-free pesto)

1 large garlic clove, smashed

3 cups dinosaur or curly green kale, stemmed and torn into large pieces (so it's easier to measure)

2 cups fresh basil leaves (or use all kale)

1/2 teaspoon fine-grain sea salt

Freshly ground black pepper

1 tablespoon freshly squeezed lemon juice

3/4 cup unrefined, cold-pressed, extra-virgin olive oil

1/3 cup grated pecorino or Parmigiano cheese (omit for vegan/DF)

Kale Pesto

MAKES JUST UNDER 2 CUPS

1. Toast the nuts, stirring frequently, in a dry skillet over medium heat until lightly golden. Remove from the heat and allow to cool. You can also skip this step and put them in the food processor raw. If using sunflower seeds, do not toast.

2. Place the nuts and garlic in a food processor fitted with the metal blade and process until very finely chopped.

3. Add the kale, basil, salt, pepper to taste, and lemon juice and pulse until chopped.

4. With the food processor running, add the olive oil in a steady stream until you achieve a smooth texture. Add the cheese and process until well combined.

5. Taste for seasoning and add additional olive oil to make a looser pesto.

6. Store in the fridge for up to seven days; pesto also freezes really well!

Kitchari

SERVES 6 · VEGETARIAN, GF, VEGAN ADAPTABLE, DF ADAPTABLE

2 tablespoons ghee (not vegan/DF) or unrefined virgin coconut oil

1 tablespoon yellow or brown mustard seeds

½ tablespoon cumin seeds

Pinch or 2 of crushed red pepper flakes

1 cup dried split yellow mung dal, rinsed

1 cup brown or white basmati rice, rinsed

2 large carrots, cut into large chunks

1½ teaspoons ground turmeric

1 teaspoon ground coriander

2 cups finely chopped kale, spinach, beet greens, or Swiss chard

½ cup chopped fresh cilantro, or more to taste

1½ teaspoons sea salt, plus more to taste

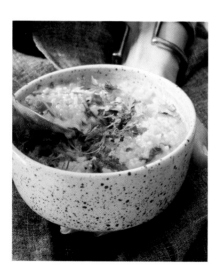

Kitchari is a very digestible and nourishing meal that is both healing and cleansing. It has a wonderful creamy consistency and earthy flavors of turmeric, cumin, and coriander. Traditionally kitchari is more of a stew than a brothy soup, but feel free to add as much water as you want to achieve the consistency you like best. Likewise, white basmati rice is always used in kitchari since it is more digestible than brown. If you prefer to use brown, do soak it in water for 8 hours and then drain before adding to the pot (see page 128 for soaking tips).

1. Heat the oil in a large pot over medium heat. Add the mustard seeds, cumin seeds, and red pepper flakes and gently sauté until the seeds begin to pop.

2. Add the dal, rice, carrots, turmeric, and coriander. Stir together a bit so the spices evenly coat the rice and dal. Add the 8 cups of water. Bring the stew to a boil, cover, and simmer over low heat for about 45 minutes for brown rice or 25 minutes for white rice (add more water, if needed). Feel free to simmer longer, if desired.

3. Once the rice and dal are cooked, add the chopped greens, cilantro, and salt. Stir until just mixed. Turn off the heat, cover, and let stand for about 5 minutes, or until the greens are tender. Kitchari will thicken as it cools, so you may need to add more water than you originally thought.

4. Taste for salt. Serve hot or warm.

5. To freeze, follow the instructions on page 20 for freezing stock.

Broccoli, Celery Root, and Spinach Soup

SERVES 6 · GF, VEGAN ADAPTABLE, VEGETARIAN ADAPTABLE, DF ADAPTABLE

This quick soup is so full of green goodness that you'll feel the nutrients bursting in every spoonful. Celery root, also known as celeriac, is actually the root of a celery plant. It has a definite celery flavor, and it helps to make this soup creamy without having to add any dairy. If you can't find celery root, you can substitute a couple of Yukon Gold potatoes. Pureed vegetable soups mostly follow the same formula: sauté onion in oil or butter, add the main vegetable with some stock and seasoning, cook until tender and puree. You can then play around with different flavor boosters, such as herbs, spices and acids. Give me this and a thick piece of avocado toast and I'm a happy camper!

1. In a large pot over medium heat, melt the butter or heat the oil. Add the onion and garlic and sauté until tender and translucent, about 6 minutes.

2. Add the broccoli, celeriac, stock, salt, and pepper to taste. Bring to a boil over high heat and then lower the heat to a simmer. Cook, partially covered, until the broccoli and celeriac are tender, about 20 minutes. Add the spinach and lemon zest and cook for another couple of minutes until wilted.

3. Puree the soup with an immersion blender or in batches in a blender. Taste for seasoning.

4. To freeze, follow the instructions on page 20 for freezing stock.

- If you are not DF, you can stir in shredded cheese before serving, garnish with grated Parmesan or pecorino, or top with grilled cheese croutons or chopped chives.

TIP: If using broccoli stalks, the outer layer of the stalk should be shaved with a vegetable peeler to remove the tough skin and any fibrous sections.

2 tablespoons unsalted butter (not vegan/DF) or unrefined cold-pressed olive oil

1 medium-size onion, chopped

1 large garlic clove, chopped

1¼ to 1½ pounds broccoli florets and/or broccoli stalks, ends trimmed and any tough woody layers removed

1 celery root, peeled and cubed

6 cups chicken (not vegan/vegetarian) or vegetable stock, preferably homemade (pages 248–249)

1 teaspoon sea salt

Freshly ground black pepper

2 handfuls baby spinach (about 4 cups lightly packed)

2 teaspoons lemon zest

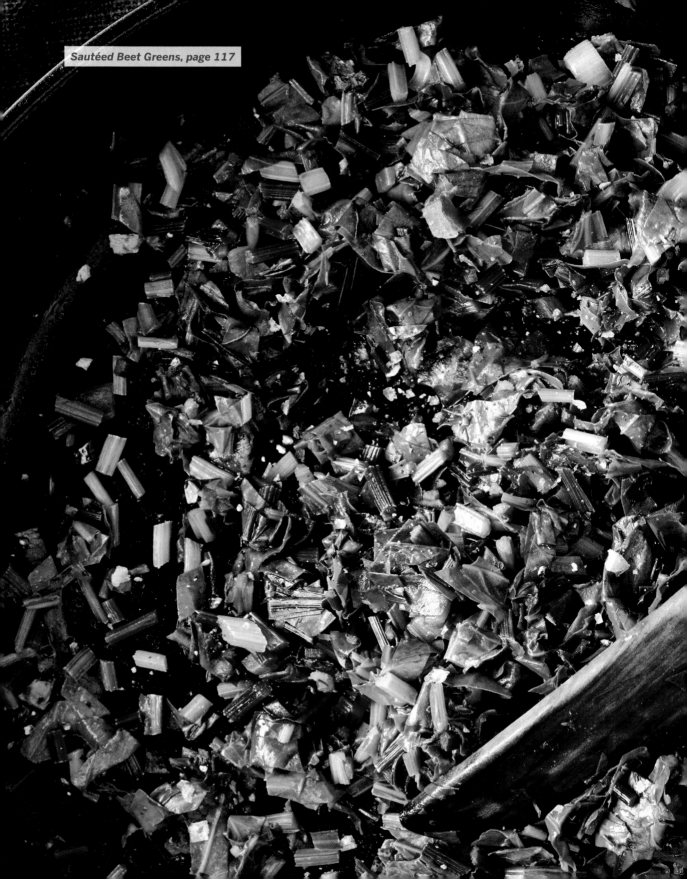

Sautéed Beet Greens, page 117

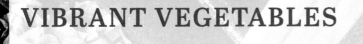

VIBRANT VEGETABLES

Whatever your relationship was with vegetables when you were a kid, it's time to kiss and make up. They are your new best friends when it comes to eating healthfully. And there's no shortage of them; I am always amazed by the incredible variety and sheer beauty the Earth produces for us every season. In fact, if you do your best to use vegetables that are in season, they will be at their peak flavor.

Vegetables contain phytonutrients, which are natural and beneficial compounds found in plants, as well as loads of antioxidants, fiber, vitamins, minerals and all for very few calories. Some vegetables are better for you than others, but all vegetables are good for you (unless of course you have an allergy to them). You don't have to like them all, but if you set one goal for yourself, make it "to eat more vegetables." Vegetables can be eaten raw, roasted, steamed, blanched, sautéed, and grilled. You don't have to be fancy, though. Even if you simply sauté or roast one vegetable a day with salt and pepper, I will be doing cartwheels for you.

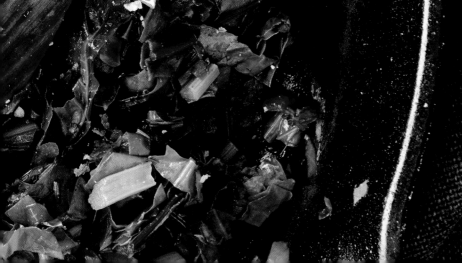

How to Roast Vegetables

My default side dish on any night of the week is roasted vegetables. Roasting brings out the vegetables' natural sugars and a deep flavor. The key to perfectly roasted vegetables is to ensure that each vegetable is caramelized. Caramelizing makes the veggie tender on the inside, crisp on the outside, and most important, brings out the natural sweetness. On pages 104–105, you'll find a chart with common veggies, best oils, roasting times, and other general info. Here, I pass along some of best tips for making perfectly roasted veggies every time.

- Make plenty of vegetables each time and save them for different dishes throughout the week: frittatas, quick lunches, simple salads, and grain bowls.

- When choosing a pan for roasting vegetables, go for a rimmed baking sheet. The rim prevents vegetables from sliding off the edge while it is low enough that the heat will circulate around the vegetables.

- Make sure that all the pieces are all cut to approximately the same size so that they will roast evenly and be finished at the same time. If you are roasting different kinds of vegetables on the same pan, make sure they have similar cooking times and oven temperatures.

- Make sure the vegetables are coated well in the proper oil (see chart for suggestions). You want each vegetable to have a light coating of oil (the oil keeps some moisture in for that interior tenderness), and not pools of oil left on the pan. Too much oil does not result in more crispy vegetables; it actually does just the opposite. A good rule of thumb is about 2 tablespoons of oil per baking sheet; toss the cut veggies with the oil.

- Once the vegetables are properly coated with oil, spread them out evenly across your baking sheet in one layer. If the vegetables are arranged too closely together or are on top of one another, they will steam, making them mushy rather than caramelized.

- Next, season with salt and pepper. This is a key step and can really make a difference in the final flavor. It is hard to give an exact measurement since saltiness really is a personal preference and can vary from vegetable to vegetable, but as a rule of thumb I like to use around ½ to ¾ teaspoon of salt per baking sheet and a few grinds of black pepper. You can always taste the vegetables when they have finished cooking and add more.

- If using only one sheet pan, the center of your oven is usually a good place to put it. When using multiple pans, always go side by side if the oven allows. If you have to roast veggies on two different racks, make sure you put the top rack in the upper third of the oven and the lower rack in the bottom third of the oven. This will allow the heat and air to circulate better to help get the vegetables tender and caramelized. If the baking sheets are only an inch or two apart, the bottom vegetables will steam.

- Another tip when using multiple pans is to rotate the pans halfway through to ensure that all veggies are getting equal exposure to the heat and have an equal chance at getting crispy and caramelized. In my experience, almost every oven has hot spots, so rotating the pans is never a bad idea.

- If you are using multiple pans, another option is to bake on convection, a setting where the heat is circulating via a fan and can produce a better allover heat. This can be very helpful when you are roasting multiple vegetables at once. However, this setting is also more drying and cooks more quickly, so a good rule of thumb is to reduce the oven temperature by 25°F when using a convection setting.

- Lastly, you can add fresh herbs, such as rosemary or thyme, to the pan for a little extra flavor. You can also toss most vegetables with a little ground turmeric for an anti-inflammatory boost. Don't forget to taste the vegetables before serving. You can always finish them with a sprinkle of flaky sea salt and more freshly ground black pepper.

- Roasted vegetables can be stored in the refrigerator for 3 to 4 days. They do not freeze well.

A Guide to Roasting Common Vegetables

VEGETABLE	PREP
Artichoke hearts	If fresh, blanched and quartered
Asparagus	Ends trimmed
Beets	Tops trimmed, scrubbed
Bell peppers	Quartered, stemmed and seeded
Broccoli	Cut into florets, stems trimmed and peeled, sliced into ¼-inch slices
Brussels sprouts	Trimmed and halved
Cabbage	Cut into wedges
Carrots	Peeled and cut into chunks
Cauliflower	Cut into florets
Eggplant	Cut into rounds or cubes
Fennel	Trimmed, cored, and cut into wedges
Garlic, whole head	Wrapped first in parchment and then in foil
Green beans	Trimmed
Kale	Leaves stripped from stems and torn into large pieces
Leeks	Halved lengthwise, washed well and dried
Mushrooms	Sliced or halved
Onions	Sliced or cut into wedges
Parsnips	Peeled and cut into chunks or "fries"
Potatoes, whole	Scrubbed or peeled and cubed
Rutabagas	Peeled and cubed
Scallions, whole	Washed and dried
Sweet potatoes	Scrubbed and cubed or sliced into rounds or "fries"
Sweet potatoes, whole	Scrubbed and wrapped first in parchment and then in foil
Tomatoes, cherry	Left whole or halved
Tomatoes, Roma	Halved
Winter squash	Peeled, seeded and cubed or cut into ½-inch wedges
Zucchini	Cut into rounds or sticks

* Preheat the oven to the recommended temperature (I am aware that olive oil should not be heated above 375°F, but

TEMPERATURE*	TIME	OIL**
400°F	20–25 minutes	olive oil
425°F	20–25 minutes	olive oil, ghee
400°F	45–75 minutes	n/a, roasted in a baking dish with ½ inch of water, covered
425°F	30–35 minutes	olive oil
400°F	30–35 minutes	olive oil, coconut oil
400°F	25–30 minutes	olive oil, coconut oil
400°F	40–45 minutes	coconut oil, olive oil, ghee
400°F	25–30 minutes	coconut oil, olive oil, ghee
400°F	30–35 minutes	coconut oil, olive oil
425°F	20–25 minutes	olive oil
425°F	35–40 minutes	olive oil
350°F	60 minutes	n/a
425°F	12–15 minutes	olive oil
350°F	12–15 minutes	olive oil
400°F	15–20 minutes	olive oil, ghee
400°F	25–30 minutes	olive oil
400°F	30–35 minutes	olive oil
400°F	25–30 minutes	coconut oil, olive oil
400°F	35–40 minutes	olive oil or unsalted butter
425°F	40–45 minutes	olive oil
450°F	12-15 minutes	olive oil
425°F	30–35 minutes	coconut oil, olive oil
400°F	45–60 minutes	n/a
400°F	15–20 minutes	olive oil
450°F	25–35 minutes	olive oil
400°F	40–45 minutes	coconut oil, olive oil, ghee
425°F	20–25 minutes	olive oil

sometimes the flavor is just more compatible). *** Butter and ghee are not vegan/DF.*

Crispy Stovetop Brussels Sprouts

SERVES 6 · VEGETARIAN, GF, VEGAN ADAPTABLE, DF ADAPTABLE

1½ pounds medium-size Brussels sprouts, ends trimmed, halved

Kosher salt

2 tablespoons unrefined, cold-pressed extra-virgin olive oil

2 tablespoons unsalted butter or ghee (not vegan/DF), or unrefined coconut oil (or all olive oil)

Sea salt and freshly ground black pepper

Lemon for squeezing over sprouts or aged balsamic vinegar (optional)

One day I arrived to teach a class only to discover the power was out in the entire neighborhood. I couldn't use the oven, which was needed to roast the Brussels sprouts. I decided to blanch them until they were tender and then sear them in a skillet to get the edges crispy. I was amazed by how much better these were than roasted sprouts. The flavor of caramelized Brussels sprouts is out of this world—sweet, nutty, and completely addictive. This is a great method to have in your back pocket during those times when oven space is limited (Thanksgiving, anyone?).

1. Bring a large saucepan of water to a boil over high heat. Add a heaping tablespoon of kosher salt and the halved Brussels sprouts. Set your timer for 6 minutes.
2. In the meantime, lay a clean kitchen towel on a large, rimmed baking sheet. After the sprouts have been in the water for 6 minutes, either drain them in a colander or remove them from the water with a slotted spoon. Transfer them to the towel to drain very well.
3. Go put on an apron if you are not wearing one, so any splattering doesn't mess up your outfit. Heat a large, heavy-bottomed skillet over medium heat. Add the olive oil and butter.
4. When the oil is foaming, add the sprouts in one layer. Sprinkle generously with sea salt and pepper to taste.
5. Allow the sprouts to brown without burning, 2 to 3 minutes, and then turn with tongs to brown on the other side. Cook until crispy on both sides. Taste for seasoning. Serve as is or with a squeeze of freshly squeezed lemon juice or a drizzle of aged balsamic vinegar.

ASK PAMELA: Why do you use kosher salt in some recipes and sea salt in others? *I use sea salt for everything except in recipes where the salt will not actually be consumed, such as water to blanch vegetables, marinades, pasta water, and so on—kosher salt's my go-to there. You certainly can use sea salt in those recipes, but it seems like a waste of money since sea salt is more expensive.*

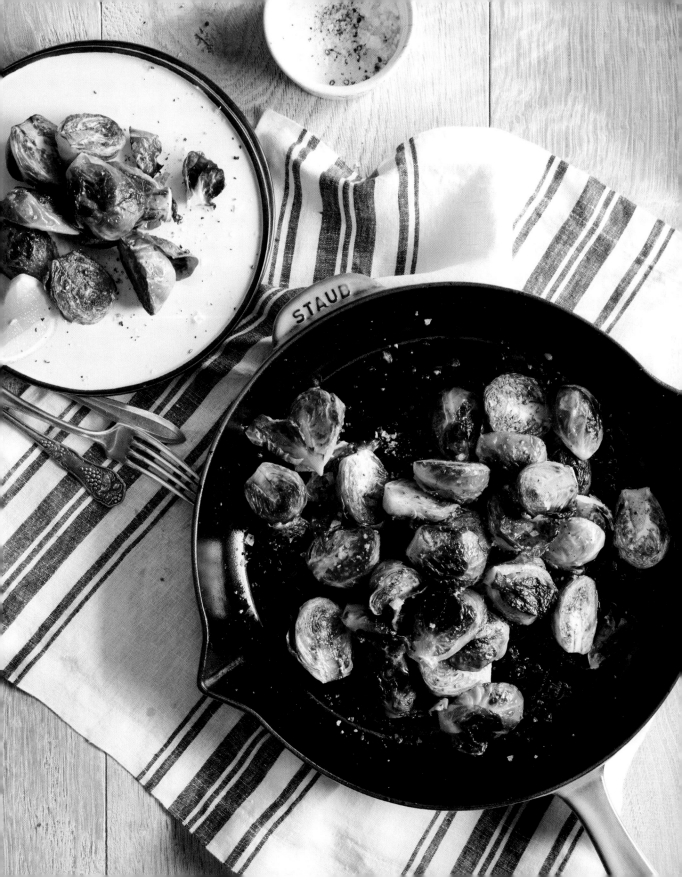

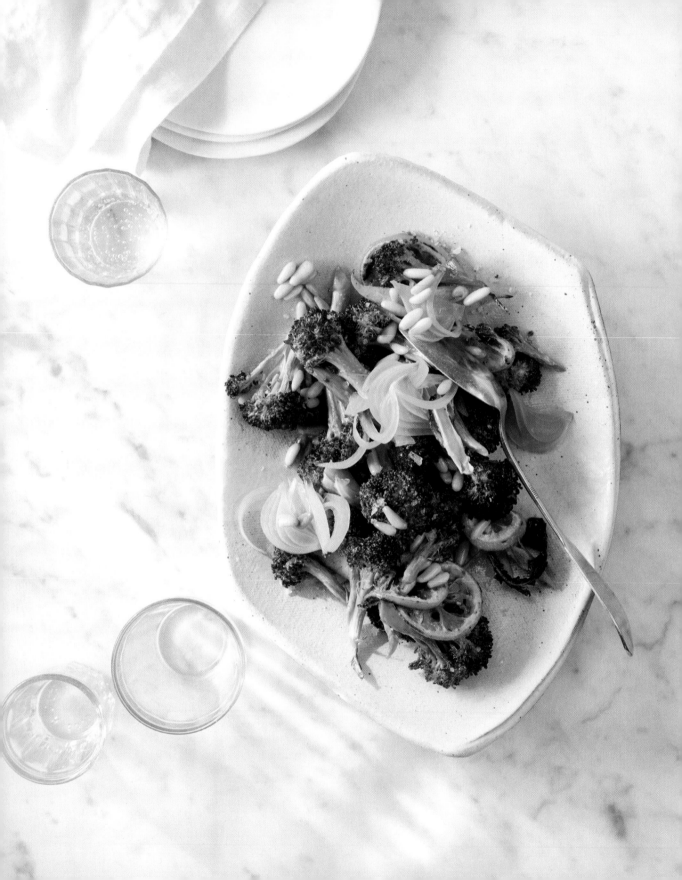

Roasted Broccoli and Lemon with Feta, Pickled Shallots, and Pine Nuts

SERVES 6 · VEGETARIAN, GF, VEGAN ADAPTABLE, DF ADAPTABLE

Broccoli is one of the most nutritious foods you can consume. Because I try to incorporate broccoli into my family's meals at least once per week, I am always looking for new ways to serve it. Roasting broccoli brings out a delicious and nutty flavor; roasting lemon slices and pickling shallots takes this to a whole new level for not much more effort. I have been known to eat half the serving bowl of this and call it a meal!

1. Preheat the oven to 425°F. Line a large baking sheet with unbleached parchment paper.
2. Place the broccoli and lemon slices on the prepared pan. Drizzle with oil and toss to combine. Spread out evenly in a single layer on the pan and sprinkle with salt and pepper to taste. Roast for 20 to 25 minutes, or until lightly golden on the edges.
3. Prepare the pickled shallots: Combine 1 cup of water and the vinegar, sugar, and salt in a small saucepan and bring to a boil. Add the sliced shallots and simmer for 15 minutes. Remove from the liquid and set aside in a bowl to cool.
4. Toast the pine nuts in a dry skillet over medium heat until toasted. Remove from the heat, drizzle with the olive oil, and sprinkle with sea salt to taste. Toss to combine.
5. Place the roasted broccoli and lemon in a bowl and top with the pickled shallots, crumbled feta, if using, and toasted pine nuts. Serve immediately or at room temperature.

ASK PAMELA: I heard grapeseed oil is the best oil to cook with. Why don't you recommend it? *Most grapeseed oil is processed with solvents, such as hexane, and other chemicals. Even if it is expeller-pressed or cold-pressed, grapeseed oil is very high in omega-6 fats, which in excess are pro-inflammatory. Ideally our diet should have a balance of omega-3 fats to omega-6 fats of around 1:1 to 1:3. But the standard American diet has a ratio of omega-3s to omega-6s that is more like 1:25 or even 1:40! If you do want to use grapeseed oil in moderation, look for dark glass bottles that are labeled "cold-pressed" or "expeller-pressed."*

1 pound broccoli crowns, cut into florets and stems sliced

1 lemon, peel on, thinly sliced crosswise (or more if you like)

3 to 4 tablespoons unrefined extra-virgin olive oil or coconut oil, melted

Sea salt and freshly ground black pepper

PICKLED SHALLOTS:

2 tablespoons red wine vinegar

1 tablespoon granulated cane sugar

½ teaspoon kosher salt

2 medium-size shallots, thinly sliced

TO ASSEMBLE:

¼ cup raw pine nuts

¼ teaspoon unrefined extra-virgin olive oil

Sea salt

2 ounces feta cheese, crumbled, preferably goat or sheep's milk (optional; omit for vegan/DF)

TIP: Try to buy feta made with either goat's milk, sheep's milk, or a blend of both, which will taste much richer than feta made with cow's milk. Furthermore, goat's and sheep's milk, which are naturally homogenized, are more digestible than cow's milk.

Turmeric Roasted Cauliflower with Raisins, Capers, and Crispy Quinoa SERVES 6 · VEGAN, GF, DF

1 large head cauliflower (about 2 pounds), cut into 2-inch florets

½ teaspoon ground turmeric

5 tablespoons unrefined virgin coconut oil or olive oil

Sea salt and freshly ground black pepper

3 garlic cloves, thinly sliced

2 tablespoons capers, drained and patted dry

⅓ cup unsulfured golden raisins

½ cup hot water

1 tablespoon white wine vinegar

¾ cup Crispy Quinoa (recipe follows)

2 tablespoons chopped flat-leaf parsley

TIP: Turmeric, a root related to ginger, is one of the most anti-inflammatory foods you can consume. It has more health bene-fits than I have room to mention. It's basically anti-anything you don't want to get! And it is so versatile! It has a pleasant pungent flavor and is available both fresh and dried. I have added ground turmeric to warm almond milk, hot porridge, pancake batter, rice, marinades, soups, and vegetables. Something to consider is that studies have found that consuming black pepper with turmeric boosts the absorption of curcumin, the anti-inflammatory substance in turmeric.

One of my favorite Sicilian-inspired dishes that my grand-mother used to make was pasta with cauliflower, raisins, capers, and toasted bread crumbs. I have dropped the pasta and bread crumbs and roasted the cauliflower with my favorite healthy spice, turmeric. To achieve the same texture that the bread crumbs provided, I use crispy quinoa, which is nothing more than cooked quinoa sautéed in oil until crunchy. If you love the quinoa topping, you can add it to sal-ads, soups and, of course, pasta. My only caveat with eating anything containing turmeric is that it stains like crazy, so don't put out your best napkins with this dish!

1. Preheat the oven to 425°F. Line two rimmed baking sheets with unbleached parchment paper.

2. In a large bowl, toss the cauliflower florets with the tur-meric and 3 tablespoons of the oil. Arrange the cauliflower in one layer on the prepared baking sheets. Season with salt and pepper to taste. Roast until the cauliflower is golden and tender, 40 to 45 minutes.

3. While the cauliflower is roasting, heat the remaining 2 tablespoons of oil in a small skillet over medium-low heat. Add the garlic and sauté, stirring occasionally, until the edges are just golden, 4 to 5 minutes. Stir in the capers and cook until they start to open up, about 3 more minutes. Remove the skillet from the heat.

4. In a medium-size bowl, soak the raisins in the hot water and vinegar until softened and plumped, about 10 minutes. Drain.

5. Transfer the roasted cauliflower to a serving bowl. Sprinkle the raisins and garlic mixture on top, then toss to combine. Taste for seasoning. Top the cauliflower with crispy quinoa and parsley.

ASK PAMELA: Is it okay to drain the whole bottle of capers if not using all at once? *Absolutely! The capers will stay good in the refrigerator with or without the brine.*

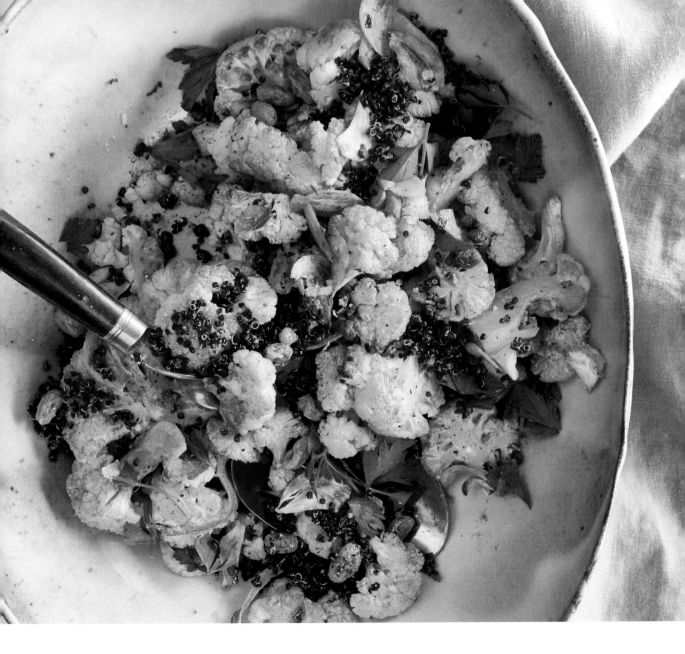

Crispy Quinoa

MAKES ¾ CUP

1. Heat the coconut oil in a skillet over medium heat. Add the quinoa and cook, stirring frequently, until crispy, 6 to 8 minutes. Can be done 1 day in advance and kept in a sealed container at room temperature.

1½ teaspoons unrefined, virgin coconut oil

¾ cup cooked quinoa

Stir-Fried Baby Bok Choy

SERVES 4 TO 5 · GF, DF, VEGAN ADAPTABLE

12 ounces baby bok choy

¾ teaspoon arrowroot powder

½ teaspoon sea salt

3 tablespoons chicken stock (not vegan) or vegetable stock (for homemade, see pages 248–249), or water

1½ tablespoons mirin

1½ teaspoons unrefined toasted sesame oil

1 tablespoon unrefined peanut oil or avocado oil

1 tablespoon peeled, minced fresh ginger (about a 1-inch piece)

2 scallions (white and green parts), thinly sliced

3 large garlic cloves, thinly sliced

Bok choy, also known as pak choi, is a type of Chinese cabbage. Not only is it supernutritious, but bok choy is also a beautiful vegetable with a delicate tulip shape. When cooked, the bottom white part stays relatively crisp, while the green tops become soft and silky. This preparation is simple, quick, and more like a sauté than "fried." Keep in mind you can use this recipe as a formula for stir-frying other quick-cooking vegetables, such as mushrooms, snow peas, and leafy greens. Always remember to have all your ingredients prepped and ready to go, since stir-fries move quickly. If you need to double this recipe, cook it in two batches and not all in one pan; otherwise the vegetables won't cook properly. Serve this with a simply roasted piece of salmon or seared tofu and steamed brown rice.

1. Trim ⅛ inch from the bottom of each head of bok choy, then cut each head into quarters. Wash well between each layer of leaves. Set aside on a clean kitchen towel to dry.

2. In a small bowl, whisk together the arrowroot, salt, chicken stock, mirin, and sesame oil.

3. Heat a wok or a large sauté pan over medium heat and add the peanut oil. Add the ginger, scallions, and garlic to the hot oil and stir-fry until fragrant, about 15 seconds. Add the bok choy and stir-fry until the leaves are bright green and wilted, 1 to 2 minutes.

4. Stir in the stock mixture and stir-fry until the bok choy is crisp tender and the sauce is slightly thickened, about 1 minute. Serve immediately.

TIPS: Sometimes I'll add a pinch or two of crushed red pepper flakes with the ginger mixture, to add a little heat.

You can peel ginger with a vegetable peeler or the tip of a spoon. You can also freeze peeled ginger. Freezing actually helps soften the tough fibers and makes it easier to chop. You might need to leave the frozen ginger on your counter for 5 minutes before cutting it.

Garlicky Kale

SERVES 4 · VEGAN, GF, DF

All vegetables are good for you, but dark green leafy vegetables really are a key superfood if you want to eat your way to better health. And the only thing more healthful than dark green leafies is dark green leafies with garlic! Both groups are very important in the prevention of cancer, and greens are off-the-charts rich in minerals and antioxidants. Garlicky kale is terrific as a side dish with practically any meal, and is especially good in grain bowls and with my Slow Cooker Italian Pot Roast (page 208).

1. Heat a large skillet over medium heat and add the olive oil.
2. Add the garlic and red pepper flakes to the oil and sauté for 30 to 60 seconds, or until fragrant but not golden.
3. Add the kale and toss to coat in the oil.
4. Add ½ cup of water and salt (start with ½ teaspoon) and increase the heat to bring to a boil. Lower the heat to a simmer and cook until the kale is tender and the water has evaporated, 6 to 8 minutes. Taste for tenderness. If the kale is tender, add salt, if necessary, and serve. If the water has evaporated but the kale is still tough, add another ¼ cup of water and simmer until all the liquid has evaporated.

TIP: To strip kale leaves from the stems, grasp the bottom of the stem end with one hand. Take your other hand and place it just above the start of the leafy part, right under your other hand. Pull your hands in opposite directions, stripping the leaves from the stem.

ASK PAMELA: Why can't I eat the kale stems? *You can eat the kale stems, if you like, but I find them to be tough and fibrous. Sometimes I will save them and use them in my juicer.*

2 tablespoons unrefined, cold-pressed extra-virgin olive oil or unrefined coconut oil

4 garlic cloves, thinly sliced

¼ teaspoon crushed red pepper flakes

2 bunches kale, any type, stems stripped and discarded, leaves chopped

Sea salt

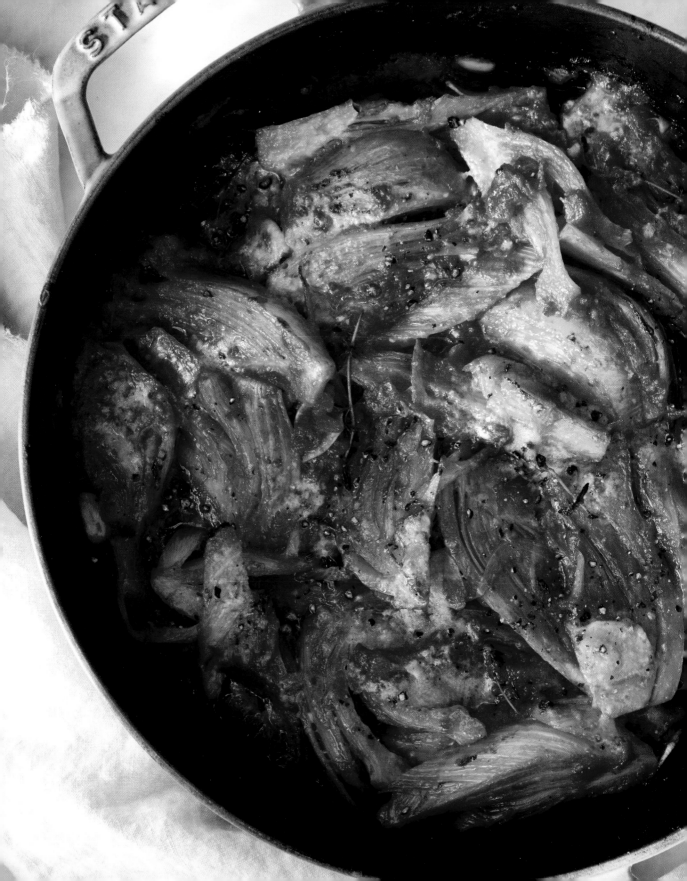

Braised Fennel with Tomatoes and Thyme

SERVES 6 · VEGETARIAN, GF, VEGAN ADAPTABLE, DF ADAPTABLE

Fennel is so underrated. We used to eat it raw in the winter-time after our big Sunday dinners, to help with digestion. I loved its subtle licorice flavor and refreshing crunch. My favorite way to prepare it, though, is by braising it with tomatoes and white wine until it is meltingly tender and almost buttery. This is divine over soft polenta, with roasted chicken, or a piece of simply baked halibut.

1. Heat a large, ovenproof skillet over medium heat and melt the ghee. Add the onion slices and sauté until tender and translucent.
2. Add the fennel wedges and cook for a few minutes on each side, until lightly browned.
3. Make some room in the pan and add the garlic and red pepper flakes. Sauté until fragrant, about 1 minute.
4. Add the white wine and simmer until reduced by half. Add the tomatoes, salt, black pepper, and thyme sprigs. Bring to a boil, lower the heat to a simmer, cover (you can use a piece of foil if you don't have a lid for the skillet), and simmer for 20 to 30 minutes, or until very tender (check this by poking the fennel with the tip of a paring knife.)
5. Position an oven rack 6 inches below the broiler unit (usually the second level in the oven). Preheat the broiler in the oven to high. Sprinkle the grated cheese, if using, evenly over the fennel and broil for 2 to 3 minutes, or until golden brown. Serve hot, warm, or at room temperature.

ASK PAMELA: Which white wines are best for cooking? *You want to cook with a dry white wine, which means one that is not sweet. I like chardonnay, pinot grigio, and sauvignon blanc for cooking. You do not need to buy an expensive wine for this or any other recipe. I usually pick a modestly priced one—it's good enough to cook with. Don't buy "cooking wine," which I think tastes awful. If you're not a white wine drinker, consider buying four-packs of smaller bottles of wine so you don't have to open a brand new bottle just for ¼ cup.*

2 tablespoons ghee (not vegan/DF) or unrefined, cold-pressed extra-virgin olive oil

½ large onion, thinly sliced

3 large fennel bulbs, bottoms trimmed and stalks removed, bulbs cut lengthwise through the core into quarters or sixths

3 large garlic cloves, thinly sliced

A big pinch of crushed red pepper flakes

¼ cup dry white wine

1 (18-ounce) jar diced tomatoes with the juice

1½ teaspoons sea salt

Freshly ground black pepper

4 sprigs fresh thyme

3 tablespoons grated pecorino or Parmesan cheese (optional, omit for vegan/DF)

Garden Veggie Patties with Herbed Yogurt Dipping Sauce

MAKES 12 PATTIES · VEGETARIAN, GF ADAPTABLE, DF ADAPTABLE

Unrefined extra-virgin olive oil, for the pan and tops of the patties

1½ cups cauliflower florets, steamed until tender and finely chopped

1½ cups broccoli florets, steamed until tender and finely chopped

1 cup grated carrot (about 2 medium-size carrots)

1 cup frozen chopped spinach or kale, defrosted, excess water squeezed out

3 scallions, thinly sliced

3 large eggs, beaten (you can even add 1 more to boost the protein)

1 cup whole wheat pastry flour, whole spelt flour, or GF flour (if necessary)

¼ cup grated pecorino or Parmesan cheese (omit for DF)

¼ cup shredded mozzarella cheese or sharp Cheddar cheese (omit for DF)

½ teaspoon garlic powder

Pinch of crushed red pepper flakes

1½ teaspoons sea salt

Freshly ground black pepper

Accompaniment: Herbed Yogurt Sauce (recipe follows) or warm Marinara Sauce (for homemade, see page 253)

It's not easy to find fun but healthful foods that appeal to kids and adults, but I've learned it's all about the presentation. My son gets "veggie patties with ranch dressing." My husband and our friends dine on "Garden Vegetable Croquettes with Herbed Yogurt Dipping Sauce." Whatever you call them, these patties are chock-full of vegetables and so, so yummy. You can adjust the mix of vegetables according to what you have on hand: leave out the cauliflower and double the broccoli, for example. I have also served the patties with a warm tomato sauce instead of the yogurt sauce, for a change of pace. These freeze beautifully. For a dairy-free version, omit the cheeses and add an extra pinch of salt and garlic powder. For a GF version, omit the flour and sub ½ cup of blanched almond flour and 2 tablespoons of coconut flour.

1. Preheat the oven to 400°F. Line a baking sheet with unbleached parchment paper and brush the paper with olive oil.

2. Place all the ingredients, except the olive oil for brushing the patties, in a large bowl and mix well to combine.

3. Using your hands or with a medium-size ice-cream scoop, form the veggie mixture into a ball slightly larger than a golf ball and place on the prepared baking sheet. Press down to form a patty. Continue with the rest of the batter and then brush the tops of the patties with olive oil.

4. Bake for 15 minutes, or until firm and golden. These can also be pan-sautéed in olive oil, coconut oil or ghee (omit for DF). Serve with herbed yogurt sauce or marinara.

TIPS: To steam the cauliflower and broccoli, cut into large florets and place in a vegetable steamer over boiling water and steam, covered, until tender, 7 to 10 minutes.

Squeeze extra water out of your spinach in a nut milk bag or a thin kitchen towel.

Herbed Yogurt Sauce

1. Place all the ingredients in a bowl and stir to combine.
2. Transfer to a container and refrigerate, covered, for at least an hour so that the flavors develop.

1 cup plain, unsweetened full-fat Greek yogurt (not DF) or Savory Cashew Cream (page 258)

1 small clove garlic, grated or minced

2 teaspoons freshly squeezed lemon juice

1/2 teaspoon sea salt

Freshly ground black pepper

Pinch of cayenne pepper

2 tablespoons chopped fresh chives, or 1 scallion, finely chopped

2 tablespoons flat-leaf parsley leaves, finely chopped

Sautéed Beet Greens

SERVES 2 · VEGAN, GF, DF

Yes, you can eat the leafy green tops of the beet plant! They are so, so good for you and they taste exactly like Swiss chard. Beet greens have a higher nutritional content than beets themselves and rival the iron content in spinach. They are incredibly high in beta-carotene and vitamins C and K, as well as calcium. The key with this recipe is taking the time to dice those stems and leaves as finely as possible. Beet greens contain a fair amount of natural sodium, so be conservative when seasoning. You can also sauté them with olive oil and garlic for a different flavor.

1. Cut the stems off the beet greens and dice finely, smaller than the size of a pea. Set aside. Chop the leaves very finely, keeping separate from the diced stems.
2. Heat a medium skillet over medium heat, add the coconut oil, and melt. Add the beet green stems and onion. Sauté until the onion is translucent and the stems are tender, 3 to 5 minutes.
3. Add the chopped leaves, plus salt and pepper to taste. Sauté until wilted, 2 to 3 minutes.
4. Drizzle with a little aged balsamic vinegar and stir. Taste for seasoning and serve.

1 bunch beet greens (from 3 large beets), washed very well

1 tablespoon unrefined virgin coconut oil or olive oil

2 tablespoons diced red onion or shallot

1/8 teaspoon sea salt, plus more to taste, if desired

Freshly ground black pepper

Aged balsamic vinegar

TIPS: Make sure you buy beets with healthy greens attached, ones that are vibrant and strong, not wilted or slimy. They go bad quickly, so try to use them up within a few days of purchase.

If you only have a small bunch of greens, mix them up with a bunch of Swiss chard—you'll have enough for the whole family.

Miso-Glazed Japanese Mushrooms

SERVES 4 TO 6 · GF, DF, VEGAN ADAPTABLE

GLAZE:

2 tablespoons mirin

2 tablespoons chicken stock (not vegan) or vegetable stock (for homemade, see pages 248–249), mushroom stock, or water

2 tablespoons unseasoned rice vinegar

1 tablespoon GF white or yellow miso

MUSHROOMS:

1 tablespoon unrefined toasted sesame oil

1 tablespoon unrefined extra-virgin olive oil or avocado oil

1½ pounds mixed mushrooms, preferably Japanese, wiped clean with a damp paper towel, then sliced

4 garlic cloves, thinly sliced

Sea salt

Freshly ground black pepper

1 green onion, sliced thinly, for serving

All mushrooms are good for you, but Japanese mushrooms are nutritional standouts. Studies show they are antitumor, antiviral, and immunity-boosting; support heart health; and can help lower cholesterol. I also think Japanese mushrooms taste better: They tend to have a more intense, meaty flavor. Shiitake, maitake, enoki, and oyster mushrooms go well together in this recipe, but you can also mix in some cremini or button mushrooms. A nice combination would be ½ pound each of maitake, shiitake, and cremini. Or if you simply cannot find Japanese mushrooms, use all standard ones.

1. Combine the mirin, stock, and rice vinegar in a small saucepan and heat over medium heat until warm. Turn off the heat and whisk in the miso until smooth.

2. Heat a large, cast-iron skillet over medium heat and add ½ tablespoon each of the sesame oil and the olive oil. Add half of the mushrooms to the hot oil and allow to sit undisturbed for a minute or two, until slightly golden brown. Sauté until just tender. Transfer to a serving bowl.

3. Add remaining ½ tablespoon each of sesame oil and 1 olive oil to the skillet with the remaining mushrooms and repeat.

4. Just before the mushrooms are tender, add the garlic and stir around the skillet until fragrant, about 30 seconds. Return the reserved cooked mushrooms to the skillet.

5. Turn off the heat, pour the miso mixture into the pan, and stir until well combined. Season with a pinch of salt and a few generous grinds of black pepper, or more to taste. Garnish with sliced green onions and serve.

TIPS: Since mushrooms are like little sponges, it is better to clean them by wiping them with a damp paper towel. If you wash them under running water or in a bowl of water, they just get waterlogged and soggy. The only time this doesn't matter is when you're using the mushrooms in a soup or a stew.

Keep in mind when you are cooking with miso, because it is a live food, you want to take care not to boil it so as to preserve the live enzymes. This is why the last step instructs you to remove the skillet from the heat and then stir in the miso mixture.

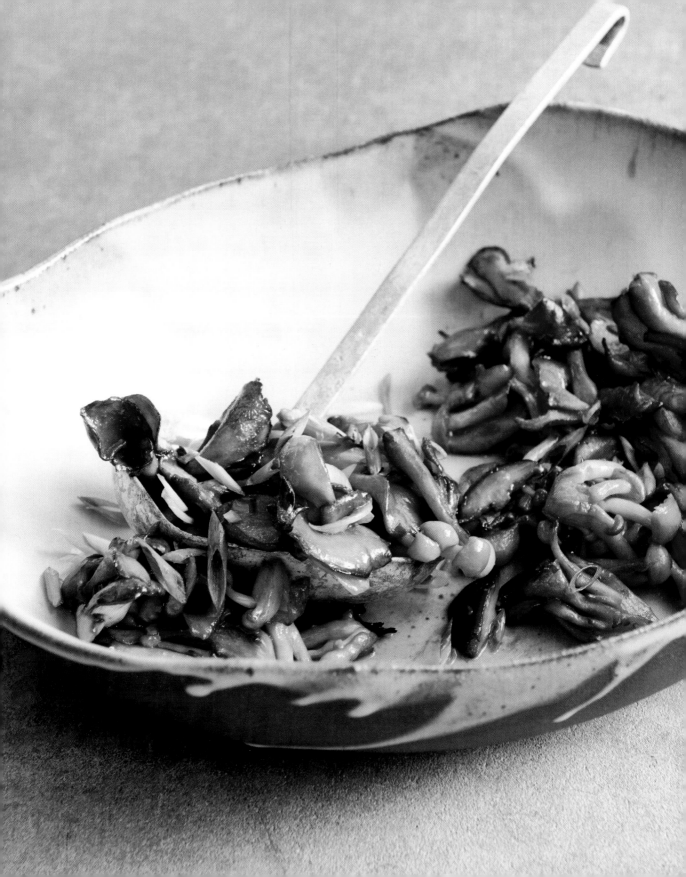

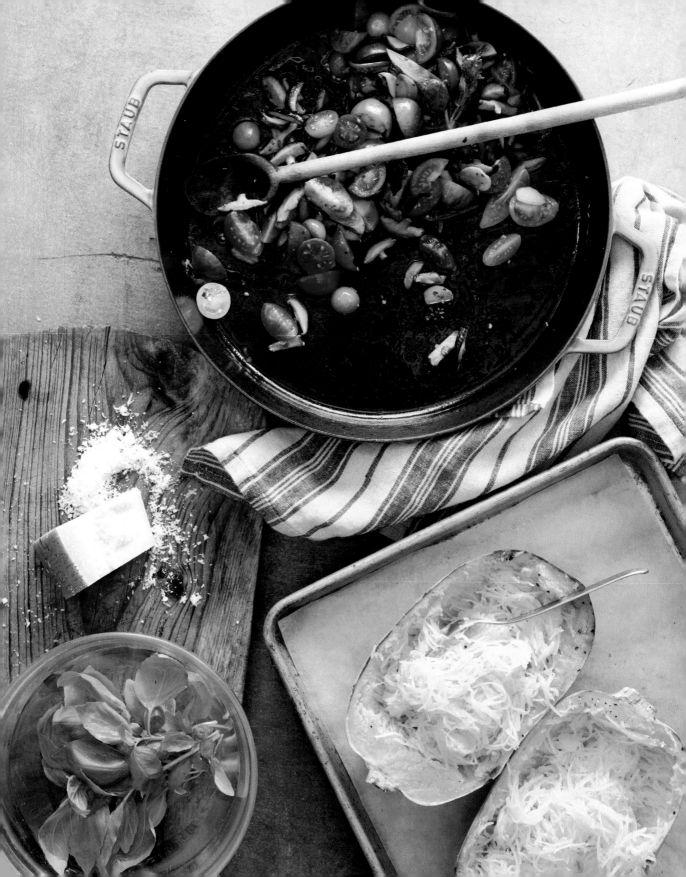

Spaghetti Squash with Cherry Tomatoes, Mushrooms, and Spinach

SERVES 4 TO 6 · GF, VEGAN ADAPTABLE, DF ADAPTABLE

I love substituting a whole food, such as squash, for a processed (and usually refined) food, such as pasta. Furthermore, I can eat a lot more spaghetti squash than pasta and not feel heavy and weighed down. While it is considered a winter squash, spaghetti squash has the water content of a summer squash. It is much lower in carbohydrates than a butternut squash, for example. All that water makes for a very mild flavor, so I always pair it with such ingredients as garlic, chiles, and lots of herbs. This heavenly mixture of vegetables, garlic, and herbs would also work well as a topping for traditional pasta. This could easily be a vegetarian main dish to which you can add cooked white beans or chickpeas and/or toasted pine nuts.

1. Preheat the oven to 375°F. Line a baking sheet with parchment paper and set aside. Cut the spaghetti squash in half lengthwise and remove the seeds. Rub the inside of each half with a drizzle of olive oil and season with ½ teaspoon of salt and black pepper to taste. Arrange, cut side down, on the prepared baking sheet and bake for 30 to 45 minutes, or until tender. Check doneness by inserting a fork between the skin and the flesh. If it is tender and you can start to create strands with the fork, then it's done.

2. Flip them over (otherwise they'll keep cooking) and set aside until they are cool enough to handle.

3. Heat the olive oil in a large sauté pan over medium heat. Add the mushrooms and sauté until caramelized and just tender, about 3 minutes.

4. Add the garlic and red pepper flakes and sauté until fragrant, 30 to 60 seconds. Add the tomatoes and two big pinches of salt, plus black pepper to taste. Cook the tomatoes, stirring, until they start to lose their shape, about 5 minutes.

continued on page 122

1 spaghetti squash (about 3¼ pounds)

¼ cup cold-pressed extra-virgin olive oil, plus more for drizzling the squash

Sea salt and freshly ground black pepper

½ pound shiitake mushrooms, stems removed, caps wiped clean with a damp paper towel and sliced

6 garlic cloves, thinly sliced

Pinch of crushed red pepper flakes

1 pound cherry tomatoes, stemmed and halved

2 big handfuls baby spinach leaves

½ cup fresh basil leaves

Grated Parmesan or Pecorino Romano cheese (optional; omit for vegan/DF)

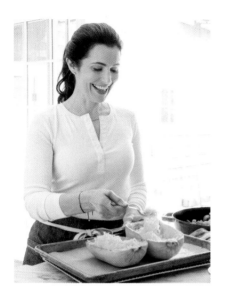

TIP: To cut a spaghetti squash, first slice off the stem end. Then insert the tip of your knife an inch or two above the round mark at the bottom of the squash and pull down, making a small cut. Move the knife another inch or two above the first cut and pull down again. Keep moving toward the center of the squash until you reach the middle, then flip the squash around and insert the knife in the middle and pull down in the opposite direction. It should split in half all the way. Scoop out the seeds with a large spoon.

5. Stir in the spinach and sauté until wilted, about 3 minutes. Tear or slice the basil leaves and stir into the mixture. Check for seasoning and remove from the heat.

6. Using a fork, pull the strands of squash crosswise (the short way) from the peel so that it resembles spaghetti. Place the strands into a serving bowl and add the sauce. If you cook the spaghetti squash in advance and it is no longer hot, add it to the sauce in the sauté pan and sauté over medium heat until warmed through. Add the Parmesan or pecorino, if using, and toss to combine. Taste for seasoning. Since spaghetti squash is rather bland, you will need to add extra salt and black pepper.

ASK PAMELA: How do I pick out a good spaghetti squash?
When they're in season, they should all be good so long as the skin is smooth and tight and there are no soft spots or bruises. I think the paler-skinned squashes make better, more separate strands. It's good to know that a smaller spaghetti squash requires less roasting time and a larger squash requires more.

Sautéed Zucchini with Shallots

SERVES 4 · VEGAN, GF, DF

My father always planted several zucchini plants every year; if we weren't paying attention, the zucchini could grow to be as large as a baseball bat. Bigger isn't better with zucchini, though; the most tender and sweet zucchini are the smallest ones. Zucchini are not meant to be peeled, and you shouldn't since that's where most of the nutrients lie. They are full of antioxidants, potassium, and B-complex vitamins and minerals. Zucchini can also help replenish the adrenal glands, which are overtaxed in many of us due to our stressful lives. Ironically, zucchini are the only vegetable my father isn't crazy about, so I came up with this recipe to change his mind. And I did! I make this dish all summer long, served with Herbed Mixed-Grain Pilaf and Grilled Lemon-Herb Shrimp (pages 149 and 201).

2 tablespoons unrefined, cold-pressed extra-virgin olive oil or avocado oil

2 medium-size shallots, peeled and sliced (about ½ cup)

1½ pounds small or medium-size zucchini, ends trimmed, sliced ¼ inch thick on the diagonal

½ teaspoon sea salt, plus more to taste

A few grinds freshly ground black pepper

⅓ cup sliced almonds

1 lemon, halved

1. Heat the oil in a large skillet over medium heat.
2. Add the shallots to the oil and sauté until just tender, 3 to 4 minutes.
3. Increase the heat to medium-high and add the zucchini, salt, and pepper. Sauté until the zucchini is tender and cooked through, 5 to 6 minutes.
4. Stir in the sliced almonds.
5. Squeeze the lemon halves over the zucchini and stir. Taste for seasoning and serve immediately. This would also be nice with some fresh mint.

ASK PAMELA: What exactly is one shallot if it is peeled and reveals two separate cloves inside? *I try to put exact measurements for shallots in my recipes, but I always consider one shallot the entire bulb, no matter how many cloves it splits into. A large shallot will yield between ⅓ and ½ cup of chopped or sliced shallot; a medium-size one, about ¼ cup; and a small one, about 2 tablespoons.*

Grilled Eggplant with Pomegranate Molasses

SERVES 4 · GF, VEGAN ADAPTABLE, DF ADAPTABLE

1 medium-size to large globe eggplant (about 1 pound), ends trimmed, or 1¼ pounds baby eggplant

2 teaspoons kosher salt (optional)

3 tablespoons unrefined, cold-pressed extra-virgin olive oil

Freshly ground black pepper

2 teaspoons pomegranate molasses

¼ cup fresh mint leaves, small ones left whole, larger ones sliced

Toasted pine nuts and/or crumbled feta (optional; omit for vegan/DF)

TIPS: If you can't find pomegranate molasses, use aged balsamic vinegar.

Salting eggplants prior to cooking them may reduce possible bitterness, but I also like to do this step because it helps soften the flesh.

Turkey's veggie-centric cuisine is a perfect blend of Mediterranean and Middle Eastern; I was in heaven when I visited. Something I noted when I was there was the liberal use of pomegranate molasses, a thick, tart syrup that is essentially reduced pomegranate juice (hello, antioxidants!). It was drizzled on things where you might expect to use aged balsamic vinegar. Check the Sources Section on where to find it. The jolt of pomegranate molasses is simply divine combined with the smokiness of grilled eggplant. This is a really easy vegetable dish which can be served warm or at room temperature. It would be perfect with Chicken Shawarma (page 188).

1. Slice the eggplant into ½-inch rounds. (If you are using baby eggplants, just halve them through the stem.) If you have time, salt the slices: arrange the slices in one layer on a baking sheet and sprinkle the tops of each slice with kosher salt. Allow to sit at room temperature for 30 to 60 minutes, until the eggplant slices have "sweated." About 15 minutes before you want to cook the eggplant, preheat a grill to medium.
2. Rinse the eggplant and squeeze dry between two paper towels. Arrange them once again on the same baking sheet. Use 2 tablespoons of the oil to brush both sides of each eggplant slice. Sprinkle with pepper to taste.
3. Place the eggplant slices on the grill and cook until golden brown, 5 to 6 minutes (it could take less time depending on temperature of your grill). Flip over and cook the other side.
4. Arrange the eggplant on a platter by slightly overlapping them. Cover the platter with aluminum foil and allow the eggplant to steam to further soften, about 10 minutes.
5. Remove the foil and drizzle eggplant with the remaining tablespoon of oil and the pomegranate molasses and garnish with mint leaves. You can also add toasted pine nuts, as well as crumbled feta.

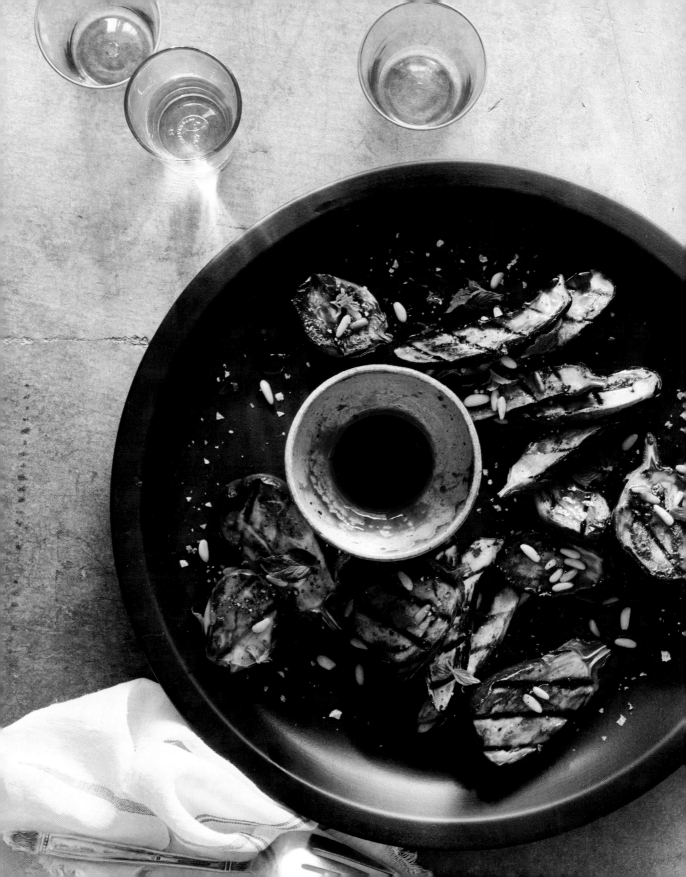

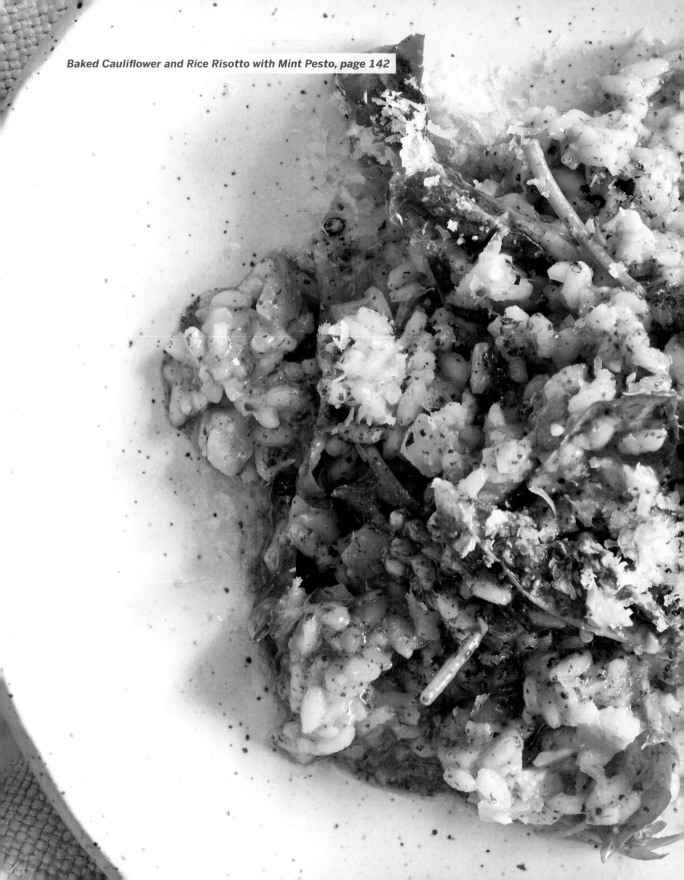

Baked Cauliflower and Rice Risotto with Mint Pesto, page 142

GREAT GRAINS AND STARCHES

Whole, complex carbohydrates are an important part of my diet. They form the basis for many meals, are inexpensive, and contain many nutrients as well as fiber. Grains and legumes have become controversial and there are people who think they are detrimental to our health—but I disagree. Certainly there are some who cannot tolerate grains and/or legumes, and they should abstain from eating them. But most people can consume both without any difficulty. It helps if you soak them (more on this in a few pages).

My family and I eat a wide variety of grains and legumes, and that is the key: variety.

There's such a rich array, plus the flavor is more interesting and satisfying in whole grains than refined. I love making big batches of different grains and legumes on the weekend to have on hand for any meal, as the basis for bowls, porridges, and stir-fries, and to be added to salads, soups, and more. They are blank canvases, ready to be enhanced in infinite ways. To expand your canvas with a totally grain-free "grain," you can switch off to Cauliflower Rice (page 251).

Whatever grains and legumes you don't consume within three days can be successfully frozen for up to three months.

How to Soak Grains and Legumes

Whole grains definitely can be part of a healthful diet, but they are much more nutritious and digestible when prepared the way our ancestors did. Whole grains and legumes contain an antinutrient called phytic acid, which can bind with certain minerals, such as zinc, calcium, and iron, and prevent them from being absorbed by the body.

Soaking, fermenting, or sprouting your grains and legumes before cooking them will neutralize the phytic acid, thus making these foods much easier to digest and making the nutrients easier to assimilate. Phytic acid can be neutralized in as little as seven hours when soaked in water with the addition of a small amount of an acidic medium such as vinegar or lemon juice. Soaking also helps to break down gluten, a hard-to-digest protein found in such grains as wheat, spelt, rye, and barley. If you've been eating whole grains and legumes for years without soaking, don't stress. A small amount of phytic acid is reduced just by the cooking process alone. But for minimal effort, you can significantly improve the digestibility and nutrition of these important foods. Fortunately, grains and legumes are very easy to soak; here are basic instructions:

1. Start the soak the night before or the morning of the day you want to eat them.
2. Pour the grains or legumes into a bowl and cover with warm or room-temperature filtered water. Add a tablespoon of something acidic, such as yogurt, raw cider vinegar, lemon juice, whey, or kefir, for example.
3. Cover and allow to sit at room temperature for at least 7 hours or longer.
4. Change the water after 24 hours if you're still soaking (see note below).
5. Drain and rinse the grains or legumes before cooking with fresh water.

Even though 7 to 8 hours is the minimum recommended for soaking, even a few hours is better than nothing. An extra benefit to soaking grains is a shorter cooking time. The longer you soak them, the less time is needed to cook and also less water. There's no formula to figuring this out, but usually if you soak 1 cup of brown rice for 8 hours, you can reduce the cooking time from 50 minutes to about 40 and use about ⅓ cup less water. For 1 cup of soaked quinoa, you can cook for about 10 minutes and use 1¼ cups of water.

If the grains or legumes have been soaking all day but you can no longer commit to cooking them, change the water and refrigerate them for up to three more days.

If you don't want to make the effort to soak, many supermarkets now carry sprouted grains (as well as sprouted flours, nuts, and seeds) that have already been soaked; you can simply follow the package directions to cook them.

How to Cook Beans from Scratch

I use beans in chili, soups, salads, pastas, veggie burgers, with braised greens, in dips, and even in desserts. Beans are quite affordable. In fact, you will save a lot of money cooking your beans from scratch. Not only that, most cans are lined with BPA, which is a carcinogen that is not easily detoxified. That said, I still keep a few BPA-free cans of cooked beans in the pantry. Here are some tips:

- Buy beans from a store with a high turnover because old beans take longer to cook.

- Plan ahead: Beans need to soak for at least 6 hours, then cook for an hour or more.

- Pick through the beans before soaking and look for any small stones or debris.

- Beans expand once cooked and usually yield about three times the amount. One pound of dried beans usually translates to four 15-ounce cans of cooked beans.

To soak: Place the beans in a large bowl or pot and cover with a generous amount (4 to 6 inches) of cold water. If you have a piece of kombu (kelp), add that to the beans for additional digestibility and alkalinity. Leave the bowl on the countertop or in the refrigerator for at least 6 hours or overnight. It is not necessary to cover the bowl, but you can. Check to make sure all the beans stay below sea level!

To cook on the stovetop: Drain the soaking liquid and transfer the beans (with kombu, if using) to a large pot. (If you're using the beans for a salad, you can add chopped onion or celery.) Fill with fresh cold water to cover by at least 4 inches and bring to a boil over high heat. Lower the heat to a simmer and skim off any foam from the top. Partially cover. Maintain a gentle, active simmer. Boiling the beans rapidly can make them lose their shape. Start to test the beans for tenderness after 50 minutes. Continue to taste them until the desired tenderness is achieved. This can take an hour or more, depending on the age of the beans.

   Turn off the heat and if you have time, add some kosher salt to the beans and allow them to cool in their cooking liquid. Drain and now they're ready to eat! Or store them in the refrigerator for up to 3 days or in the freezer for up to 3 months.

To cook in a slow cooker: A 6½-quart slow cooker can cook up to 2 pounds of beans.
   Drain the soaked beans and place in the slow cooker. Do not add kombu to the slow cooker as it will impart a seaweed flavor to the beans. Fill as high as you can with fresh water. Set the slow cooker to low for 6½ hours. Taste for tenderness and add more time, if necessary.

continued on page 130

To cook in a pressure cooker: A 6- to 8-quart pressure cooker can cook up to 1 pound of beans. Drain the soaked beans and place in the pressure cooker with or without the kombu. Add a tablespoon of olive oil to help keep the foam down (which can clog the pressure valve) and only enough water to fill the pressure cooker halfway. Secure the lid and set the heat to high. When it reaches pressure, lower the heat and cook for 20 minutes for small beans, 25 minutes for medium-size beans, and 30 minutes for very large beans. Release the pressure cooker using the natural method. Taste for tenderness.

How to Cook Basic Quinoa

MAKES 3 CUPS · VEGAN, GF, DF

1 cup regular or sprouted quinoa, rinsed in a fine-mesh sieve

Pinch of sea salt

TIP: To cook quinoa that has been soaked for 6 to 12 hours, use 1¼ cups of water and time it for 10 to 12 minutes.

Quinoa is a weekly staple in my home, where it finds its way into salads, breakfast porridges, grain bowls, and variations of Not-Fried Rice. I'll make a big batch on Sundays to have during the week, but you can also make it every month and freeze what you won't use in one week. Technically a seed, quinoa cooks up much more quickly than most whole grains and is a complete protein, which is not easy to find in the plant world. The most common quinoa is a natural-colored one, but you can also find red, black, and a mix of all three colors. I think the natural color turns out the fluffiest, but the red and black have more antioxidants and can add a beautiful color to whatever dish they accompany.

1. Place the quinoa, 1¾ cups of water, and the salt in a medium-size saucepan and bring to a boil. Cover, lower the heat to a simmer, and cook, covered, for 15 minutes, or until all the water is absorbed. Turn off the heat and allow to sit, covered, for 5 to 10 minutes. Fluff with a fork and serve.

ASK PAMELA: Do I have to rinse quinoa? *Technically, you don't have to rinse quinoa. It will cooked perfectly well without having been soaked or rinsed. But there is a natural bitter coating on the outside of the grains that can be removed with a simple rinse under water, ensuring a better flavor.*

How to Cook Basic White and Brown

Believe it or not, I am probably asked more questions about how to make rice than about anything else. The good news is that there are not that many variables in cooking rice: rice, water, the pot, and the cook.

First, the ratio of water to rice is almost always 2 to 1. Next, make sure to use the correctly sized pot. Too big a pot and the water evaporates before the rice becomes tender. Too small, the rice can get mushy. A 1½-quart saucepan is perfect for 1 cup of rice. Next, do not stir the rice or it will become sticky, and do not lift the lid while it is cooking because you need all that steam to make the rice tender.

1. Place all the ingredients in the pot, add 2 cups of water (or 1¾ cups if the rice has been soaked), and bring to a boil over high heat.
2. Lower the heat to low, cover, and simmer for 18 minutes for white rice (or 15 minutes if it has been soaked) and 50 minutes for brown rice (or 40 minutes if it has been soaked). Do not peek and do not stir until the time is up. Check to make sure all water has been absorbed and allow to sit, covered, for an additional 10 minutes, if possible. Fluff with a fork and serve, or cool to room temperature and refrigerate for up to 4 days, or freeze for up to 3 months.

ASK PAMELA: Is it true there is arsenic in rice? *Consumer Reports published findings about "troublesome" levels of arsenic in rice and rice products, from baby cereal to pasta. Arsenic exists in two different forms: organic, which is naturally occurring and not quite toxic to our body, and inorganic, which is man-made. The inorganic arsenic is toxic to our body, and also the form that is present in rice.*

To avoid arsenic, a few steps that you can take include buying imported rice, soaking your rice (see Tips), and cooking rice in copious amounts of water, like cooking pasta. If you aren't able to follow any of these practices, use white rice rather than brown as the outer bran layer has been removed from white.

1 cup long- or sho
brown rice (ba:
etc.), rinsed in a fine-mesh sieve
(or soaked for 1 to 8 hours and
drained) or sprouted brown rice,
which doesn't need soaking

2 teaspoons unrefined extra-virgin
olive oil or unsalted butter
(optional)

¾ teaspoon sea salt (optional)

TIPS: Alternatively, you can use the "pasta" method by bringing a large stockpot of water to a boil, placing your rice (unsoaked or soaked and drained) in the pot, and boiling gently for 20 to 30 minutes, or until tender. Drain well.

To soak rice, place the desired amount in a bowl with lots of water to cover. Allow to sit at room temperature for 1 to 8 hours. Drain and proceed to the cooking steps.

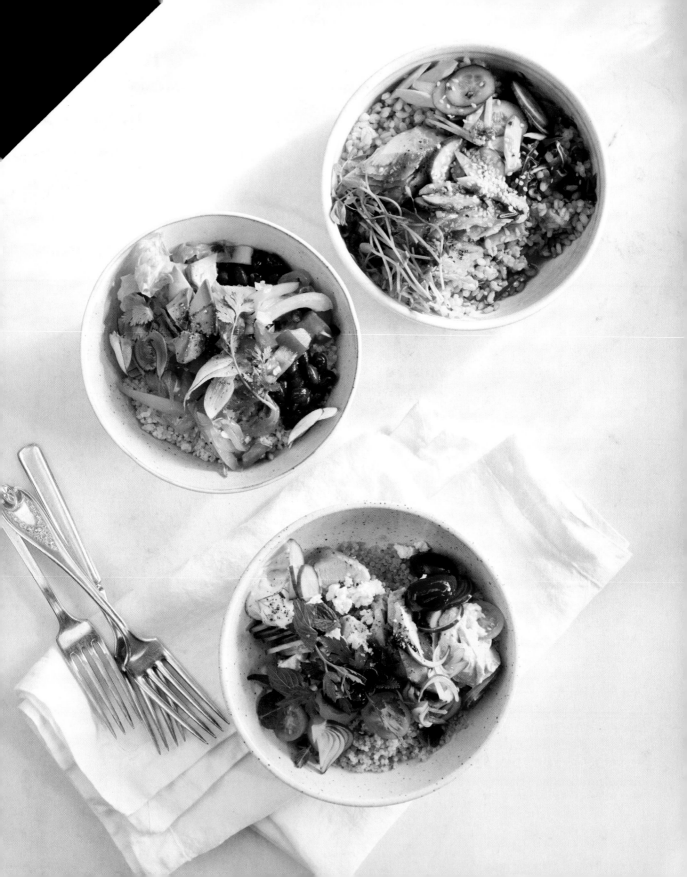

Grain Bowls

SERVES 4 · VEGAN ADAPTABLE, GF ADAPTABLE, DF ADAPTABLE

Bowls, both sweet and savory, are all the rage—and for good reason. They're so delicious, filling, and infinitely customizable. Nothing is more satisfying and nourishing than a warm scoop of whole grains with loads of vegetables in a bowl with a simple dressing or sauce to pull it all together. They're easy enough to make for a spontaneous lunch at home or for a simple weeknight dinner. To make a simple grain bowl, first start with the base of any cooked grain or legume. Add sautéed, steamed, or roasted vegetables (see page 104 for a guide to roasting vegetables). You can also include your favorite protein and/or fermented vegetables. Top off the bowl with your favorite sauce or condiments. I am sharing my family's favorites below.

BASE (USE ABOUT 1 CUP GRAINS OR LEGUMES PER BOWL):

4 cups cooked grains or legumes: brown rice, millet, quinoa, farro (not GF), lentils, barley (not GF), wheat berries (not GF)

VEGGIES (USE ABOUT 1½ CUPS VEGGIES PER BOWL):

8 to 10 cups mixed cooked vegetables: broccoli, cauliflower, carrots, Brussels sprouts, sweet potatoes, beets, kale, Broccolini, parsnips . . .

Or raw vegetables, such as thinly sliced or julienned radishes, tomatoes, microgreens, avocado, carrots

SAUCE/CONDIMENTS (USE ABOUT 2 TABLESPOONS SAUCE PER BOWL):

Kale Pesto (page 97)

Cilantro Tahini Sauce (page 134)

Green Sauce (from South American Roast Chicken recipe on page 187)

Guacamole and salsa for a burrito bowl

Tzatziki for a Mediterranean bowl

Asian Bowl

Any grain or legume or Cauliflower Rice (page 251)

Broccoli, carrots, cabbage, onions, bok choy, mushrooms, avocado

Top with sesame seeds or gomasio, and crumbled nori

Can add broiled or seared salmon, or seared tofu

ASIAN SAUCE

VEGAN, DF, GF ADAPTABLE

1 garlic clove, minced, or 1 scallion, thinly sliced

2 tablespoons peeled and grated fresh ginger (use a large Microplane)

2 tablespoons soy sauce (not GF), tamari, or coconut aminos

2 tablespoons pure Grade A or B maple syrup

1 teaspoon unrefined toasted sesame oil

½ teaspoon crushed red pepper flakes

1. Puree all the sauce ingredients plus 2 tablespoons of water in a blender until smooth. Will keep for 4 days in the fridge.

Thai Red Curry Bowl

Any grain or legume or Cauliflower Rice (page 251)

Roasted or steamed broccoli, carrots, onions, mushrooms, asparagus, winter squash, avocado, cilantro

THAI RED CURRY SAUCE

VEGAN, DF, GF ADAPTABLE

½ (14-ounce) can culinary coconut milk

½ to 1 tablespoon red curry paste

½ tablespoon shoyu (not GF), tamari, or coconut aminos

½ tablespoon pure Grade A or B maple syrup

Freshly squeezed lime juice

1. In a small saucepan, whisk together all the ingredients, adding lime juice to taste, and warm over medium heat. Keeps for 3 to 4 days in the fridge.

Burrito Bowl

Any grain or legume or Cauliflower Rice (page 251)

Sautéed bell peppers, zucchini, onions, raw radishes, chopped romaine lettuce, thinly sliced red cabbage, tomatoes or salsa

Guacamole or avocado and fresh cilantro (try the Green Sauce, page 187)

Black beans or cooked chicken, steak, or shrimp

Greek Bowl

Any grain or legume or Cauliflower Rice (page 251)

Romaine lettuce, spinach, tomato, cucumber, red onion, fresh parsley, dill and/or mint, avocado

Feta, and/or grilled chicken or shrimp (pages 176 and 201)

Tzatziki and/or hummus

Pesto Bowl

Any grain or legume or Cauliflower Rice (page 251)

Raw or cooked cherry tomatoes, cooked asparagus, mushrooms, green beans, onions, broccoli, eggplant, or zucchini

White beans or chickpeas

Kale Pesto (page 97), Basil-Parsley Pesto (page 252), or your favorite pesto

Cilantro-Tahini Bowl

Any grain or legume or Cauliflower Rice (page 251)

Raw or cooked cherry tomatoes, cooked green beans, onions, broccoli, cauliflower, carrots, eggplant, zucchini, bell peppers, beets

CILANTRO-TAHINI SAUCE

VEGAN, DF, GF

1 cup lightly packed cilantro leaves and tender stems

2 tablespoons freshly squeezed lemon juice (from about ½ lemon)

1 garlic clove, grated or minced

3 tablespoons raw tahini (roasted tahini is fine, but raw is a little milder)

3 tablespoons unrefined, cold-pressed, extra-virgin olive oil

½ teaspoon sea salt + more to taste

Pinch of cayenne pepper (optional)

1. Puree all the sauce ingredients plus 3 tablespoons of water in a blender until smooth. Taste for salt. Will keep for 4 to 5 days in the fridge.

Millet and Cauliflower Mash

SERVES 6 · GF, VEGAN ADAPTABLE, DF ADAPTABLE

When I planned this millet and cauliflower mash several years ago, I knew there would be skeptics in my classes. At the time, cauliflower wasn't the "it" vegetable it is today and very few people knew what millet was. Millet is a small, gluten-free grain with a mild, nutty, almost cornlike flavor and light and fluffy texture when cooked. Easier to digest than most grains, it also contains a fair amount of protein and iron. I sold this to my skeptical students as a healthful alternative to mashed potatoes; they agreed that this comforting mash provided the same creamy, buttery goodness. You can serve this with anything that would go well with mashed potatoes. Leftovers firm up in the refrigerator, but you can easily loosen the mash up with some warm water.

1. In a large saucepan, heat the olive oil. Add the onion and sauté over medium heat until tender and translucent, 3 to 4 minutes.

2. Add 3 cups of water and the millet, cauliflower, garlic, and salt. Bring to a boil over high heat, cover, and simmer for 25 to 30 minutes, until the vegetables are soft and the millet is cooked.

3. Remove from the heat. Transfer to a food processor and blend until smooth or mash with a potato masher until the desired consistency is achieved. The food processor will make this much smoother.

4. Transfer to a serving bowl and sprinkle with chives, if you like. You can also stir in a little unsalted butter for a creamy finish (omit for vegan/DF), but it's delicious without.

1 tablespoon unrefined extra-virgin olive oil, unsalted butter (not vegan/DF), or unrefined virgin coconut oil

1 medium-size onion, chopped

1 cup millet, rinsed

3 cups cauliflower florets

3 garlic cloves

2 teaspoons sea salt

1 tablespoon chopped chives (optional)

1 to 2 tablespoons unsalted butter (optional, omit for vegan/DF)

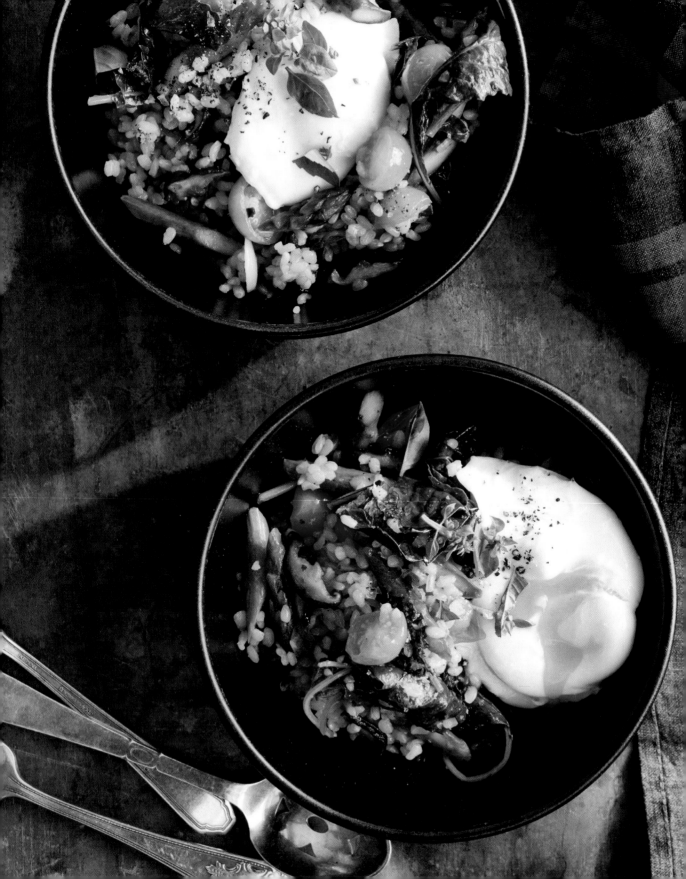

Not-Fried Rice and Vegetables

SERVES 4 · DF, VEGAN ADAPTABLE, GF ADAPTABLE

Fried rice makes a very nutritious, inexpensive, and delicious meal. But rather than being fried, these ingredients are quickly sautéed with a minimal amount of oil. It is typically made with leftover cold rice and whatever other bits are in the fridge, from veggies to cooked meat. Any cooked grain, lentils, or chickpeas can be subbed for the rice, keeping in mind which grains contain gluten, if that is important to you.

1. Heat a large skillet over medium heat. Add the olive oil, then add the garlic and red pepper flakes to the warmed oil. Sauté until the garlic is just starting to turn golden on the edges, 30 to 60 seconds.

2. Add the cherry tomatoes, asparagus, mushrooms, and a pinch of salt and black pepper and sauté until the tomatoes just start to lose their shape and the asparagus and mushrooms are tender, 5 to 6 minutes.

3. Add the cooked rice, greens, and another pinch of salt and pepper and sauté until the rice is warmed through and the greens are wilted. If the rice and vegetables are sticking to the pan, add a splash of stock or water. Serve immediately with or without the suggested accompaniments.

▪ Other quick-cooking vegetables, such as diced zucchini, shredded carrot, very small cauliflower florets, peas, or scallions, also work really well here.

▪ Italian version: Add a few leaves of thinly sliced basil at the end and finish with grated Parmesan or pecorino cheese (omit for vegan/DF)

▪ Tex-Mex: Substitute chopped bell pepper for the asparagus and add ¼ cup of chopped cilantro; top with chopped avocado.

▪ Greek: Add ½ teaspoon of dried oregano in step 2. Add ¼ cup of chopped flat-leaf parsley or dill at the end and top with crumbled feta or tzatziki (omit for vegan/DF).

▪ Indian curry: Add 1 teaspoon of curry powder in step 2, stir in ¼ cup of chopped fresh cilantro at the end.

▪ Turmeric: Add ½ teaspoon ground turmeric in step 2.

2 tablespoons unrefined, cold-pressed extra-virgin olive oil or avocado oil

4 garlic cloves, thinly sliced

A pinch of crushed red pepper flakes (optional)

½ pint cherry tomatoes, halved

½ bunch asparagus, cut into 1-inch pieces

1 to 2 cups shiitake mushrooms, stemmed, caps wiped clean with a damp paper towel and sliced thinly

Sea salt and freshly ground black pepper

3 to 4 cups cold cooked short-grain brown rice or quinoa, millet, farro (not GF), freekeh (not GF), or lentils

2 to 3 cups baby leafy greens, such as chard, kale, and spinach, or 6 kale stalks, stemmed and leaves chopped

Chicken stock (not vegan) or vegetable stock (for homemade, see pages 248–249), or water, if necessary

Optional accompaniment ideas: poached or fried egg (omit for vegan); toasted, chopped nuts; hot sauce

The Perfect Baked Potato

SERVES 6 · VEGETARIAN, GF, VEGAN ADAPTABLE, DF ADAPTABLE

6 medium-size russet or Idaho baking potatoes (6 to 8 ounces each)

6 teaspoons unsalted butter (not vegan/DF), at room temperature, or olive oil

Coarse kosher salt

Favorite toppings: sour cream (not vegan/DF), crème fraîche (not vegan/DF) or Greek yogurt (not vegan/DF), chopped fresh chives or scallions, steamed vegetables such as broccoli, cauliflower, or spinach, chili, salsa, Vegan Mac and Cheese sauce (page 214) or shredded cheese (not vegan/DF), sautéed onions

Potatoes get a bad rap because they are so often cooked as chips, fries, or as slices swimming in cream and cheese and with the skin—the most nutritious part—removed. Granted, potatoes are high in starch, but they are actually reasonably low in calories and high in fiber, B vitamins, and antioxidants. Enter baked potato night: potatoes are a perfect foil for lots of nutrient-dense vegetables, such as broccoli and cauliflower, or a scoop of your favorite chili. Cooking potatoes on a bed of kosher salt is the best method I have ever used. The salt ensures a light and fluffy interior, while the skin (my favorite part!) turns a little crispy and also supertasty.

1. Preheat the oven to 400°F.
2. Scrub the potatoes, blot dry, and rub each with 1 teaspoon of butter. Pour a layer of salt on the bottom of a shallow baking dish or cookie sheet; 1½ cups is perfect for a 9 x 13-inch dish.
3. Place the potatoes 2 inches apart on top of the salt and bake for 50 minutes, or until tender. Squeeze one with a kitchen towel to make sure.
4. When each potato is removed from the baking dish, rub off any salt clinging to the bottom of the potato. Split open lengthwise and top as desired. You can save the kosher salt and reuse it, if you like.

TIP: Leftover baked potatoes make the best home fries. Just cube them and sauté in a skillet with ghee, onions, a little paprika, salt, and pepper.

One-Pot Barley with Melted Cabbage

SERVES 6 AS A SIDE DISH OR 4 AS A MAIN DISH · VEGAN ADAPTABLE, VEGETARIAN ADAPTABLE, DF ADAPTABLE

It doesn't get much easier than layering a bunch of nutritious ingredients into a pot and simmering them until done. Cabbage is highly underappreciated. A member of the cruciferous family (one of the most healthful of all the vegetable groups), it is inexpensive, available all year round, and nutrient dense. But cabbage is also incredibly versatile. You can eat it raw, sautéed, roasted, or grilled. When it is sautéed, it takes on a luxurious, buttery flavor. This recipe is so simple and very satisfying. I love using the barley and cabbage as a vegetarian entrée paired with a green salad or as a bed for a simply roasted piece of salmon or chicken.

1. Place all the ingredients, except the cheese, in a medium saucepan in the order listed, with the barley first, then the onion, etc. Bring to a boil over high heat, lower the heat to a simmer, and cover. Stir occasionally. After 30 minutes, the barley should be tender. Turn off the heat and keep covered until ready to serve. The longer it sits, the plumper the barley becomes.

2. Serve warm with Parmesan or pecorino cheese, if desired.

TIPS: If you stir the barley more often, it becomes like a risotto.
   You can stir the cheese into the barley before serving or grate it on top of each person's portion.

ASK PAMELA: What's the deal with all the different types of barley? *Barley is available hulled which means the bran and germ layer are still present as is all the fiber. But hulled barley takes a verrrry long time to cook. Other options include Scotch barley (in between hulled and pearled), semipearled barley (minimally polished, and it still has a light brown color) and fine pearled barley (almost white, like white rice). Some brands, such as Bob's Red Mill and Arrowhead Mills, are labeled "pearled," but they are truly semipearled as evidenced by the light brown color of the grains and the presence of 8 grams of fiber and 5 grams of protein in a mere ¼ cup dried.*

1 cup semipearled barley

1 small onion, cut into quarters and thinly sliced

2 garlic cloves, thinly sliced

Pinch of crushed red pepper flakes

1¾ teaspoons sea salt

A few grinds of freshly ground black pepper

1 tablespoon unrefined, cold-pressed, extra-virgin olive oil

1 tablespoon unsalted butter (not vegan/DF), or use all olive oil, but I like it better with the butter

4 cups sliced green cabbage (about ½ large head)

2 cups water or chicken stock (not vegetarian), or a combination

Accompaniments, if desired: grated Parmesan or pecorino cheese (recommended; omit for vegan/DF)

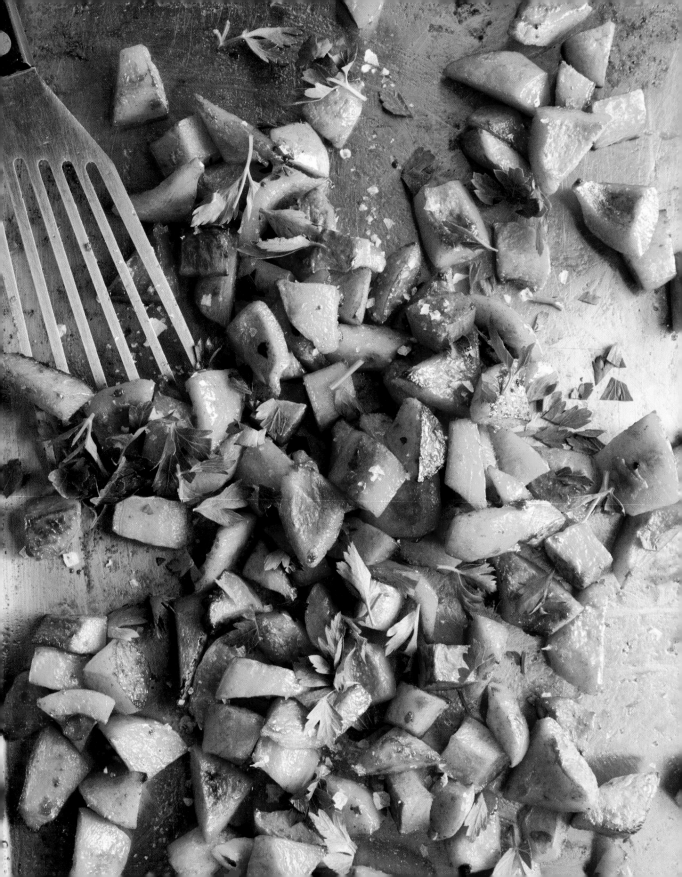

Moroccan Spiced Butternut Squash

SERVES 6 · VEGAN, GF, DF

Just a word of caution—this butternut squash is highly addictive! I have to control myself from consuming the entire pan myself. I love foods with a lot of flavor and this recipe includes some of my favorite spices, most of which have amazing anti-inflammatory effects on the body. I am using the label "Moroccan" very liberally here; the flavors reminded me of Moroccan dishes that I have enjoyed. You can also substitute sweet potatoes, delicata squash, or carrots for the butternut, or put together a mix of these vegetables. This recipe is fantastic with Sautéed Beet Greens (page 117).

1. Preheat the oven to 400°F. Line a baking sheet with unbleached parchment paper.
2. Place the squash in a large bowl and add the salt, spices, oil, maple syrup, and orange juice. Toss to combine and pour onto prepared baking sheet.
3. Roast in the oven until tender, 30 to 40 minutes, tossing halfway to ensure even browning. Garnish with the parsley and serve hot, warm, or at room temperature.

TIP: You need a very strong vegetable peeler to remove the skin of a butternut squash. If yours isn't getting the job done, cut the squash into two sections—the neck and the bulb. Slice a little off the bottom of the bulb so you can stand it up safely on the cutting board. Use a sharp knife to cut away the skin.

1 large butternut squash (about 2¾ pounds), peeled, seeded, and cut into 1-inch pieces

1 teaspoon sea salt

1 teaspoon ground cinnamon

½ teaspoon ground cumin

½ teaspoon ground turmeric

Pinch of cayenne pepper

A few grinds freshly ground black pepper

2 tablespoons unrefined virgin coconut oil, melted

2 tablespoons pure grade A maple syrup

Juice of 1 orange (about 6 table-spoons)

2 tablespoons flat-leaf parsley, chopped

Baked Cauliflower and Rice Risotto with Mint Pesto

SERVES 6 · GF, VEGETARIAN ADAPTABLE

2 tablespoons unrefined, cold-pressed extra-virgin olive oil

1 cup finely chopped onion

1 cup Arborio rice

1 teaspoon sea salt

Freshly ground black pepper

1 cup uncooked Cauliflower Rice (page 251)

½ cup dry white wine

2¾ to 3 cups very hot light chicken stock (not vegetarian), vegetable stock, or water (or a combo of stock and water) (see homemade stocks on pages 248–249)

2 tablespoons unsalted butter

1 cup grated Parmesan or pecorino cheese

1 cup baby spinach leaves (optional)

⅓ cup mint pesto (recipe follows)

I'll admit, the title of this recipe isn't supercatchy—but the flavor and ease more than make up for that. If you've ever made risotto, you know that it is typically a dish that requires a lot of stirring. This version is virtually hands-free, but with the same lush and creamy consistency as traditional risotto. It's a great, easy recipe for beginners and the result is restaurant-worthy. It's superadaptable; the mint pesto is great but you can adapt your favorite risotto into this one or stir in your favorite pesto. If you want to time this perfectly for guests, you can complete the recipe through step 6 up to an hour ahead of time and leave it off the heat, covered. Five minutes before you want to eat, place over medium heat and proceed with the rest of the recipe.

1. Preheat the oven to 350°F.
2. Heat the olive oil in a large, ovenproof saucepan or Dutch oven over medium heat. Add the onion and sauté until tender and translucent, about 6 minutes. Do not let it brown.
3. Add the Arborio rice, salt, and pepper and stir to combine, coating all the rice with the oil. Sauté the rice for 3 to 4 minutes, or until some of the grains become translucent.
4. Stir in the cauliflower rice and sauté for 2 minutes.
5. Pour the wine into the pan, bring to a simmer, and cook until it has been absorbed, about 3 minutes.
6. Pour in 2 cups of the very hot stock or water, bring to a simmer, cover, and place the pan in the oven. Bake until most of the liquid is absorbed but the rice is still slightly undercooked, about 15–16 minutes.
7. Remove the pan from the oven and set on the stovetop over medium heat. Add ¾ cup of superhot stock or water and cook the rice, stirring constantly, for 2 to 3 minutes. Taste the rice for doneness. Ideally, it is a little al dente and the risotto creamy. Stir in the butter, ¾ cup of the Parmesan, the spinach, if using, and the pesto. Adjust the consistency with additional stock, if needed; season with salt and pepper to taste.
8. Serve immediately with additional Parmesan on the side.

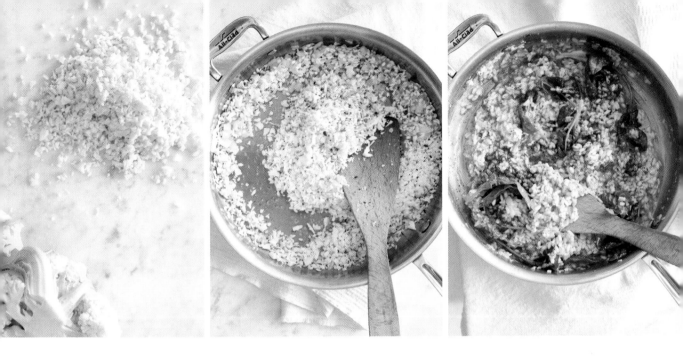

Mint Pesto

MAKES ⅓ CUP · VEGAN, GF, DF

1. Process the nuts and garlic in a mini food processor until finely chopped.
2. Add the mint, salt, and pepper to taste and pour the oil on top. Process until well blended.

ASK PAMELA: How do I know when all of the wine is evaporated? *Drag the end of a wooden spoon across the bottom of the saucepan. If any liquid seeps in, it has not evaporated.*

   Do I rinse Arborio rice? *Never rinse Arborio rice. The reason you use this type of rice for risotto is that it is very high in starch, which releases into the water and gives risotto its creamy texture. Rinsing the rice washes away some of that starchiness and your risotto won't be as creamy.*

2½ tablespoons blanched almonds (see page 25 for substitutions)

1 medium-size garlic clove

2 cups packed fresh mint leaves

½ teaspoon sea salt

Freshly ground black pepper

3 tablespoons unrefined, cold-pressed, extra-virgin olive oil

Soft Polenta with Mushroom Ragout

SERVES 6 · GF, VEGAN ADAPTABLE, VEGETARIAN ADAPTABLE

MUSHROOM RAGOUT:

8 cups mushrooms, any variety, but a mix is nice (about 1¼ pounds)

2 to 4 tablespoons unrefined, cold-pressed extra-virgin olive oil

½ teaspoon sea salt

Freshly ground black pepper

3 garlic cloves, chopped

¼ cup dry white wine

1 cup chicken stock (not vegan) or vegetable stock, preferably homemade (pages 248–249), or mushroom stock

1 teaspoon arrowroot powder

POLENTA:

1½ teaspoons sea salt

1 cup quick-cooking polenta

1 to 3 tablespoons unsalted butter (not vegan), unrefined extra-virgin olive oil, or vegan organic butter, such as Earth Balance (I prefer dairy butter)

¼ cup grated Parmesan or pecorino cheese (optional; omit for vegan)

2 tablespoons flat-leaf parsley leaves, chopped, for serving

This is my idea of comfort food at its best. Soft, creamy polenta is a wonderful base for any saucy vegetable. My favorite topping is mixed sautéed Japanese and cremini mushrooms, but use whatever you can find. If I'm not serving this to my youngest child, I'll also add a few pinches of crushed red pepper flakes for some bite. This recipe plus Garlicky Kale (page 113) are all I need. My husband loves soft polenta with Slow Cooker Italian Pot Roast (page 208).

1. Prepare the mushroom ragout: Wipe the mushrooms clean with a damp paper towel and slice ¼ inch thick.
2. Heat a large skillet over medium heat and add 2 tablespoons of the olive oil. Add to the warmed oil only enough mushrooms to cover the bottom of the skillet in one layer. Season with salt and pepper to taste. Allow the mushrooms to sit undisturbed for a few minutes until the undersides develop some golden color. Sauté until tender, 4 to 5 minutes. If you cook only some of the mushrooms, transfer them to a bowl. Add the remaining 2 tablespoons of olive oil and repeat with the remaining mushrooms. Transfer them to the bowl.
3. Add the garlic to the skillet and cook until fragrant, about 60 seconds.
4. Return the reserved mushrooms to the skillet and add the white wine. Cook, stirring occasionally, until most of the wine has been absorbed.
5. Whisk the arrowroot with the stock in a medium-size bowl or measuring cup and pour into the skillet. Simmer until the sauce is slightly thickened, about 5 minutes.
6. Prepare the polenta: Bring 5 cups of water to a boil in a medium-size, heavy-bottomed saucepan. Add the salt, then slowly add the polenta to the pot, whisking constantly. Lower the heat to low and cook, stirring constantly, until the mixture thickens and the polenta is tender, 2 to 3 minutes.
7. Stir in the butter and cheese, if using. The polenta should be pourable and creamy. If it's too thick, stir in more liquid.
8. Spread the polenta on a platter, top with the mushroom ragout, and garnish with parsley. Eat immediately.

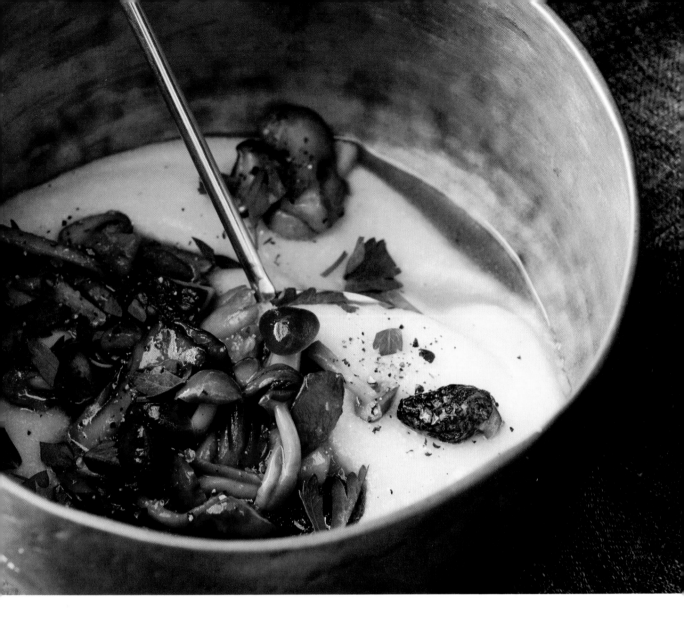

■ Other options: For extra richness, you can stir in ½ cup of whole milk (not vegan/DF) or plain, unsweetened hemp milk at the end, or some mascarpone (not vegan/DF), regular or vegan cream cheese, or fontina (not vegan/DF).

TIP: I like the de la Estancia brand of polenta that cooks in 1 minute, but is not considered instant, processed or precooked. This polenta is made from a unique, low-starch, high-protein variety of corn, which is also organic and non-GMO. Check the Resources section for where to buy. Otherwise, feel free to use any organic polenta you like, but note that the cooking times will vary. Refer to the instructions on the packaging to be sure.

Braised Lentils with Brussels Sprouts and Creamy Dijon Cashew Drizzle SERVES 4 · GF, DF, VEGAN

3 tablespoons unrefined extra-virgin olive oil

1 large onion, diced

1 garlic clove, finely chopped

1 cup dried black or French lentils, rinsed

6 tablespoons dry white wine

2½ cups vegetable stock (for home-made, see page 248)

¾ teaspoon sea salt

A few grinds of freshly ground black pepper

¾ pound Brussels sprouts, trimmed, halved, and thinly sliced

DIJON-CASHEW DRIZZLE:

¼ cup raw unsalted cashews, soaked for 4 to 6 hours in water and drained, or ¼ cup raw cashew butter

1 tablespoon Dijon mustard

1 medium-size garlic clove

1 teaspoon white wine vinegar

¼ teaspoon sea salt

Freshly ground black pepper

TIP: There are many different types of lentils, but I find French lentils hold their shape the best. There seems to be a wide variety of lentil cooking times. Whole Foods' 365 brand takes about 30 minutes, but I have used some imported varieties that take up to 50 minutes.

When I was a vegetarian, I lived on lentils, which are a rich source of protein, fiber, and iron. Turns out, lentils also have the second-highest antioxidant capacity among legumes and are anti-inflammatory as well. The combination here of savory, nutty lentils laced with leafy Brussels sprouts is so satisfying and this drizzle, this drizzle! I could eat it with a spoon, there's so much flavor in this creamy dressing. The secret to this recipe? Raw cashews. Soaked and blended with a little liquid, they become über-creamy, like heavy cream. A high-powered blender, such as a Vitamix, does the best job of making this sauce perfectly smooth, but a food processor is absolutely acceptable. If you are using precooked lentils, taste them for seasoning and proceed with the recipe from step 4.

1. In a medium-size to large saucepan, heat 1 tablespoon of the oil over medium heat. Stir in the onion and garlic and sauté until tender and translucent.

2. Add the lentils and wine and simmer until the wine has been absorbed.

3. Pour in the stock. Bring to a boil over high heat, lower the heat to a simmer, cover, and cook until the lentils are tender, 30 to 55 minutes, depending on the type of lentils and the brand. If the lentils seem too liquidy, simmer for a little longer uncovered. Taste the lentils and season with ¼ teaspoon of the salt and pepper as needed.

4. While the lentils are cooking, heat the remaining 2 table-spoons of oil in a large skillet over medium heat. Add the Brussels sprouts, season with the remaining ½ teaspoon of salt and pepper to taste and sauté until just tender, 3 or 4 minutes.

5. Prepare the cashew sauce: Place 6 tablespoons of water and all the ingredients, including pepper to taste, in a blender or food processor and process until completely smooth.

6. Stir the Brussels sprouts into the lentils and drizzle with the Dijon-cashew sauce. Serve as is or toss to combine.

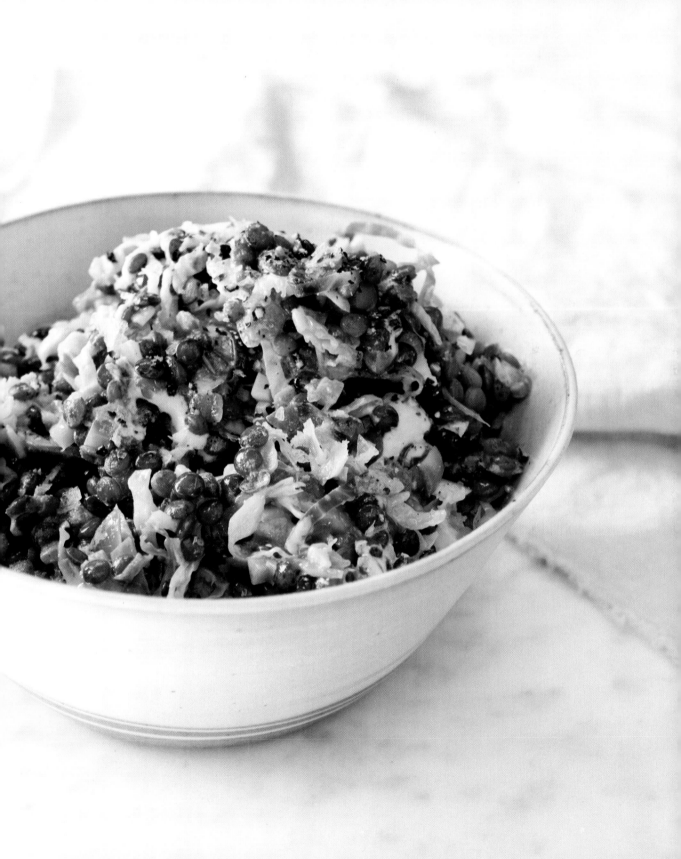

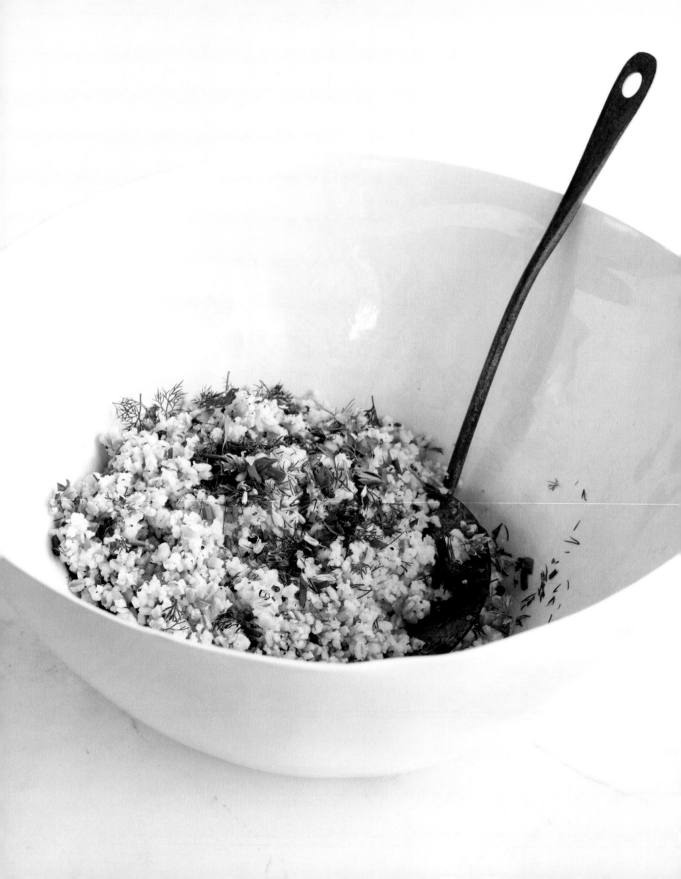

Herbed Mixed-Grain Pilaf

SERVES 4 TO 6 · VEGETARIAN, VEGAN ADAPTABLE, DF ADAPTABLE

Everyone needs a good, basic, starchy side dish that is a step above just plain steamed rice. This pilaf is that for me and a staple in my repertoire. It goes with everything, is simple to put together, and tastes a little fancy. This is not a true pilaf because it is cooked in water rather than broth and you won't find the cooked onion that's often in a pilaf. But no matter, it's still an upgrade from basic grains. I use my favorite combination of herbs in the recipe, but other herbs that are lovely here are cilantro, mint, and chervil. Use what you've got or adapt this to whatever else you are serving.

1. In a medium-size saucepan, bring 3 cups of water to a boil. Add the grains, oil, butter, garlic, and salt. Once the water comes back to a boil, cover, lower the heat to low and cook until the grains are tender and the water has been absorbed, about 30 minutes.
2. Remove the saucepan from the heat and leave covered for 10 minutes.
3. Fluff the grains with a fork and stir in the herbs. Serve.

TIP: Leftovers can be turned into Not-Fried Rice (page 137).

¹/₃ cup millet, rinsed

¹/₃ cup farro, rinsed

¹/₃ cup semipearled barley, rinsed

1 tablespoon unrefined cold-pressed extra-virgin olive oil

1 tablespoon unsalted butter (not vegan/DF), or use all olive oil

2 large garlic cloves, crushed with the flat side of a knife

³/₄ teaspoon sea salt

¹/₃ cup mixed fresh tender herbs, finely chopped (I like equal parts chives, parsley, and dill)

Pasta with Kale, Walnuts, and Ricotta

SERVES 4 TO 6 · VEGETARIAN, VEGAN ADAPTABLE, GF ADAPTABLE, DF ADAPTABLE

1½ pounds any type of kale (about 2 large bunches), washed well and stemmed

Kosher salt

1 pound whole-grain pasta, such as fusilli or strozzapreti, or GF pasta of choice

½ cup raw walnuts (see page 25 for substitutions)

¼ cup unrefined, cold-pressed extra-virgin olive oil, plus more for drizzling

6 large garlic cloves, thinly sliced

¼ teaspoon crushed red pepper flakes, plus more if you want it spicy

Zest of 2 lemons (about 1 tablespoon)

Sea salt and freshly ground black pepper

1 cup high-quality ricotta cheese (not vegan/DF) or vegan ricotta

Since I grew up in a 100 percent Italian home, it was impossible for me to write a cookbook without a pasta recipe. As a child, we probably ate pasta three or four times a week, and I can't say I didn't love that. However (and my father might like to challenge me on this), pasta is a high-carbohydrate, processed food and one that is very easy to overeat. So, my strategy these days is to use whole-grain or legume-based pasta and incorporate a ton of vegetables into the dish. I cook pasta al dente, which means "to the tooth" and calls for pasta to have a little resistance when bitten, and not be overly soft. Al dente pasta also has a lower glycemic index than overcooked pasta. You can also adapt this recipe to spaghetti squash.

1. Bring a large pot of water to a boil. Add a heaping tablespoon of salt and the kale. Cook the kale until tender, about 6 minutes. Using tongs, pull the kale from the water and place in a colander to drain. When cool enough to handle, squeeze out the excess moisture from the kale using a thin kitchen towel or a fine-mesh sieve and the back of a large spoon, and chop the kale on a cutting board.

2. Bring the water back to a boil and add the pasta. Start stirring the pasta immediately and continue to stir until the water comes back up to a boil. Lower the heat to medium-high and cook until al dente, according to the package directions. Usually this is 9 to 11 minutes. Remove 1 cup of pasta water and reserve. Drain the pasta.

3. In a large, dry skillet over medium heat, toast the walnuts until fragrant, 5 to 8 minutes. Do not leave the walnuts alone! Transfer to a cutting board and chop.

4. In the same skillet in which you toasted the walnuts, heat the olive oil over medium heat and add the garlic and crushed red pepper flakes. Lower the heat to medium-low and cook until fragrant but not golden, 30 to 60 seconds. Add the lemon zest and toasted walnuts and turn off the heat.

5. Add the chopped kale to the garlic mixture, along with ¼ teaspoon of salt plus a few grinds of black pepper.

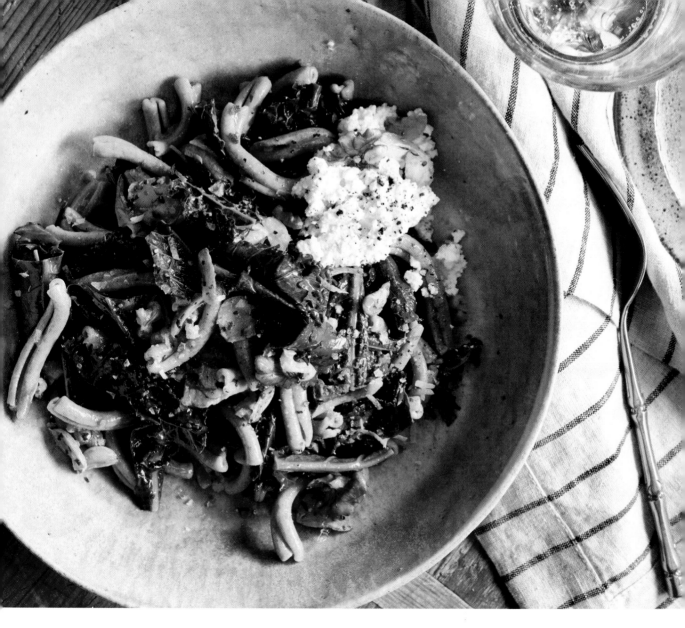

6. Add the pasta to the skillet and toss to coat. Add a little reserved pasta water to moisten the pasta. Start with ¼ cup.

7. Finish the pasta with a drizzle of olive oil and either stir in the ricotta or pass it on the side.

ASK PAMELA: How do I prevent my pasta from sticking?
Adding olive oil to the pasta water does not *keep pasta from sticking. Once you add the pasta to boiling water, you must stir it constantly until the water comes back to a boil and then stir occasionally until done.*

TIP: The finished dish can be drizzled with plain olive oil or lemon-infused olive oil.

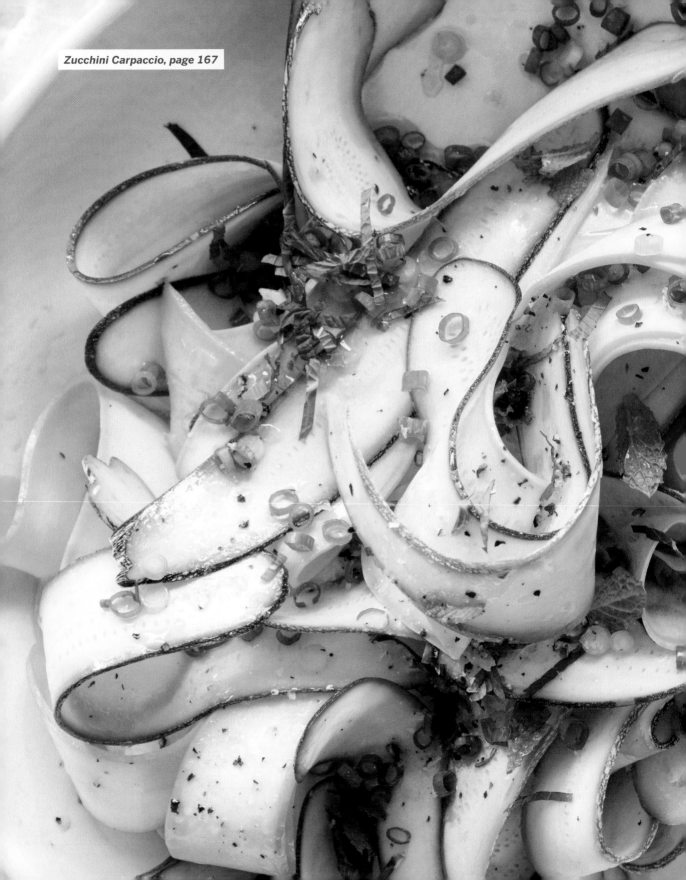

Zucchini Carpaccio, page 167

BEYOND THE LEAF SALADS

I have always been fairly obsessed with salads. When I was in second grade, I asked my mother whether she could pack me a bottle of oil and vinegar in my lunch box so I could drink it. Okay, that's not really a salad, but they go hand in hand and I loved vinaigrettes, too. To me, salads can be so much more interesting than lettuce with tomato and cucumber. I love mixing different foods together, especially different colors, textures, and flavors. Sometimes I use lettuces, sometimes not. A salad can have all raw ingredients or some raw and some cooked. Salads are about showcasing what's in season, no matter how simple the ingredients. My everyday salads are created using what's in my kitchen, but it is important to use fresh, flavorful ingredients because there's nowhere for them to hide.

As long as you have a great vinaigrette, you can pull together an infinite number of salads. Looking for an easy way to get more veggies onto your plate? Every week I make two bottles of the Everyday Salad Dressing (page 255), thereby allowing me to have a default side dish at a moment's notice.

Typically, a vinaigrette for a salad with lettuces is one part acid (such as vinegar or lemon juice) to three or four parts oil, depending on your taste. Add salt and pepper and you're done. To take it one step further, you can add other flavors, such as Dijon mustard, honey, shallots or garlic, or fresh herbs. A vinaigrette for a grain-based salad would be a little different, more like one part acid to one part oil.

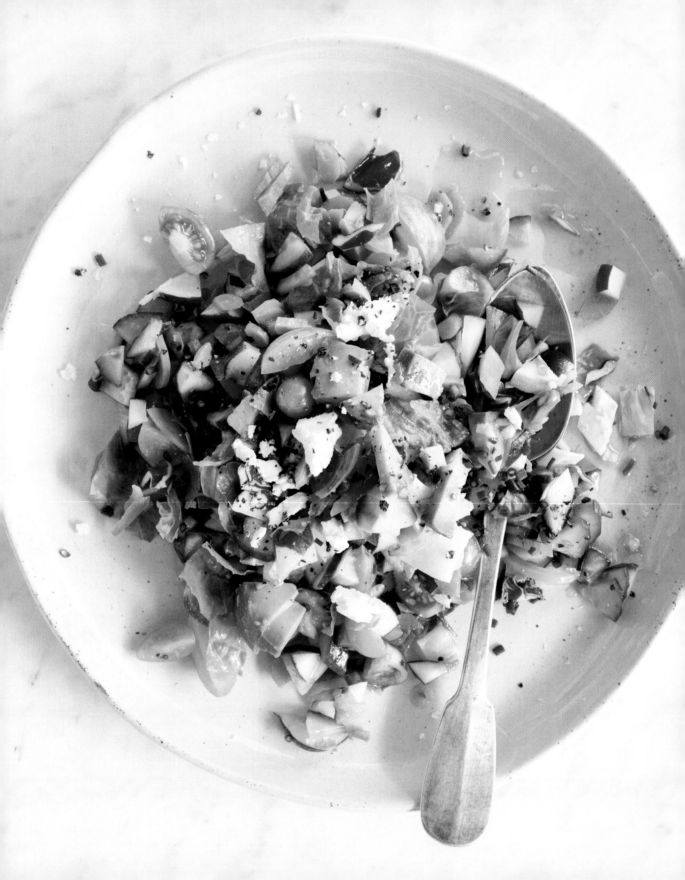

Saturday Chopped Salad

SERVES 6 · VEGETARIAN, GF, VEGAN ADAPTABLE, DF ADAPTABLE

One Saturday at lunchtime, I took some leftover undressed salad and chopped it all into the smallest pieces I could, transferred it to a big bowl, and tossed it with my "house dressing." It was the most addictive salad I have ever eaten, and it was the first salad my son (who is not the biggest consumer of vegetables) inhaled enthusiastically. I started making a chopped salad every Saturday for lunch. I can't say I've ever made a chopped salad the same way twice, nor do you really need a recipe, but this is a good place to start. I'm sure you see that the goal in preparing the vegetables is to cut them about the size of a pea. I use my Everyday Salad Dressing here because it goes with anything and everything.

1. Combine the lettuce and cabbage in a large bowl. Add the radishes, cherry tomatoes, pickled shallots, chives, cucumbers, and carrots. Toss with enough dressing to coat lightly. Add the avocado and feta and drizzle with a small amount of dressing. Toss very gently with your hands to incorporate into the salad without smearing avocado and feta everywhere.

- Other variations:
- Chopped oranges instead of tomatoes and toasted sunflower seeds instead of cucumbers in the winter and spring;
- Radicchio and endive in place of some of the romaine;
- Fresh or grilled corn in place of the carrots.

1 head romaine lettuce, finely chopped (about 6 cups)

3 cups diced red cabbage (or a mix of cabbage and chopped endive)

3 radishes, finely diced

½ pint cherry tomatoes, quartered (optional)

⅓ cup pickled shallots, diced (page 109) or 5 pepperoncini, seeded and finely chopped

½ bunch chives, finely chopped

2 Persian cucumbers, finely diced

2 carrots, finely diced or julienned and finely chopped

⅔ cup Everyday Salad Dressing (page 255)

1 avocado, peeled, pitted, and diced

3 ounces feta, preferably goat's milk feta, crumbled (omit for vegan/DF)

Additional protein: quinoa, diced cooked chicken (not vegan), tuna in olive oil (not vegan), canned salmon (not vegan), chopped hard-boiled egg (not vegan), chickpeas

Raw Kale Salad with Citrus Vinaigrette

SERVES 6 · VEGAN, GF, DF

2 medium-size bunches kale
    (12 to 14 ounces), washed and
    dried (I like dinosaur and green
    curly kale)

DRESSING:

2 teaspoons minced shallot

½ teaspoon sea salt

A few grinds of freshly ground black
    pepper

2 tablespoons freshly squeezed
    lemon juice or unseasoned rice
    vinegar

2 tablespoons freshly squeezed
    orange juice or any fresh fruit
    juice, such as apple or pome-
    granate

2 teaspoons pure Grade A maple
    syrup

6 to 7 tablespoons unrefined, cold-
    pressed extra-virgin olive oil

*Optional add-ins: Toasted pine nuts
or sunflower seeds, pomegranate
seed, dried cranberries, crumbled
feta (omit for vegan/DF), chopped
avocado, cooked quinoa, chopped
red cabbage*

This salad has converted many kale skeptics into kale lovers. Even though I first created this recipe many, many years ago, I still continue to make it regularly for potlucks, school lunches, traveling on a plane, or just to add to our weekday dinners. Kale has been very hyped over the last decade and for good reason. One cup of kale contains over 600 percent of the RDA of vitamin K, 200 percent of vitamin A, and over 100 percent of vitamin C. It is rich in anticancer phytonutrients and has more anti-inflammatory compounds than any other leafy green vegetable. Kale is also a better source of bioavailable calcium than a glass of milk!

1. Strip the kale leaves from the stems and compost or discard the stems. Finely slice the leaves with a sharp knife. Place in a serving bowl.

2. Prepare the dressing: Whisk all the remaining ingredients, except the optional add-ins, in a small bowl until emulsified or place in a glass jar with a lid and shake until emulsified.

3. Add enough dressing to coat the kale lightly. Massage the dressing into the kale leaves with your hands to soften the leaves. This is the most important step. You must take your hands and actually squeeze the kale with the dressing. Add your favorite salad fixings. The salad can be made a day or even 2 days ahead.

Italian White Bean and Tuna Salad with Capers

SERVES 4 TO 6 · GF, DF, VEGAN ADAPTABLE

This is one of my go-to summer salads for lunch before the beach or on Sunday nights, to go with grilled pizzas. It doesn't look like much, but I promise the fragrant basil dressing is insanely good, especially with these humble ingredients. If you can find a high-quality wild tuna in olive oil, that's what you want to use here. Omit the tuna if you are vegetarian and replace it with more white beans, or with shaved Parmesan cheese or bocconcini (not DF).

1. Place the basil, vinegar, salt, pepper, and olive oil in a blender and process until smooth. Set aside.
2. Place the greens in a salad bowl and scatter the tomatoes, onion, white beans, and capers on top. Drizzle with most of the dressing and lightly toss.
3. Flake the tuna, using a fork, and mound in the center of the salad. Drizzle the tuna with remaining dressing.

TIP: If the tuna is packed in water, drizzle with a little extra olive oil. If the tuna is unsalted, sprinkle with an extra pinch of sea salt.

1/3 cup fresh basil leaves

2 tablespoons white wine vinegar

1/2 teaspoon sea salt

A few grinds of black pepper

6 tablespoons unrefined, cold-pressed extra-virgin olive oil

8 cups mixed greens (butter lettuce, arugula, romaine lettuce)

12 cherry or grape tomatoes, halved

1/4 cup finely diced red onion

1 cup cooked white beans, such as great northern or cannellini, drained and rinsed if canned

1/4 cup capers, drained

1 (6- to 7-ounce) can or jar of tuna, preferably packed in oil (omit for vegan)

Superfood Salad

SERVES 4 TO 6 · GF, DF, VEGAN ADAPTABLE, VEGETARIAN ADAPTABLE

DRESSING:

1 medium-size garlic clove, minced

½ teaspoon sea salt

Freshly ground black pepper

½ teaspoon Dijon mustard

2 teaspoons pure Grade A or B maple syrup or raw honey (not vegan)

2 tablespoons raw cider vinegar

6 tablespoons unrefined, cold-pressed extra-virgin olive oil

8 cups baby spinach leaves (about 5 ounces)

1½ cups cooked quinoa

2 cups finely chopped red cabbage

1 cup blueberries or pomegranate seeds (whichever is in season)

¼ cup chopped Brazil nuts

1 cup broccoli sprouts or sprouts of choice (about 2 ounces)

1 (6- to 7-ounce) can wild salmon, preferably without bones (optional; omit for vegan/vegetarian)

1 large avocado, peeled, pitted, and cubed

TIP: To make 1½ cups of cooked quinoa, start with ½ cup dried. See "How to Cook Basic Quinoa" on page 130.

There is no universal agreement as to which foods fit the "superfoods" bill. In my opinion, a superfood is a nutritional powerhouse that contains a crazy amount of antioxidants, vitamins, minerals, and phytonutrients. There are a lot of superfoods, and by no means does this mean you should eat as many of them as you want in one sitting or that you should limit your diet to so-called superfoods. It's important to have variety in what we eat. My solution? I decided to take my favorite "superfoods" and put them all into a salad—for an incredibly delicious result. I think you'll not only enjoy this salad, but you'll feel energized and healthier after eating it.

1. Prepare the dressing: Whisk together the dressing ingredients in a medium-size bowl or shake in a jar with a screw-top lid.

2. Combine all the remaining ingredients in a large bowl and toss to coat with the dressing.

ASK PAMELA: What are your top ten superfoods?

Garlic: Boosts immune system, antibacterial

Spinach: Contains phytonutrients that have anti-inflammatory and anticancer properties

Quinoa: Contains all nine essential amino acids

Cabbage: Contains sulfuric compounds that aid in detoxifying

Blueberries: High in antioxidants that fight free radicals

Brazil nuts: Rich in selenium, which aids in detoxifying heavy metals

Sprouts: Superhigh levels of enzymes and vitamins

Wild salmon: High in brain-boosting, anti-inflammatory omega-3 fatty acids

Avocado: High in vitamin E and monounsaturated fats, which help absorption of nutrients

Turmeric: Anti-inflammatory, anticarcinogenic, and can help improve cognitive function

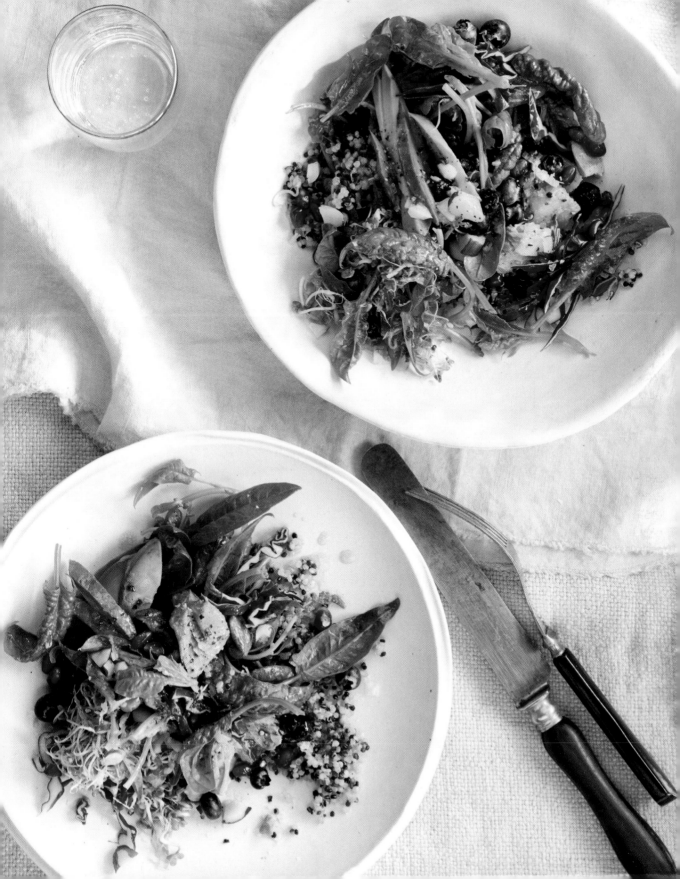

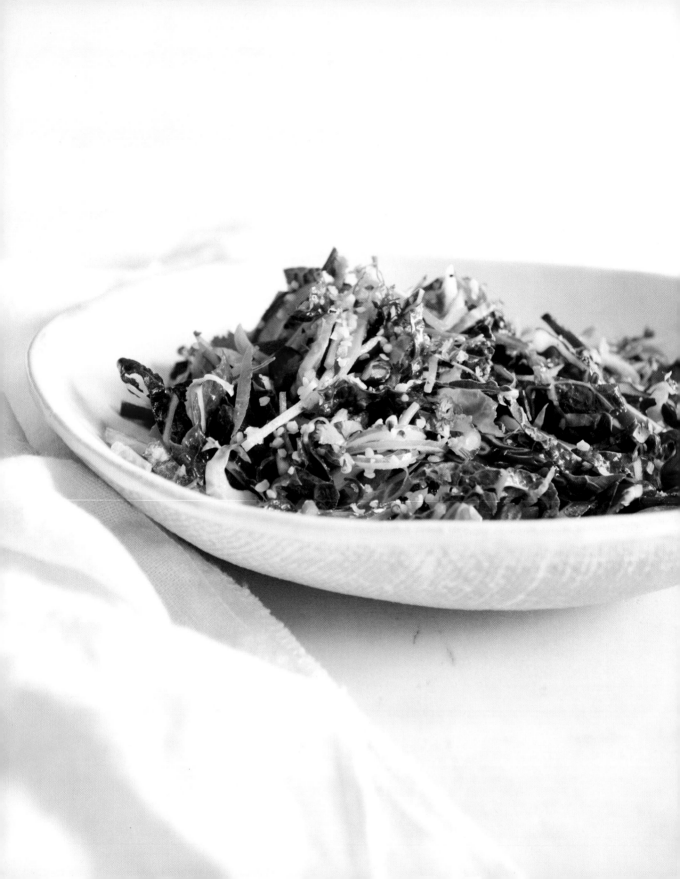

Winter Vegetable Slaw with Ginger and Lime

SERVES 4 · VEGAN, GF, DF

Sometimes the wintertime can be lacking for fresh vegetables and vibrant colors. This slaw changes all that. Slaw does not need to be a sloppy mess of mayonnaise and cabbage. This bright, crunchy slaw is light and fresh with a punchy ginger-lime dressing. I love serving this with salmon or shrimp or mixed with quinoa for a vegan entrée.

1. Combine the vegetables and cilantro in a large bowl.
2. Whisk the ginger, lime juice, and olive oil together. Pour the mixture and salt on top of the vegetables and toss to coat. Top with the almonds and hemp seeds.

TIPS: Soaking the onion slices in ice water for 10 minutes cuts the harshness.

To easily mince peeled ginger, use a medium Microplane.

ASK PAMELA: What is the best way to toast nuts? *If your oven is already on, you can place the nuts in a dry pie plate or a baking dish and put them in a 350°F oven or toaster oven for 8 to 12 minutes, or until lightly golden brown. Alternatively, you can place the nuts in a dry skillet over medium-low heat and stir regularly until fragrant and golden. Do not step away from the skillet since nuts can go from pale to burned in seconds! Once toasted, drizzle with ¼ teaspoon of olive oil and toss with a pinch of sea salt.*

3 cups thinly sliced purple cabbage

3 cups thinly sliced green cabbage, Brussels sprouts, or kale (discard the stem)

3 cups julienned or grated carrot

¾ cup thinly sliced red onion

¼ cup finely chopped cilantro or parsley leaves and tender stems

4 teaspoons peeled and minced fresh ginger

¼ cup freshly squeezed lime juice

¼ cup unrefined, cold-pressed extra-virgin olive oil

1 teaspoon sea salt

½ cup chopped toasted almonds

2 tablespoons hemp seeds

Green Goddess Chicken Salad

SERVES 6 · GF, DF ADAPTABLE

3 bone-in, skin-on chicken breasts
  (about 12 ounces each)

½ small onion, peeled

4 large garlic cloves, peeled and
  smashed

1 tablespoon kosher salt

1 tablespoon whole peppercorns

DRESSING:

½ cup unsweetened, plain, whole-
  milk Greek yogurt (not DF; see
  headnote for DF version)

1 cup fresh flat-leaf parsley leaves

3 tablespoons chopped fresh chives

2 tablespoons fresh basil leaves

2 tablespoons fresh dill

1 scallion, chopped

2 tablespoons freshly squeezed
  lemon juice

1 teaspoon anchovy paste, or 2
  anchovy fillets

½ cup unrefined, cold-pressed,
  extra-virgin olive oil

¾ teaspoon sea salt

Freshly ground black pepper

1 head Baby Gem lettuce, leaves
  washed, dried, and left whole, or
  2 cups chopped romaine lettuce

1 Persian cucumber, chopped

2 celery stalks, sliced

¼ cup diced red onion

¼ cup capers, drained

This salad is undeniably green from an abundance of fresh herbs and green veggies. Think of it as a healthified, updated, and upgraded chicken salad. I tend to not toss the whole salad in dressing since it will look like an indistinguishable mass of green. Instead I just coat the lettuce lightly with dressing and pass the rest on the side. Although Green Goddess dressing feels most appropriate for spring when green herbs are coming into season, I make it all year long. It also doubles as a lovely dip for crudités. For a dairy-free version, use ½ cup of silken tofu in place of the yogurt and increase the lemon juice to 3 tablespoons.

1. Place the chicken in a saucepan with the onion, garlic, salt, and peppercorns and add water to cover.

2. Bring to a boil over high heat, lower the heat to low, cover, and gently simmer until the chicken is just cooked through, about 25 minutes.

3. Remove from heat and allow the chicken to cool in the poaching liquid for 20 minutes.

4. Remove the skin and bones and shred the meat into large, bite-size pieces. Set aside in a large bowl.

5. Prepare the dressing: Place all the dressing ingredients, except the oil, salt, and pepper, in a blender or food processor. With the motor running, slowly pour in the olive oil. Taste for salt and pepper and add accordingly.

6. Toss the lettuce with enough dressing to coat lightly. Add the remaining salad components on top of the lettuce and serve with extra dressing on the side.

■ You can replace half of the chives with green onions.

TIPS: You can use a rotisserie chicken and remove skin and bones and shred the meat into large bite-size pieces. You should have 4 to 5 cups of shredded meat.

The original Green Goddess dressing that this recipe departs from contains lots of tarragon. Feel free to experiment with other different fresh green herbs, such as tarragon, cilantro, chervil, or mint.

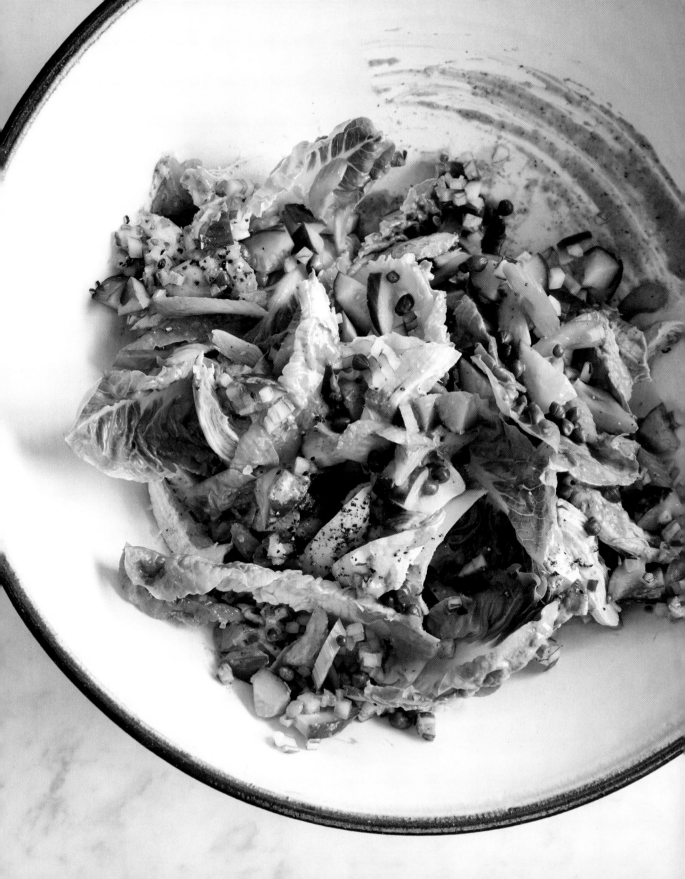

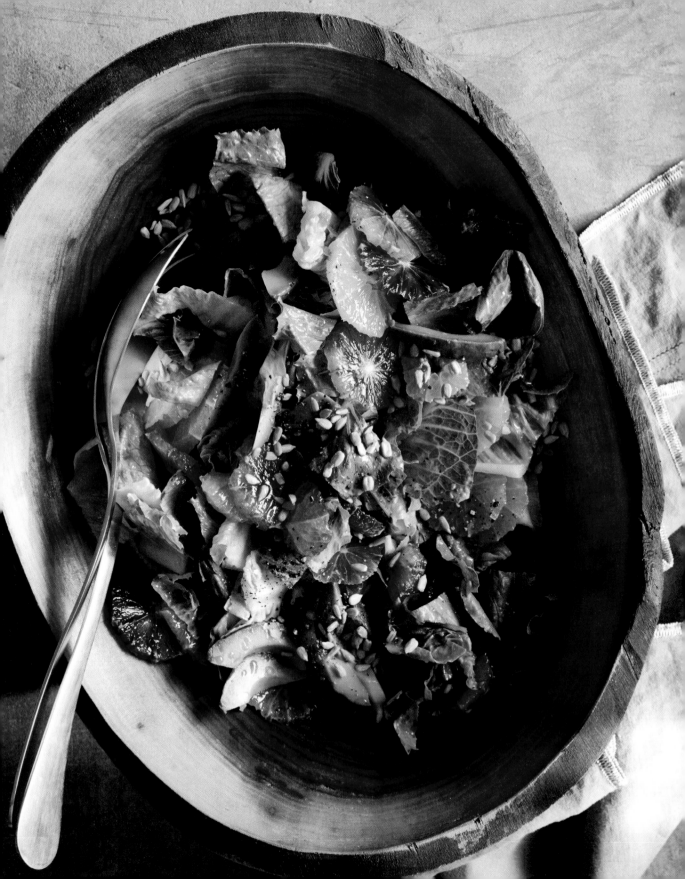

Asian Green Salad with Avocado and Oranges

SERVES 6 · VEGAN, DF, GF ADAPTABLE

This is a vibrant and flavorful salad that can either complement a meal with Asian flavors or add some punch to a meal of a simple piece of fish. Salads can be complicated or simple, but I want them all to be like this one—clean, fresh, bright, and with an interplay of interesting textures. Crisp lettuce, juicy citrus, creamy avocado, and crunchy nuts all come together with a light sesame dressing. I have also made this as an entrée salad, cutting back on some of the lettuce and adding cooked quinoa or salmon.

1. In a medium-size bowl, whisk together the vinegar, maple syrup, shoyu, ginger, mustard, and the sesame and olive oil. Or shake vigorously in a screw-top jar.

2. To supreme the oranges: Using a very sharp knife, slice a bit off the top and the bottom of each orange so it sits flat on a cutting board. Starting at the top of the orange, cut the peel away from the fruit, following the natural curve of the fruit down towards the cutting board. The idea is to take off the peel, white pith, and membrane, but not to remove too much of the fruit. Continue around the entire orange until no more peel remains. Take the orange in one hand positioned over a bowl (to catch the juices) and the knife in the other hand. Identify the white lines in the orange that separate the segments from each other and slice as close to the white line as possible, cutting down to the center of the fruit. Cut alongside the membrane holding the segment and wedge the piece out with the knife. Continue with the remaining segments. Or cut away the peel and slice the fruit crosswise into pinwheels.

3. Place the lettuce in a serving bowl and toss with enough dressing to coat lightly.

4. Add the fruit, avocado slices, and almonds to the bowl. Drizzle with the remaining dressing. Sprinkle with sea salt and pepper to taste.

3 tablespoons unseasoned rice vinegar

1 tablespoon pure Grade A or B maple syrup

2¼ teaspoons shoyu (not GF), tamari, or coconut aminos

⅜ teaspoon ground ginger

⅜ teaspoon Dijon mustard

1½ tablespoons unrefined toasted sesame oil

1½ tablespoons unrefined extra-virgin olive oil or avocado oil

3 small oranges or tangerines

10 cups romaine lettuce (about 1 large head), cut into bite-size pieces

1 to 2 firm but ripe avocados, peeled, pitted, and thinly sliced

⅓ cup sliced almonds or sunflower seeds

Sea salt and fresh ground black pepper

TIP: Whatever salad you are making, be sure all the ingredients that have been washed (e.g., lettuce, herbs, vegetables) are dry. Otherwise, the dressing will not cling to the ingredients (oil and water don't mix) and it will be diluted.

Mexican Chopped Salad with Spicy Cilantro Dressing

SERVES 6 · GF, VEGETARIAN, VEGAN ADAPTABLE, DF ADAPTABLE

DRESSING:

½ cup soy-free Vegenaise or good-quality mayonnaise

½ cup unsweetened, plain, whole Greek yogurt

½ cup buttermilk or kefir (see page 24 for substitutions)

1 tablespoon freshly squeezed lemon juice

½ teaspoon Dijon mustard

1 medium-size garlic clove, grated or minced

½ jalapeño pepper (keep the seeds for extra heat)

1 teaspoon sea salt

Freshly ground black pepper

2 pinches of cayenne pepper

Several dashes of hot sauce

2 tablespoons chopped fresh chives, or 1 scallion, finely chopped

2 tablespoons fresh cilantro, finely chopped, or more if you like

SALAD:

1 head butter or romaine lettuce, chopped (about 8 cups)

2 cups chopped red cabbage

1½ cups cooked pinto beans, or 1 (15-ounce) can, drained and rinsed

2 cups diced cucumbers (I like Persian), unpeeled, large seeds scooped out

1 pint cherry tomatoes, halved

3 small or 2 large avocados, pitted, peeled and cubed

½ cup toasted pepitas

I never serve dinner without a nonstarchy vegetable side dish or a salad or both. This salad often appears on taco night and I sometimes eat it as my whole meal since it is so filling and has plenty of protein from the beans and pepitas. You can easily adjust the heat in the dressing by omitting all of the spiciness—jalapeño, cayenne, and hot sauce. Or just use half of what's listed and taste to see whether it's at your tolerance level. You can prep this whole salad, with the exception of the avocado, in the morning and assemble at the end of the day. See page 7 for an image of this gorgeous salad.

1. Prepare the dressing: Place all the ingredients, except the fresh herbs, in a blender and puree until you have a smooth mixture. Stir in the herbs. Transfer to a container and refrigerate, covered, for at least an hour so that the flavors develop.

2. Prepare the salad: Combine the lettuce and cabbage in a large bowl. Add the pinto beans, cucumber, and cherry tomatoes. Toss with enough dressing to coat lightly. Drizzle a little dressing on the avocado and gently mix into the salad. Sprinkle the pepitas on top. If you have additional dressing, save in the refrigerator for up to 3 days.

To make the dressing dairy-free and vegan, make the following substitutions: Combine ¼ cup of soy-free Vegenaise (instead of the ½ cup of Vegenaise or mayonnaise), 2 tablespoons of freshly squeezed lemon juice (instead of 1 tablespoon), omit the yogurt, and use a nondairy substitute for the buttermilk. Add 1 cup of water and ¾ cup raw cashews, soaked for 4 to 6 hours in water and drained. The other dressing ingredients stay the same. A high-powered blender does a good job blending the cashews until they're creamy. If you don't have one, do this in a food processor and process for at least a few minutes.

TIP: Toast pepitas in a dry skillet until fragrant. Drizzle with ¼ teaspoon of olive oil and sprinkle with a pinch of sea salt.

Zucchini Carpaccio

SERVES 4 TO 6 · VEGETARIAN, GF, VEGAN ADAPTABLE, DF ADAPTABLE

Raw zucchini may sound unusual, but paper-thin ribbons of this summer squash drizzled with good olive oil and lemon juice is about the most refreshing salad you'll find. Zucchini can be bland, so that just means it needs a little help from some supporting ingredients. I make this raw salad two ways—either with basil and Parmesan, or with mint and feta or goat cheese. If you have the time, some toasted pine nuts or sliced almonds make this even better.

Zucchini is not usually thought of as a nutrient-dense vegetable, but it has its benefits: rich in potassium and B-complex vitamins, zucchini is also rich in naturally occurring salts, which help replenish the adrenal glands. Unfortunately, most zucchini in the United States is genetically modified, so it is advisable to seek out organic varieties.

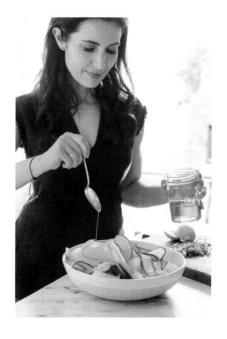

1. Layer the zucchini slices on a platter or place in a bowl. Top with the scallions and mint.
2. Squeeze lemon juice over the platter. Drizzle with olive oil and season to taste with sea salt and pepper.

TIP: It's easy to thinly slice zucchini with a mandoline, but this can also be accomplished with a very sharp knife or a vegetable peeler.

4 small zucchini (a combination of yellow and green is nice), sliced lengthwise as thinly as possible

4 small scallions, thinly sliced

Several fresh mint leaves, finely julienned

2 ounces feta, thinly sliced, or goat cheese, crumbled (omit for vegan/DF)

½ lemon

Unrefined, cold-pressed extra-virgin olive oil, for drizzling

Flaky sea salt

Freshly ground black pepper

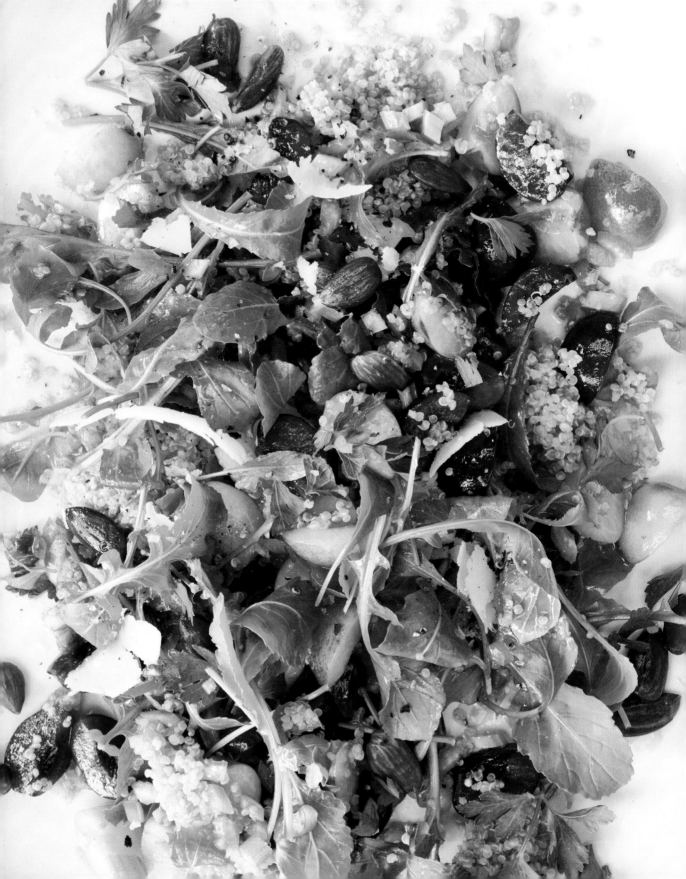

Quinoa Salad with Cherries, Almonds, Celery, and Pecorino

SERVES 6 · VEGETARIAN, GF, VEGAN ADAPTABLE, DF ADAPTABLE

I'm on a mission to get everyone eating quinoa. It has a delightful bouncy and springy texture and the flavor is nutty and quite pleasant. Plus it is one of the only nonanimal foods that contains all eight essential amino acids, so it's perfect if you're looking to cut back on meat (hint, hint). Quinoa also never weighs me down like meat does, but instead makes me feel energized and light. If you've tried quinoa and haven't fallen in love yet, will you please give it another chance and make this salad? If cherries aren't in season, you can substitute strawberries, diced nectarines, or quartered figs. Another option is to make this salad reversed as an arugula salad with only a handful of quinoa tossed in.

1. Place the quinoa and 1¾ cups of water in a medium-size saucepan and bring to a boil over high heat. Cover, lower the heat to a simmer, and cook for 15 minutes, or until all the water has been absorbed. Allow to sit, covered, off the heat for at least 10 minutes, but longer if possible. Transfer to a serving bowl and fluff with a fork. Set aside to cool.

2. Add the arugula, cherries, celery, parsley, almonds, and pecorino, if using, to the quinoa.

3. Prepare the dressing: Combine all the dressing ingredients in a screw-top jar and shake until emulsified or whisk in a bowl.

4. Pour enough dressing over the salad to coat everything lightly. Add more as needed.

TIPS: Toast the almonds in a skillet with a smidge of olive oil and a pinch of salt. For a nut-free option, use toasted sunflower seeds.

I prefer using raw almonds for their high enzyme content. But almonds grown in the United States can actually be labeled "raw" even if they've been steamed or pasteurized, which is not technically raw. The word "raw" should really be replaced with "not roasted." To buy truly raw almonds, seek out a source that sells imported raw almonds or buy directly from your local grower. Check the Resources section for my recommendations (page 263).

1 cup quinoa, rinsed

4 cups lightly packed arugula leaves

2 cups cherries, pitted and quartered (use a cherry pitter to make this job easier)

2 celery stalks, diced

½ cup flat-leaf parsley leaves and tender stems, chopped

⅓ cup raw almonds, toasted, chopped

Pecorino, shaved with a vegetable peeler (about ½ cup shaved pieces) (omit for DF)

DRESSING:

3 tablespoons freshly squeezed lemon juice

2 tablespoons freshly squeezed orange juice

2 teaspoons minced shallot

2 teaspoons pure Grade A maple syrup or raw honey (not vegan)

3 tablespoons unrefined, cold-pressed, extra-virgin olive oil

½ teaspoon sea salt

Freshly ground black pepper

Shaved Vegetable Salad

SERVES 4 TO 6 · GF, DF, VEGAN ADAPTABLE

DRESSING:

1 tablespoon finely chopped shallot, or 1 teaspoon minced garlic

1 teaspoon lemon zest (do not omit this—it makes the salad!)

2 tablespoons freshly squeezed lemon juice

1 tablespoon raw honey (not vegan) or pure Grade A maple syrup

1 teaspoon whole-grain or Dijon mustard

6 tablespoons unrefined, cold-pressed extra-virgin olive oil

1 teaspoon sea salt

Freshly ground black pepper

2 small raw golden or striped beets, peeled and thinly sliced

3 medium-size carrots, peeled and thinly sliced lengthwise

5 radishes, trimmed and thinly sliced

2 large fennel bulbs, core removed and thinly sliced, fronds saved

4 cups torn butter lettuce

½ cup microgreens

Heirloom varieties of vegetables make me happy! When I see rows of differently colored carrots, beets and radishes, I want to buy them all. If you can find multiple colors of any of these vegetables, this salad will look like a rainbow in a bowl. By shaving the vegetables thinly, the flavors become very fresh and delicate. I've had people tell me they don't like beets, but they love this salad! Sometimes I'll add a little feta or ricotta salata for some protein (omit for vegan/DF).

1. Prepare the dressing: Combine all the dressing ingredients in a glass jar and shake to emulsify.

2. Place the beet, carrot, radish, and fennel slices and lettuce in a large bowl. Toss with just enough dressing to coat lightly. Top with the microgreens and a few fennel fronds.

TIP: I use my slicing disk on the food processor set to just under the 1 mm mark to slice the vegetables. Otherwise you can use a mandoline or a vegetable peeler, or do your best with a sharp knife.

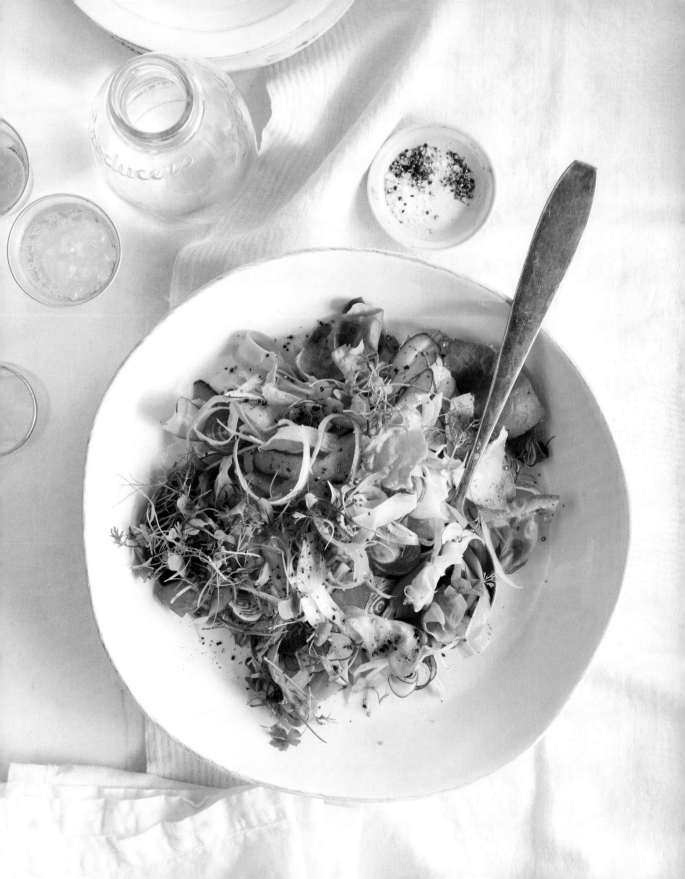

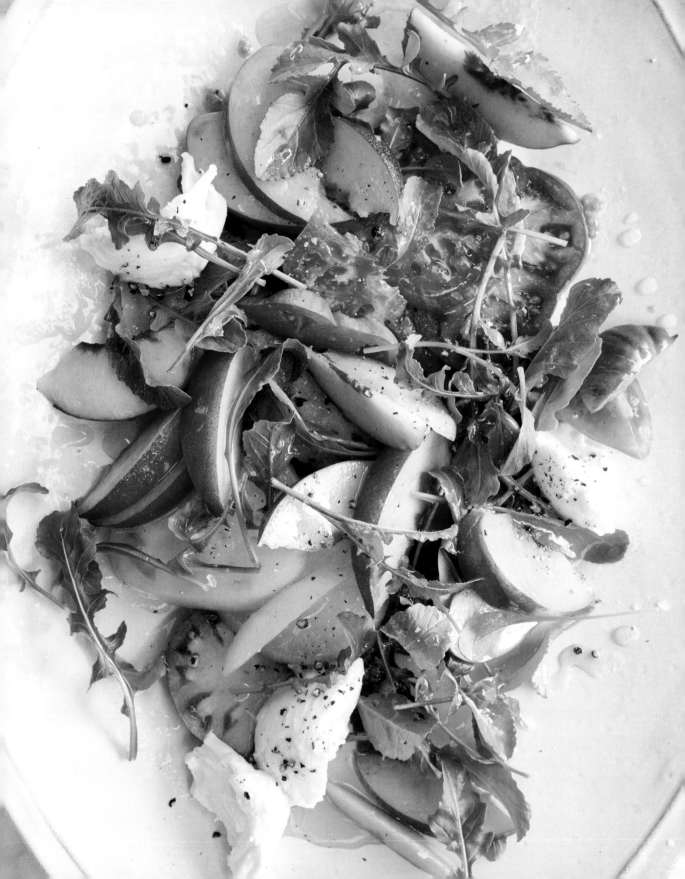

Arugula Salad with Nectarines, Tomatoes, and Fresh Mozzarella

SERVES 6 · VEGETARIAN, GF, VEGAN ADAPTABLE, DF ADAPTABLE

This version of a Caprese salad is what I make when my girlfriend calls me at five p.m. and says, "Why don't we meet at the beach for dinner at six?" No problem! The only key to this recipe is that you must use perfect, in-season tomatoes and nectarines, because those are the stars of the show. For a nondairy version, avocado is a wonderful sub for the mozzarella. Although I love the peppery flavor of arugula, if you need a milder version of this salad, blend a little arugula with some mixed greens, or just use a handful. If you can find aged white balsamic vinegar, use it to keep the salad looking clean. But traditional dark aged balsamic is perfectly wonderful, too.

1. Place the arugula in a large bowl and drizzle with the ¼ cup of balsamic vinegar and the olive oil. Toss to coat. Arrange the arugula on a platter and sprinkle with a few pinches of sea salt.

2. Tuck the fruit wedges into the arugula, evenly spacing them throughout the platter. Do the same thing with the tomatoes and mozzarella.

3. Drizzle the entire salad with equal parts additional balsamic vinegar and olive oil. Sprinkle with several pinches of sea salt.

4. Taste for seasoning. Using enough salt is key to bringing out the sweetness of the tomatoes and nectarines, so don't be afraid to add another pinch.

ASK PAMELA: How do I know if my balsamic vinegar is aged or not? *Traditionally, balsamic vinegar has been an aged vinegar with a thick, syrupy consistency. To get the seal of approval, balsamic vinegar needs to have been aged for at least twelve years. If a recipe specifies "aged balsamic," tilt the bottle and make sure the vinegar is coating the glass. If it has the consistency of red wine vinegar, then it is not aged. Do not use "balsamic glaze," which is often a cheap imitation of aged balsamic with such additives as caramel coloring, gums, and sugar.*

- 10 ounces arugula (I prefer the baby leaves that don't need to be chopped)
- ¼ cup aged white balsamic vinegar (the thick and syrupy kind), or the traditional aged kind, plus more to finish
- ¼ cup unrefined, cold-pressed extra-virgin olive oil, plus more to finish
- Maldon sea salt (flaky) or regular sea salt
- 2 large firm but ripe nectarines or peaches, each cut into 8 wedges
- 2 large tomatoes (I use heirlooms, but use whatever tastes fantastic), each cut into 8 wedges
- 2 balls fresh mozzarella (about 8 ounces total, often packed in water), each cut into 8 wedges (not vegan/DF), or sliced avocado

TIP: You can also make the salad with less arugula, if you like. Use 5 ounces of arugula and halve the amount of balsamic vinegar and oil.

Spinach Salad with Roasted Red Onions and Shiitakes

SERVES 6 · VEGAN, GF, DF

12 medium-size to large shiitake mushrooms, stemmed, caps wiped clean with a damp paper towel and cut into ¼-inch slices (about 10 cups sliced)

2 small red onions, cut into ¼-inch wedges

2 tablespoons unrefined, cold-pressed extra-virgin olive oil

1½ tablespoons fresh thyme leaves

Sea salt and freshly ground black pepper

9 ounces baby spinach (13 to 14 cups)

Seaweed gomasio, for sprinkling (optional, but if not using, finish the salad with a couple of pinches of flaky salt)

DRESSING:

½ cup unrefined, cold-pressed extra-virgin olive oil

3 tablespoons white wine vinegar

½ teaspoon sea salt

Freshly ground black pepper

I make very few warm salads, although I love them in the fall and winter. This salad is a take on a classic spinach and mushroom salad, but I think roasting the mushrooms and onions makes them so much more interesting and flavorful. Ten cups may seem like a crazy amount of mushrooms, but they will shrink down to a fraction of that. You can definitely roast them several hours ahead and leave them at room temperature until you're ready to assemble the salad. If you want a protein and flavor boost, add some chopped turkey bacon. I love serving this with Lickety-Split Chicken (page 185) or Roasted Salmon (page 203).

1. Preheat the oven to 400°F. Line three baking sheets with unbleached parchment paper. Arrange the mushrooms and onions on baking sheets, drizzle with oil, and toss to coat. Sprinkle evenly with thyme leaves and season with salt and pepper to taste. Bake for 20 to 25 minutes, until the mushrooms are slightly golden and the onions are caramelized.

2. Prepare the dressing: Place all the dressing ingredients in a glass jar, adding salt and pepper to taste, and shake until well emulsified.

3. To assemble the salad, place the spinach in a bowl. Add the roasted onions, mushrooms, and gomasio. If you are adding veggies, you can add them to the spinach warm or at room temperature. Drizzle with enough dressing to coat lightly. Toss and serve immediately. Extra dressing can be kept in the refrigerator or a cool, dark place for up to a week.

TIPS: Even if you fall in love with kale, don't forget about spinach! It is incredibly nutritious, teeming with antioxidants, vitamins, and minerals (especially potassium, magnesium, B vitamins, and folate). Spinach is also one of the best plant sources of iron.

You can save cleaned mushroom stems in a container in the freezer for the next time you make vegetable stock.

Curried Chickpea Salad

MAKES 2 QUARTS; SERVES 6 AS AN ENTRÉE · VEGETARIAN, GF, VEGAN ADAPTABLE, DF ADAPTABLE

The classic curried chicken salad just got a vegetarian makeover, and I promise, you won't miss the meat. With chickpeas filling in for chicken, this salad still has the same sweet, salty, tangy, and earthy flavors you love in a good curried chicken salad with the perfect crunch. Eat this salad the same way you would the original—tucked between two slices of whole-grain bread or scooped into lettuce cups (my favorite). Fiber-rich legumes, such as chickpeas, are well known for helping to reduce cholesterol when consumed regularly. They are a fantastic source of inexpensive, low-fat protein. If you struggle with digesting legumes, try soaking them and then cooking them yourself. To make this vegan/DF, omit the yogurt and use a vegan/DF mayonnaise.

4½ cups cooked chickpeas, or 3 (14-ounce) cans, drained and rinsed

2 celery stalks, diced

2 scallions, white and green parts, chopped

1 cup cored and chopped unpeeled apple (about 1 medium-size apple) or grapes, halved

¼ cup unsulfured golden raisins (or dark raisins, if you prefer)

½ cup roasted, salted cashews, chopped (slivered almonds are also good)

½ cup plain, whole Greek yogurt (not vegan/DF) or use all mayonnaise

¼ cup mayonnaise (I like soy-free vegan/DF Vegenaise) or use all Greek yogurt (not vegan/DF)

5 tablespoons apricot or peach preserves, preferably no sugar added like St. Dalfour

1½ tablespoons curry powder

2 teaspoons white wine vinegar

½ teaspoon sea salt, plus more to taste

¼ teaspoon ground ginger

Pinch of cayenne pepper

Butter lettuce leaves or (vegan/DF, if necessary) whole-grain sandwich bread, for serving

1. Reserve ½ cup of the chickpeas. Place the remaining 4 cups of the chickpeas in a large bowl and mash with a potato masher or a fork to create a coarse puree.

2. Add the reserved chickpeas, celery, scallions, apple or grapes, raisins, and cashews to the mashed chickpeas.

3. In a medium-size bowl, combine the yogurt, mayonnaise, preserves, curry powder, vinegar, salt, ginger, and cayenne.

4. Pour on top of the chickpea mixture and combine to coat well with the dressing. Adjust the seasonings to taste. Serve on butter lettuce leaves as a wrap or on sandwich bread.

5. Store leftovers in the refrigerator for up to 3 days.

ASK PAMELA: Is there a difference nutritionally between canned beans and home-cooked? *Not really, but there can be a difference in sodium. So, if you are purchasing canned beans, look for no-salt-added varieties. Another important consideration is the container in which the beans are packaged. Buy beans in glass jars or only select cans that are unlined or BPA-free. However, beans are such a nutritious food that arguably any negative from the packaging would be outweighed by their health benefits.*

Grilled Summer Salad with Chicken and Spicy Cashew Dressing

SERVES 6 · GF, DF, VEGAN ADAPTABLE

SPICY CASHEW DRESSING:

¼ cup raw cashews, soaked for 4 to 6 hours in water and drained, or ¼ cup raw cashew butter

2 tablespoons unseasoned rice vinegar

2 tablespoons unrefined, cold-pressed extra-virgin olive oil

2 teaspoons Dijon mustard

1½ teaspoons pure Grade A maple syrup or mild raw honey (not vegan)

1 medium-size garlic clove

½ teaspoon sea salt, plus more to taste

A few grinds of black pepper

Pinch of cayenne pepper

1½ pounds boneless skinless chicken breasts (about 2 medium-size) (see headnote for vegan substitution)

Unrefined olive oil for brushing chicken, peaches, and corn

½ teaspoon paprika

1 teaspoon sea salt

Freshly ground black pepper

3 medium-size firm but ripe peaches, pitted and quartered

3 ears sweet corn, husked and silks removed

6 to 7 ounces baby romaine lettuce, butter lettuce, or mixed greens (about 8 cups)

4 green onions, green and white parts, thinly sliced

1 large or 2 small avocados, peeled, pitted, and cubed

⅓ cup DF sweet and spicy pecans or candied pecans, such as Trader Joe's prepared pecans

Peaches, corn, and avocados may not sound like a traditional combination, but they are amazing together. For a vegetarian version of this salad, drop the chicken and substitute ½ pound of blanched green beans. This dressing is so good, you'll certainly find multiple uses for it, including making up your own seasonal salad or platter of roasted vegetables.

1. Prepare the dressing: Place ¼ cup of water and all the dressing ingredients in a high-powered blender or food processor and blend until smooth and creamy. This will take a little longer in a food processor. Taste for seasoning. Refrigerate until ready to use. The dressing will thicken as it sits, especially if refrigerated overnight.

2. Heat a grill to medium to medium-high heat, about 400°F. Alternatively, you can use a cast-iron grill pan. Brush the chicken lightly with oil and season with paprika, salt, and pepper. Place the chicken on the grill and flip when the sides of the breasts are white and they can be released easily from the grill. Continue to cook on the other side until the chicken reaches an internal temperature of 160° to 165°F. This should take around 7 minutes per side. Set the chicken aside to rest. This can be done up to 1 day ahead of time and the chicken refrigerated.

3. Brush the peaches and corn lightly with oil. Grill until the peaches and corn have light grill marks, turning occasionally. This should only take a minute or two on each side. Set aside to cool, then slice the peaches crosswise into thirds or fourths and cut the corn kernels off the cob.

4. Slice the chicken crosswise into ½-inch slices or as desired.

5. Place the mixed greens in a bowl. Add the corn and green onions, drizzle with the dressing to lightly coat and toss. Arrange on a platter and top with the peaches, avocado, and pecans. Drizzle with some additional dressing and serve. Leftover dressing can stay in the refrigerator for up to a week.

TIPS: You could use a precooked rotisserie chicken or cooked, cold leftover chicken.

A small spoon can help remove stubborn peach pits.

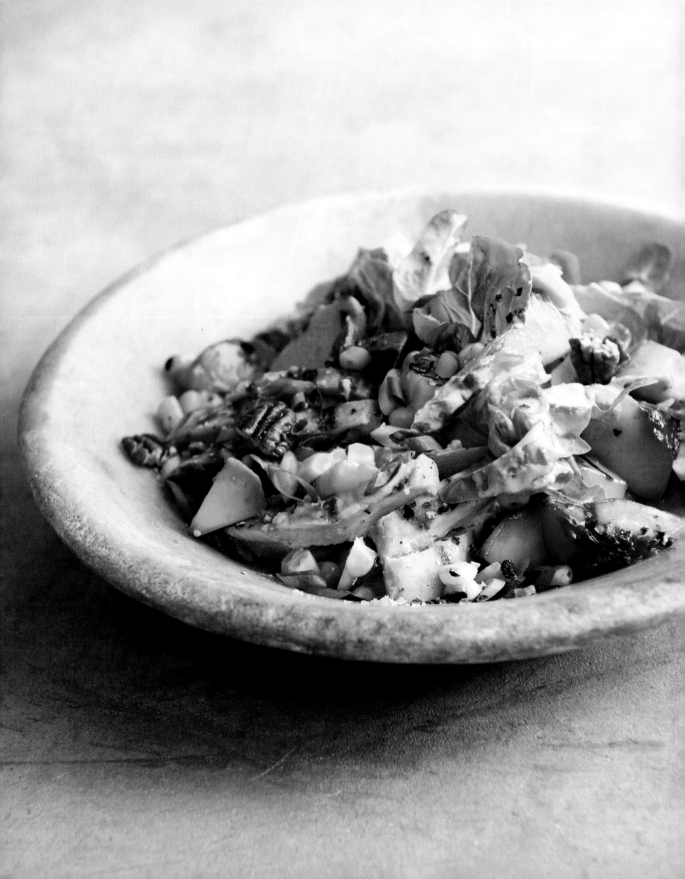

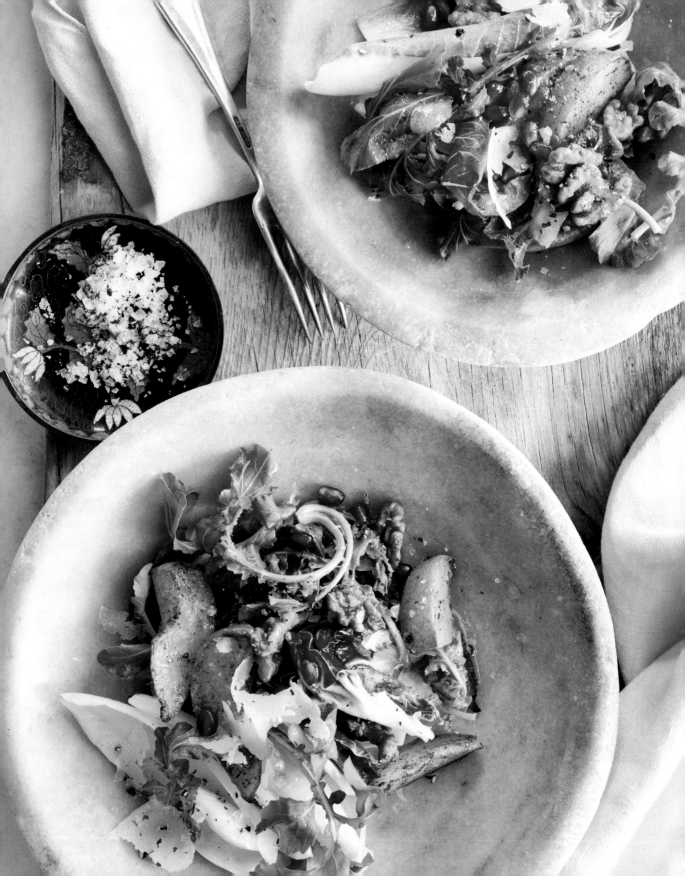

Fall Salad with Pumpkin Pie–Spiced Roasted Pears, Manchego, and Walnuts

SERVES 6 · GF, VEGETARIAN, VEGAN ADAPTABLE, DF ADAPTABLE

Although I taught this salad in one of my Thanksgiving classes, it became a regular addition to my table whenever I entertained friends during the fall and winter months. The combination of a seasonal fruit, plus crunchy nuts and a complementary cheese, is always an easy, classic and delicious salad. I prefer using at least some bitter lettuces in a salad containing fruit just so there's a contrast in flavors. They have numerous health benefits, too. Arugula, for example, has a high antioxidant profile and detoxifying compounds. Its phytonutrients can help prevent cholesterol from sticking to the arteries, and decrease inflammation and blood pressure. If the flavor of arugula is too peppery, substitute your favorite lettuce because this salad is too good not to try!

1. Preheat the oven to 425°F and line a large baking sheet with parchment. In a large bowl, gently toss the pears, oil, and pumpkin pie spice. Spread out the pears in a single layer on the prepared baking sheet and season with salt and pepper to taste. Roast until just tender and fragrant, about 25 minutes. Remove from the oven and allow to cool.

2. Prepare the dressing: Either whisk the dressing ingredients together in a small bowl or place in a glass jar with a lid and shake until emulsified.

3. Place the lettuce on a platter and toss with just enough dressing to coat lightly. Separately drizzle the roasted pears with some dressing and add to the greens. Sprinkle with the pomegranate seeds, walnuts, and Manchego, if using.

TIP: No pumpkin pie spice? No problem—use the following combination of spices:
- ½ teaspoon ground cinnamon
- ¼ teaspoon ground ginger
- ⅛ teaspoon ground cloves
- ⅛ teaspoon ground nutmeg

- 2 firm but ripe pears (I like Bartlett), cored and sliced into ½-inch wedges
- 2 teaspoons unrefined, cold-pressed extra-virgin olive oil or unrefined melted coconut oil
- 1 teaspoon pumpkin pie spice
- Sea salt and freshly ground black pepper

- 8 ounces mixed greens, including some bitter greens, such as radicchio and arugula
- ½ cup fresh pomegranate seeds
- ⅓ cup regular or candied walnuts (Trader Joe's sells good ones)
- 2 to 3 ounces Manchego cheese, shaved thinly with a vegetable peeler (omit for vegan/DF)

DRESSING:

- 2 tablespoons cider vinegar, preferably unpasteurized
- ¾ teaspoon sea salt
- A few twists of freshly ground black pepper
- 1 teaspoon Dijon mustard
- 2 teaspoons pure Grade A maple syrup
- 6 tablespoons unrefined, cold-pressed extra-virgin olive oil

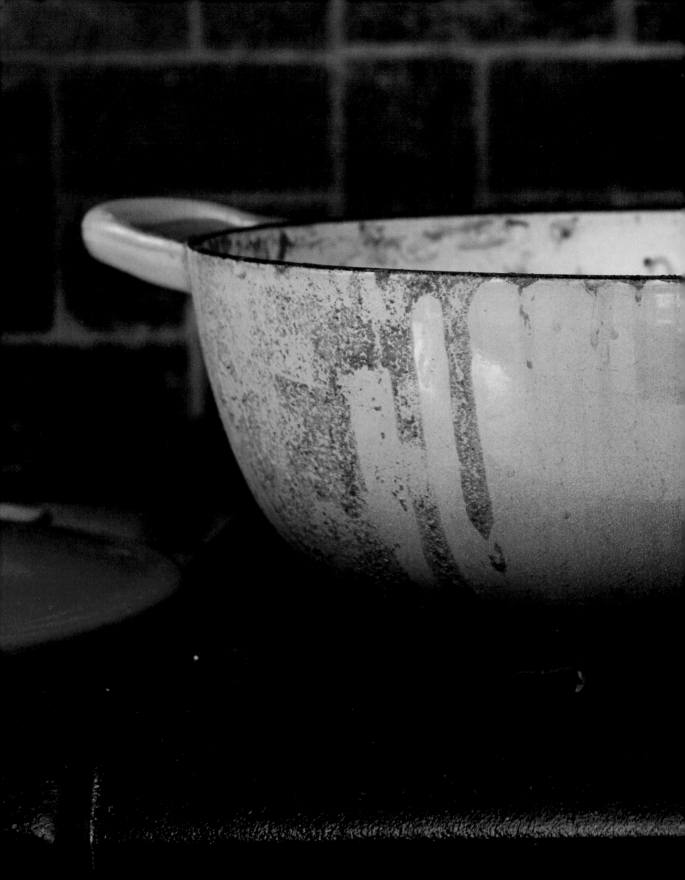

MAIN DISHES

"What should I make for dinner?" is a question that nags most people at the end of the day; I've seen it in my classes, where main dish recipes are in high demand. The recipes in this section have a variety of protein options, from beef to poultry to seafood to vegetarian foods. Whereas I do think animal protein is a whole food, I opt to eat it in moderation and I always select the most healthful and sustainable choices that I can.

Even though I have titled this section "Mains," I like to think of animal protein as a side dish which takes a backseat to plant foods. This chapter is a mix of poultry, fish, meat, and vegetarian recipes. Furthermore, animal products in most of these recipes can be replaced with a vegan option, such as tofu, tempeh, or cooked lentils. The recipes are not complicated, but well flavored and draw their inspiration from both the cooking I grew up with and my favorite international cuisines. If nothing else, I aim to make clean recipes that are also delicious and these will not disappoint.

Among my students' favorites are the South American Roast Chicken with a green sauce that you will flip for; Chipotle Shrimp Tacos and Pineapple Slaw that will satisfy your spicy and sweet cravings; aromatic and flavorful Chicken Shawarma, which is great on its own or with all the fixings; and Eggplant "Meatballs" that you won't believe are meatless. But not every dinner has to have the "wow" factor. There are plenty of terrific basic recipes in this chapter, including how to master wild salmon seven ways!

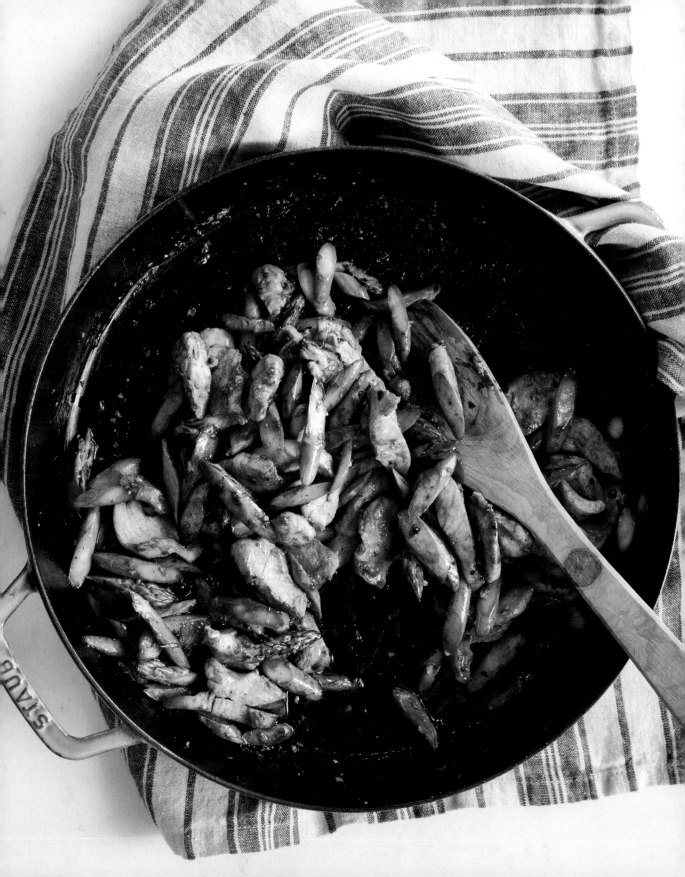

Skillet Chicken with Asparagus

SERVES 6 · DF, GF ADAPTABLE

I always plan my dinners in advance, but life is unpredictable and sometimes I need a Plan B. This simple chicken recipe is my default dinner when I need something simple to prep and quick to cook. Asparagus is just one vegetable of many that will work here. Broccoli, cherry tomatoes, zucchini, and sugar snap peas are all good alternatives. I like to serve this with rice, Millet and Cauliflower Mash (page 135), or roasted sweet potatoes (see chart on page 104).

1. Pat the chicken dry with paper towels and season with salt and pepper.

2. In a small bowl or liquid measuring cup, whisk together the arrowroot powder and chicken stock. Add the vinegar and shoyu. Set aside.

3. Heat a large skillet over medium heat and add 1 tablespoon the olive oil, or enough to just coat the bottom of the pan lightly. (If you use too much oil, the chicken won't brown well.) Add to the pan as many chicken pieces as will fit in one layer without crowding. Brown the chicken on both sides and until almost cooked through, 3 to 4 minutes. Transfer the chicken to a bowl. Repeat with the remaining chicken, and once browned on both sides, transfer to the bowl of cooked chicken.

4. Add the remaining tablespoon of oil to the skillet and toss in the asparagus. Sauté until crisp-tender, about 3 minutes. Add the garlic and oregano and sauté until fragrant, 30 to 60 seconds.

5. Add the chicken back to the skillet with the chicken stock mixture. Bring to a simmer and scrape the bottom of the skillet with a wooden spatula to dislodge any bits stuck to the pan.

6. Sauté until the chicken is cooked through, another minute or two.

3 boneless, skinless chicken breasts (about 2 pounds), cut into 1/2-inch slices, or 2 pounds boneless, skinless thighs

1 1/2 teaspoons sea salt

A few grinds of black pepper

2 teaspoons arrowroot powder

1/2 cup chicken stock, bone broth, or vegetable stock (for homemade, see pages 248–250)

3 tablespoons balsamic vinegar (not aged)

1 tablespoon shoyu (not GF), tamari, or coconut aminos

2 tablespoons unrefined, cold-pressed extra-virgin olive oil or coconut oil

2 bunches asparagus, bottom ends snapped off, stalks cut into bite-size pieces

4 garlic cloves, chopped

1/2 teaspoon dried oregano

Lickety-Split Chicken

SERVES 6 TO 8 · GF, DF

If you are looking for a quick-prep meal that is chock-full of flavor or if you have yet to master cooking chicken, this recipe is your go-to. I prefer to use bone-in, skin-on pieces when I roast chicken breasts because it helps keep the meat moister and more flavorful than boneless, skinless pieces. Yes, bone-in takes longer to cook, but if you can find the time, it's worth it. If you're averse to bone-in pieces of chicken, I also include my technique for boneless and skinless, which I adapted from one I originally saw at TheKitchn.com. There are three different spice rub options here, giving you three different flavors.

4 bone-in, skin-on chicken breasts (about 3 pounds), or 1 (4-pound) chicken, cut into parts

2 teaspoons sea salt

2 teaspoons smoked paprika

Freshly ground black pepper

1 teaspoon fennel seeds, coarsely chopped

1 teaspoon garlic powder

16 sprigs fresh thyme

Unrefined cold-pressed extra-virgin olive oil

1. In one small bowl, combine 1 teaspoon of the salt, 1 teaspoon of the smoked paprika, a few grinds of black pepper, the teaspoon of chopped fennel seeds, and the teaspoon of garlic powder. Set aside.

2. In a second small bowl, combine the remaining teaspoon of sea salt, the remaining teaspoon of smoked paprika, and a few grinds of black pepper. Set aside.

3. Divide the contents of the first small bowl (the one that contains the fennel seeds) among the underside of the chicken pieces. Place the chicken, skin side up, in a 9 x 13-inch casserole dish or a small, rimmed baking sheet. The chicken pieces should not be touching one another.

4. Insert 4 thyme sprigs under the skin of each piece of chicken.

5. Rub the skin with a little olive oil and then with the mixture in the second bowl. It is ideal if you can season the chicken a day or at least several hours in advance. If not, don't worry about it. But do allow the chicken to sit out of the refrigerator for 30 minutes before baking, if possible. Otherwise it may not cook evenly.

6. Preheat the oven to 375°F.

7. Roast the chicken for 35 to 40 minutes, or until a meat thermometer inserted in the thickest part of the breast registers 165°F.

8. Switch the oven to the broil setting. Then, broil the chicken on the second level in the oven (leave it in the baking dish) for 30 seconds, or until golden brown.

9. Remove from the oven and allow to rest for 5 to 10 minutes, covered. Remove the thyme sprigs from under the skin. Remove the meat from the bone and carve, spooning the pan juices on top. One nice option is to serve the warm chicken and the juices over fresh arugula.

Sweet and Smoky Lickety-Split Chicken

2 teaspoons sea salt

1 teaspoon chili powder

A few grinds of black pepper

2 teaspoons garlic powder

1½ teaspoons paprika

½ teaspoon chipotle chile powder

2 teaspoons muscovado sugar or brown sugar

1. Mix all together and rub on both sides of all the chicken pieces.

Mediterranean Lickety-Split Chicken

BOTTOM:

1 teaspoon salt

1 teaspoon oregano

1 teaspoon dried thyme

1 teaspoon garlic powder

1 teaspoon lemon zest

Freshly ground black pepper

TOP:

1 teaspoon salt

Freshly ground black pepper

Unrefined cold-pressed extra-virgin olive oil

16 sprigs fresh thyme (under skin)

1. Follow steps 1 -5 in the main recipe while using the Mediterranean ingredients.

Boneless, Skinless Version

1. Grease a 9 x 13-inch casserole with olive oil.
2. Combine the herbs and spices in two bowls, as directed in steps 1 and 2 of the recipe for bone-in chicken.
3. Divide the contents of the first small bowl (the one that contains the fennel seeds) among the underside of the chicken pieces (where the tender is.) Place the chicken, spice mixture side down, in the prepared baking dish.
4. Place the 4 thyme sprigs under each piece of chicken, on the baking dish.
5. Rub the top of the chicken breasts with a little olive oil and then with the mixture in the second bowl. Grease a piece of unbleached parchment paper with olive oil and place the parchment paper directly on the chicken, greased side down. Tuck the parchment around the chicken pieces. Allow the chicken to sit out of the refrigerator for 30 minutes before baking, if possible.
6. Preheat the oven to 400°F.

7. Roast the chicken for 25 to 30 minutes, or until a meat thermometer inserted in the thickest part of the breast registers 165°F.
8. Switch the oven to the broil setting. Remove the parchment paper. Then, broil the chicken on the second level in the oven (leave it in the baking dish) for 30 seconds, or until golden brown.
9. Remove from the oven and allow to rest for 5 to 10 minutes, covered. Remove the thyme sprigs from under the chicken, if using. Serve the chicken breasts with the pan juices. One nice option is to serve the warm chicken and the juices over fresh arugula.

TIPS: The bones in the chicken are most efficiently removed by hand, as opposed to a knife. I wear rubber gloves to make this task quick and easy.

If you have time, definitely season the chicken as early as you can, preferably when you bring it home from the market. The flavors will penetrate the meat and it will taste so much better.

ASK PAMELA: I freak out when I cook chicken because I am always afraid it will turn out underdone, but then I overcook it. How do I cook chicken so that it's done, but not dry? *You definitely do want to cook chicken thoroughly, but there is no reason to stress out. Go out and buy a meat thermometer. It is the only way you will know for sure whether the meat is cooked to the proper temperature, which is between 160° and 165°F. Do not be intimidated by using one. You have used thermometers before, just on human beings. Another simple rule to follow is to allow bone-in pieces of chicken and larger pieces of meat to sit out of the refrigerator for 30 minutes before roasting, so they cook evenly throughout.*

South American Roast Chicken with Green Sauce

SERVES 4 TO 6 · GF, DF ADAPTABLE

5 garlic cloves, very finely minced or grated

2 teaspoons sea salt, plus more for seasoning

2 tablespoons smoked paprika

1½ tablespoons ground cumin

½ teaspoon dried oregano

Juice of 1 lime (2½ to 3 tablespoons)

½ cup dry white wine

¼ cup white wine vinegar

¼ cup unrefined cold-pressed olive oil

1 whole (4- to 5-pound) chicken, backbone removed (you can save it for stock)

Green sauce, to serve (recipe follows)

Note: You can also do this with chicken parts, but cook for 35 to 45 minutes. Or a whole, uncut bird for 1 hour 10 minutes to 1 hour 30 minutes.

This is another very tasty chicken recipe for minimal effort. Bonus: This is also fabulous for entertaining since you do all the work ahead of time. Make sure you are using a good, fragrant smoked paprika for this, otherwise the flavor will be just eh. My favorite brand is Chiquilin. If you marinate this overnight, the meat will be falling off the bones. Even better than the chicken is this green sauce, which I adapted from a recipe found on seriouseats.com. I always make extra of the green sauce because I love it all week long on scrambled eggs, breakfast tacos, grain bowls, and sliced tomatoes.

1. In a small bowl, combine the garlic with the sea salt to make a paste; set aside.
2. In a large bowl big enough to fit the whole chicken, whisk together the smoked paprika, cumin, oregano, lime juice, wine, vinegar, and olive oil.
3. Carefully separate the skin from the chicken breast meat, sliding your fingers to separate the skin as far down as you can go, but trying not to tear the skin. Rub the garlic paste under the loosened skin and directly onto the meat as evenly as possible. Sprinkle the underside of the chicken with a pinch of salt.
4. Place the chicken in the bowl and toss to coat with the marinade. Cover the bowl and refrigerate for at least 6 hours or overnight.
5. Preheat the oven to 425°F.
6. Place the chicken, breast side up, in a roasting pan or rimmed baking sheet that is just big enough to fit it and pour the marinade over the chicken. (If your roasting pan is too large, the pan juices will burn up before the chicken is done.) Sprinkle the chicken with a pinch of salt. Roast the chicken for 50 to 60 minutes, or until the temperature of the breast is 160°F. If the juices are drying up or starting to burn, you can add ½ cup of water or stock to the pan. Allow to sit, covered, out of the oven for 5 to 10 minutes.
7. Carve the roasted chicken and serve with the green sauce.

Green Sauce

MAKES 1 CUP · VEGETARIAN, GF, VEGAN ADAPTABLE, DF ADAPTABLE

1 to 2 jalapeño peppers, seeds and ribs removed (I use 1½ with no seeds)

1 cup fresh cilantro leaves and tender stems

2 tablespoons grated pecorino or Parmesan cheese (omit for vegan/DF)

1 medium-size garlic clove

1 tablespoon unrefined, cold-pressed extra-virgin olive oil

1 teaspoon white wine vinegar

1½ tablespoons freshly squeezed lime juice (from about ½ lime)

½ cup soy-free Vegenaise or your favorite mayonnaise (not vegan)

½ teaspoon sea salt

Freshly ground black pepper

1. Place all the ingredients in a blender, adding black pepper to taste, and blend until smooth.

ASK PAMELA: Should I wash my chicken before cooking it? *Technically, no, you should not wash your chicken. You are not reducing harmful bacteria on the chicken by washing it. You need to cook your chicken thoroughly to do that. Instead, studies have shown that when people rinse poultry, they end up splashing water with raw chicken juices to different parts of the sink, countertop, and clean dishes. And they don't know it! That said, if you are using chicken that was wrapped in plastic and seems overly wet, you might find it desirable to carefully rinse off the chicken, taking extra care to disinfect the sink area afterward.*

Chicken Shawarma

SERVES 6 · GF, DF ADAPTABLE

MARINADE:

¼ cup unrefined, cold-pressed extra-virgin olive oil

¼ cup freshly squeezed lemon juice (from about 2 lemons)

2 teaspoons kosher salt

2 teaspoons ground cumin

2 teaspoons paprika

½ teaspoon ground turmeric

⅛ teaspoon ground cinnamon, or more to taste

⅛ teaspoon cayenne pepper, or more if you want it to be spicy

Several grinds of black pepper

4 garlic cloves, minced

2 pounds boneless, skinless chicken thighs, trimmed of excess fat

White sauce (recipe follows) or store-bought tahini sauce

Suggested accompaniments:
GF lavash, lettuce, tomato, pickled vegetables, onion, olives

WHITE SAUCE:

⅔ cup plain whole Greek yogurt (not DF) or plain DF yogurt

⅓ cup good-quality mayonnaise or soy-free Vegenaise

3 garlic cloves, minced

1 tablespoon freshly squeezed lemon juice

⅛ teaspoon sea salt

⅛ teaspoon paprika

Freshly ground black pepper

Shawarma is a Middle Eastern dish of meat roasted on a spit and shaved into sandwiches. I obviously don't have a revolving spit in my kitchen, but that hasn't stopped me from making a crazy good version of classic shawarma. For very little effort, you can enjoy an incredibly flavorful dish with a variety of possibilities. My kids love shawarma as a sandwich and I usually turn it into a rice bowl or big salad.

1. Prepare the marinade: Combine all the marinade ingredients in a nonreactive bowl (e.g., glass). Add the chicken and toss to coat. Marinate at room temperature for 1 hour or in the refrigerator for several hours or up to overnight.
2. Remove the chicken from the refrigerator 30 minutes before cooking. Preheat the oven to 400°F or a heat a grill to medium heat. If you are baking, line a baking sheet with parchment paper.
3. Grill until cooked through, about 7 minutes on each side, or bake on the prepared baking sheet for 35 minutes, or until cooked through. If the chicken was baked, you may slice it thinly and sauté the slices in a skillet in coconut oil or olive oil, to get some crispy edges. You don't have to do this step since the chicken is already cooked, but the crispy edges somewhat mimic traditional shawarma shaved off the spit. I also like to sprinkle with a pinch of sea salt, too.
4. Slice thinly and serve with your desired accompaniments.

White Sauce

1. Mix all the ingredients together in a bowl, adding black pepper to taste. Refrigerate until ready to serve. Can be made 1 day in advance. Stir before serving.

ASK PAMELA: Can you use boneless, skinless chicken breasts? *Why do so many people insist on breast meat all the time? Okay, fine. Yes, of course you can. Breasts take about the same amount of time. I still prefer this recipe with thighs, though, because they have more flavor and aren't as susceptible to drying out.*

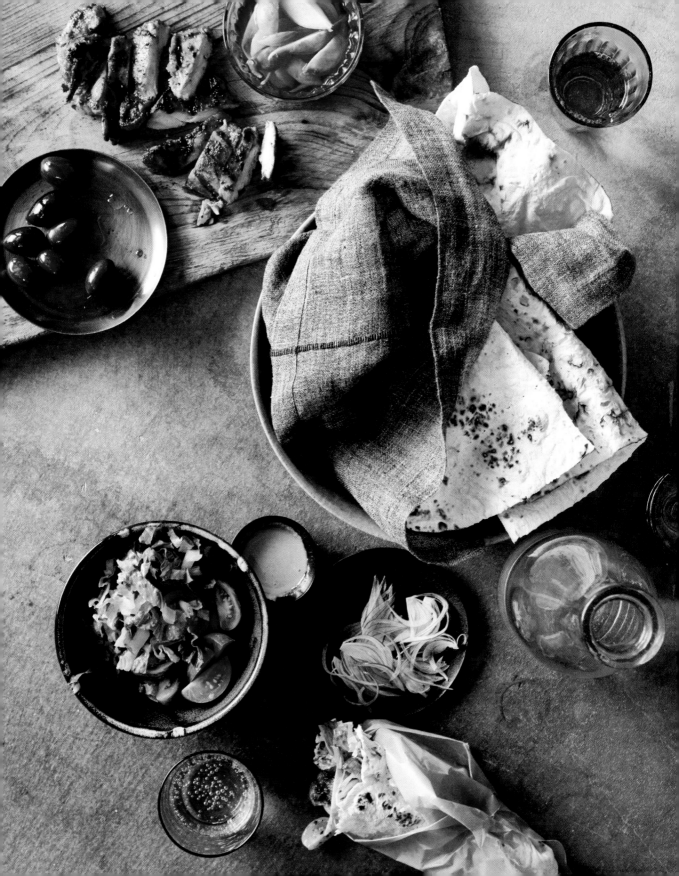

Slow Cooker Chicken Tacos

SERVES 6 · GF, DF

2 pounds boneless, skinless chicken breasts and/or thighs (I use 2 breasts and 3 thighs)

1 teaspoon chili powder

1 teaspoon ground cumin

½ teaspoon chipotle chile powder

1 teaspoon sea salt

¼ teaspoon freshly ground black pepper

4 garlic cloves, finely chopped

½ cup prepared tomato salsa (I use pico de gallo) + more for serving

Suggested accompaniments: GF corn tortillas, guacamole, salsa, shredded lettuce

Everyone wants recipes that are quicker than quick. And although I can't teach my students to cook in no time, I do have a few good recipes that take just a few minutes of prep. This is one of them. Obviously the chicken needs time to cook, but it's inactive time. I toss everything into the slow cooker before I leave for work in the morning and I come home to the aroma of a Tex-Mex fiesta. This recipe is one of the most popular on my blog and an absolute staple. You can double the recipe (no extra cooking time needed) and make a big batch of this chicken for parties. All you need are some great toppings and tortillas. I like to use a big lettuce leaf instead of a tortilla for a lighter meal. Leftovers are great in enchiladas, quesadillas, or a grain bowl.

1. Place the chicken in a slow cooker and sprinkle with chili powder, cumin, chipotle powder, salt, and black pepper. Add the garlic and salsa and rub around to combine. Cover; cook on high for 4 hours or low for 6 to 7 hours.

2. Either shred the chicken with two forks right in the slow cooker or transfer to a plate to shred. Moisten the chicken with the cooking juices and serve as desired with tortillas or taco shells and the suggested toppings.

■ Grain bowl idea: Shredded chicken over rice with lettuce, avocado, and fresh cilantro

■ Oven method: Preheat the oven to 350°F. In step 1, place all the ingredients (except the accompaniments) in a 5-quart Dutch oven or ovenproof pot with a tight-fitting lid. Add 2 cups of water or chicken stock. Cover and bake until the chicken is fork-tender, about 2 hours. Proceed with step 2.

Chipotle Shrimp Tacos with Pineapple Slaw

SERVES 4 · GF, DF, VEGAN ADAPTABLE

I love these shrimp tacos so much that I make ten times the spice mixture and put it in a bottle so that I can whip up these spicy morsels any time the craving hits. To me, the perfect taco has a combination of textures and flavors—crunchy, creamy, spicy, sour, and don't forget juicy. These shrimp tacos hit all the right notes. Chipotle powder definitely gives the shrimp a little kick, but you can adjust the amount to suit your taste. Not into spicy? Substitute smoked paprika to get the smokiness without the heat. The pineapple slaw is the perfect topping to round out these tacos, but there's enough here if you wanted to turn this into a salad and top it with the sizzling shrimp. For a vegan version, which I enjoy just as much if not more, substitute 3 cups of bite-size cauliflower florets, steamed. Toss them with a drizzle of olive oil and the spice mixture and sauté in olive oil until caramelized. So incredibly good, you'll have a hard time not eating the entire pan.

1. Rinse the shrimp and pat dry with paper towels. Set aside.
2. In a medium-size bowl, combine the spices, sugar, salt, and black pepper to taste. Add the shrimp and toss to coat.
3. In a large skillet, heat the olive oil over medium heat. Add the shrimp in one layer and cook until cooked through, 5 to 8 minutes, turning when halfway done.
4. If the shrimp are very large, chop them into bite-size pieces before serving. Season with an extra pinch of salt and serve with tortillas and desired accompaniments.

Pineapple Slaw follows on page 193

- 1 pound medium-size peeled and deveined wild shrimp, tails removed
- ½ teaspoon chipotle chili powder, or less to make it less spicy
- ½ teaspoon garlic powder
- ½ teaspoon natural cane sugar, brown sugar, or maple sugar
- ¼ teaspoon paprika
- ¼ teaspoon ground cumin
- ¼ teaspoon chili powder
- ¾ teaspoon sea salt, plus more for sprinkling
- Freshly ground black pepper
- 1 tablespoon unrefined, cold-pressed, extra-virgin olive oil
- 8 warm corn tortillas (GF/DF, if necessary) or large lettuce leaves
- Pineapple Slaw (recipe follows) or shredded cabbage, sliced avocado, and lime

TIP: If your market only offers one type of wild shrimp, do purchase that rather than farm-raised, regardless of size. Farmed shrimp is fed antibiotics, chemicals, preservatives, and antifungal agents. If the wild shrimp you are working with are very large, they can always be halved after they are cooked. Shrimp are a low-fat source of protein that is also high in vitamin D as well as three powerful antioxidants—selenium, astaxanthin, and copper.

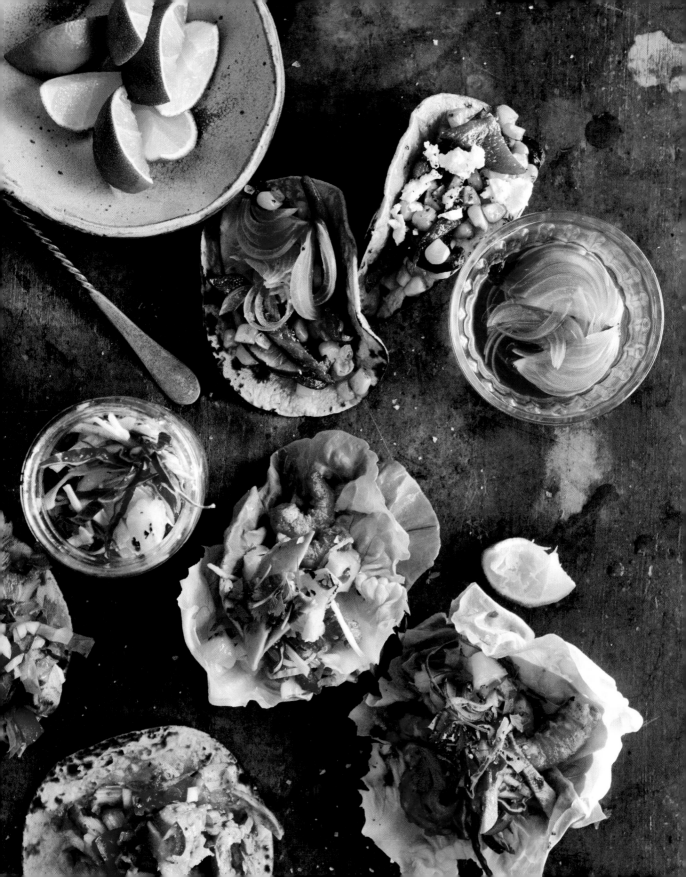

Pineapple Slaw

SERVES 6 · VEGAN, GF, DF

1. Preheat a grill to medium-high heat. Brush the pineapple with coconut oil and sprinkle with a pinch each of salt, black pepper, and chili powder. Grill until you achieve grill marks on all sides. Set aside.

2. Place the cabbage, radish, onion, and jalapeño in a serving bowl.

3. Dice the pineapple and add to the bowl.

4. Add the lime juice, olive oil, ½ teaspoon of salt, and black pepper to taste and toss to combine. Arrange the avocado slices on top and mound the cilantro in the center.

¼ whole pineapple, skin and core removed

Melted coconut oil, for brushing pineapple

Sea salt

Freshly ground black pepper

Chili powder

4 cups thinly sliced green or red cabbage (or a mix)

2 large watermelon radishes, julienned, or any smaller variety, thinly sliced (about 2 cups)

½ small red onion, diced or thinly sliced

½ jalapeño pepper, seeded and minced

2 tablespoons freshly squeezed lime juice

2 tablespoons unrefined, cold-pressed extra-virgin olive oil

1 avocado, peeled, pitted, and sliced

¼ cup fresh cilantro leaves and tender stems

From top to bottom: Portobello and Poblano Tacos with Charred Corn (page 194), Chipotle Shrimp Tacos with Pineapple Slaw (page 191), and Slow Cooker Chicken Tacos (page 190)

Portobello and Poblano Tacos with Charred Corn

SERVES 6 · GF, VEGAN ADAPTABLE, DF ADAPTABLE

4 poblano peppers (often labeled as "pasilla" peppers)

2 tablespoon unrefined, cold-pressed extra-virgin olive oil

4 portobello mushrooms, thickly sliced (about ½ inch thick)

1 cup frozen fire-roasted corn or regular sweet corn kernels, preferably organic, thawed or freshly cut from the cob

Sea salt

Freshly ground black pepper

½ teaspoon ground cumin

Accompaniments: vegan/GF corn tortillas, pickled onions, crumbled feta (omit for vegan/DF)

Mushrooms are another one of my secret substitutes for meat. They have that awesome umami flavor that satisfies our taste for protein. White button, cremini, and portobello mushrooms are actually all the same mushroom, just at different stages of development. White is the youngest and with the least flavor and portobello is the most mature with the most complex flavor. You can really use any mushrooms here, but portobello will have the most interesting flavor and when it's cut into strips resembles meat. Roasted poblanos are incredible—a little smoky, a touch spicy, and really earthy. If you don't have time to roast them (although you can do that step a few days before,) just slice them up raw and sauté them until tender.

1. Preheat the broiler to high and position a rack 6 inches below the heat source. This is usually the second level. Place the poblanos on a baking sheet and broil until blackened on all sides, turning every couple of minutes. Set aside in a bowl and cover for at least 15 minutes, or until cool enough to handle. Rub off the skin, remove the seeds, and slice thickly (about ½ inch thick).

2. In a large skillet, heat the olive oil over medium heat. Add the portobellos and sauté until tender, 5 to 6 minutes. Add the corn, sliced poblanos, a sprinkle of salt and black pepper to taste, and the cumin. Sauté until the corn is warmed through. Taste for seasoning. Serve with warmed tortillas and your desired accompaniments.

Wild Halibut Burgers

MAKES 4 TO 5 PATTIES · DF, GF ADAPTABLE

I love to sink my teeth into a good burger loaded with all the fixin's. But my burger of choice is this moist and tender patty made from wild halibut. Even my husband, a loyal beef fan, has described these as "surprisingly satisfying." Halibut is very mild-tasting, which is great for those who are pickier about fish, but that also means it needs a flavor boost. The collective tang from the Dijon mustard, lemon, and cayenne infuses the halibut with a much-welcomed punch. Even though these burgers are perfectly tasty on their own, that doesn't stop me from smothering them with a fabulous home-made tartar sauce and some spicy arugula.

1. Cut one fourth (i.e., about 4 ounces) of the halibut into 2-inch pieces. Place those pieces in a food processor fitted with the metal blade and add the egg, mustard, lemon zest and juice, and cayenne. Use the pulse button and process just until a paste is made. Transfer to a large mixing bowl.
2. Cut the remaining halibut into ¼-inch pieces. Add to the processed halibut mixture.
3. Add the minced shallot, panko, parsley, garlic powder, salt, and black pepper to taste and gently stir until combined. The mixture will seem like a sloppy mess. It's okay.
4. Line a platter or a baking sheet with parchment paper or waxed paper so you can get the burgers off the platter easily later. Form the mixture into four or five 4-inch-wide, ¾-inch-thick patties. Cover and refrigerate for at least 30 minutes, up to 12 hours ahead. This step helps bind the burgers.
5. Heat the olive oil in a large, cast-iron skillet over medium-high heat or to 375°F on a griddle. Add the patties (in batches, if necessary) and cook until browned on the bottom, 4 to 5 minutes, adjusting the heat if necessary. Turn and cook until the other side is browned and the patties feel firm in the center, 4 to 5 minutes. Serve immediately with your desired accompaniments.

Tartar Sauce follows on page 197

1 to 1¼ pounds wild halibut fillet, skinless, pin bones removed

1 large egg, or ¼ cup mayonnaise or soy-free Vegenaise

2 tablespoons Dijon mustard

½ teaspoon grated lemon zest

1 tablespoon freshly squeezed lemon juice

⅛ teaspoon cayenne pepper

1 small shallot, minced

¼ cup DF panko bread crumbs (GF, if necessary) or certified-GF oat flour

¼ cup fresh parsley leaves and tender stems, finely chopped (dill is also nice)

½ teaspoon garlic powder

½ teaspoon sea salt

Freshly ground black pepper

2 tablespoons unrefined, cold-pressed extra-virgin olive oil

Accompaniments: toasted buns (GF, if necessary), arugula, avocado, garlic aioli, or tartar sauce (recipe follows)

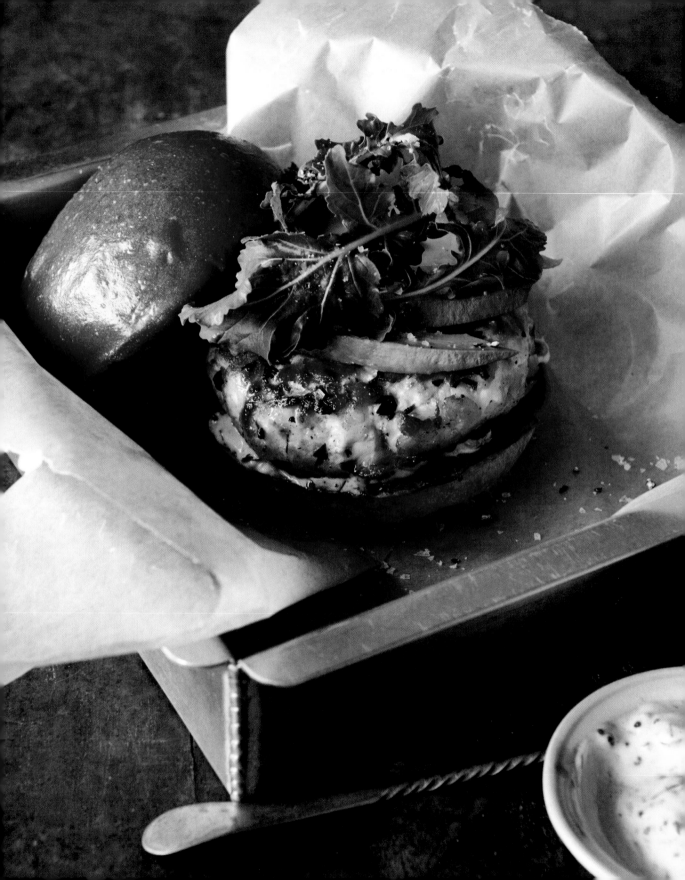

Tartar Sauce

MAKE ABOUT ¾ CUP SAUCE · VEGAN, GF, DF

1. Place all the ingredients in a small bowl and stir to combine. Keep refrigerated. Can be made 2 to 3 days ahead. Stir before serving.

TIP: Fish and veggie burgers benefit from some advance prep. By your forming the burgers and refrigerating them early, they hold their shape much better. That said, these burgers do much better cooked on a skillet or a flat-top griddle than on a grill unless your grill is impeccably clean.

1 tablespoon finely chopped dill pickles or cornichons

1 tablespoon finely chopped fresh flat-leaf parsley

1 tablespoon capers, drained and finely chopped

1 teaspoon freshly squeezed lemon juice

1 teaspoon coarse-grain mustard

½ cup soy-free Vegenaise, mayonnaise (not vegan), or plain Greek yogurt (not vegan/DF)

A dash of hot sauce, such as Tabasco

Pinch of sea salt

Pinch of freshly ground black pepper

Broiled Fillet of Sole with Lemon and White Wine   SERVES 6 · GF, DF ADAPTABLE

Unrefined cold-pressed olive oil, for pan and brushing on fish

6 (5- to 6-ounce) fillets wild sole or any thin, mild white fish, such as Petrale sole

1¼ teaspoons paprika

¾ teaspoon sea salt

Freshly ground black pepper

3 garlic cloves, thinly sliced

1 lemon, sliced into thin rounds

2 to 3 tablespoons dry white wine

1½ tablespoons unsalted butter, melted (optional; omit for DF)

1½ tablespoons fresh flat-leaf parsley, chopped

If you are trying to eat more fish, but are intimidated to cook it, this recipe will boost your confidence. Broiled sole is about as uncomplicated as it gets, but the reward is a beautiful, clean-tasting, and elegant dish that you can serve to wow your friends or have in your back pocket for a very quick weeknight meal. Since this fish cooks so quickly, wait until five minutes before you want to serve it before you put it in the oven. I like to serve this with sautéed spinach or other greens, Baked Cauliflower and Rice Risotto (page 142) or One-Pot Barley with Melted Cabbage (page 139)

1. Place an oven rack 6 inches from the heat source. This is usually the second level. Preheat the broiler to high.
2. Grease a large, rimmed baking sheet with olive oil. (I use a full sheet pan. Use two small ones if you don't have one that will accommodate all the fish.) Pat the fish dry with paper towels and arrange in one layer in the prepared baking pan. Brush the fish with olive oil and sprinkle evenly with paprika, salt, and pepper. Arrange the garlic and lemon slices around the fish. Add the wine and butter to the pan around the fish, not on top of the fish.
3. Broil for 3 minutes, or until the fish flakes easily when you insert a fork into the fish and twist gently. If the flesh separates or "flakes" easily, then it's done. The cooking time will depend on thickness of the fish.
4. Arrange the fish and lemon slices on a platter. Pour the juices from baking sheet on top of the fish and sprinkle with the parsley. Serve immediately.

ASK PAMELA: Should I leave the oven door open when I use the broiler? *My mother used to leave the oven door open a few inches, since things can burn very easily under the broiler. Fast-forward several decades and most modern ovens are closed-door broilers, although you should consult your manual to be sure. If your oven is gas, you should definitely be broiling with the door closed. My oven manual says quite plainly not to leave the door open, as it will damage the exterior knobs.*

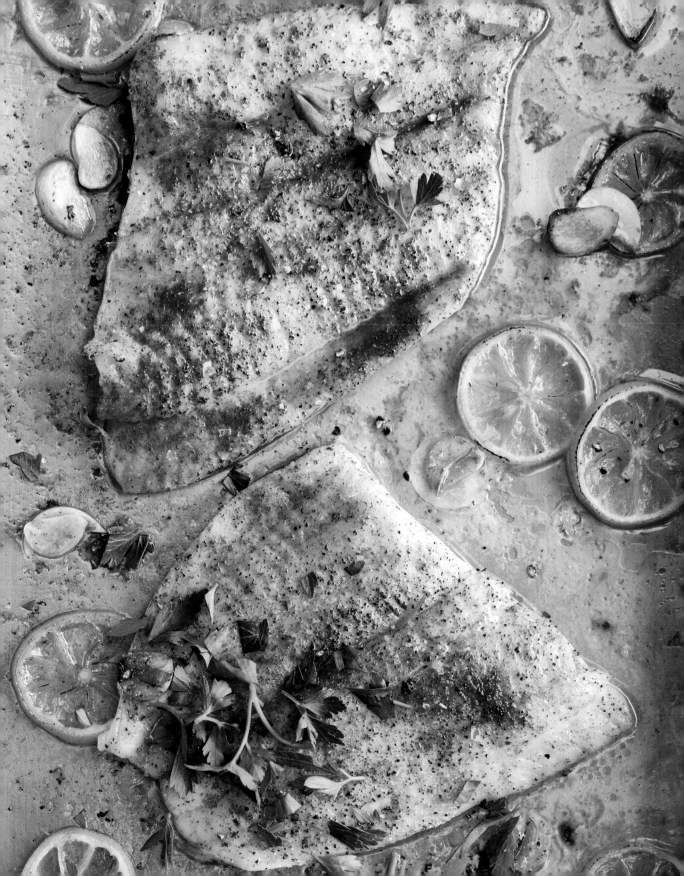

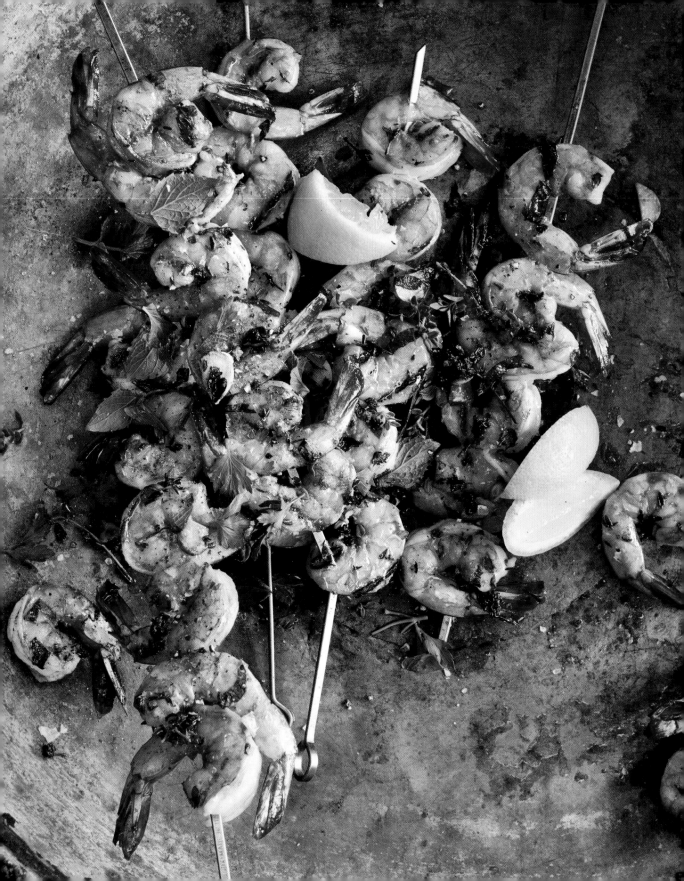

Grilled Lemon-Herb Shrimp

SERVES 6 TO 8 · GF, DF

These shrimp skewers are perfect for a busy weeknight or for guests you want to impress. This simple marinade is clean and bright and does double duty as a chicken marinade, too. You don't want to marinate any longer than the recommended thirty minutes, otherwise the lemon juice might "cook" the shrimp, which basically means the protein structure of the shrimp has changed similar to the way heat from cooking affects it. I serve these over Herbed Mixed-Grain Pilaf (page 149) and Sautéed Zucchini with Shallots (page 123) or off the skewers on top of a big salad.

¼ cup freshly squeezed lemon juice

¼ cup cold-pressed extra-virgin olive oil

4 garlic cloves, thinly sliced

¼ cup chopped mixed fresh herbs (mint, parsley, and thyme is a good combo)

1 teaspoon sea salt

Freshly ground black pepper

1½ pounds large wild-caught, peeled and deveined shrimp, rinsed and patted dry

1. Mix together all the ingredients, except the shrimp, in a shallow, nonreactive container (e.g., glass), adding pepper to taste. Add the shrimp and toss to coat well. Cover and refrigerate for 30 minutes.

2. Have ready eight skewers. If using wooden or bamboo skewers, soak them in water while the shrimp marinate.

3. Thread four or five shrimp on each skewer.

4. Preheat the grill to medium heat. Grill the shrimp about 3 minutes on each side, or until cooked through.

Wild Salmon 7 Ways

Wild salmon is the ultimate anti-inflammatory food with its substantial stores of omega-3 fats. I am not as big a fan of farm-raised salmon; it is higher in contaminants than wild and the fish are fed soy and food coloring, decreasing the nutritional benefits. I would opt for wild as much as possible. Keep in mind, "Atlantic" salmon always implies farm-raised and "Alaskan" is always wild. (I also avoid GMO salmon.) Wild salmon has a season, which is usually from about May to October. (If you see "fresh" wild Alaskan salmon being sold in the winter months, it is probably farm-raised.) But there is no reason to avoid eating fish if you can only find frozen/defrosted varieties available. Here are seven different basic techniques to cook wild salmon. Note that wild salmon is often thinner than farm-raised and will cook more quickly, so if you are using the following recipes with farm-raised, you may have to add some extra time. Salmon is a very versatile fish that can be the base of a lovely meal. I love pairing it with Herbed Mixed-Grain Pilaf (page 149), Baked Cauliflower and Rice Risotto (page 142), and any vegetable or salad recipe in this book.

Basic cooking tips: When prepared properly, salmon needs very few supporting flavors; it really shines on its own in the simplicity of a little bit of oil, salt, and pepper. However, nothing can really strip salmon of its delicious flavor, texture, and nutrition faster than overcooking it. A good rule of thumb when cooking salmon is to cook it for 4 to 6 minutes for every ½ inch of thickness. If you are using a high-heat method, such as broiling, grilling, or pan-searing, you will use the lesser time. For moderate heat methods, such as baking, poaching, and slow-roasting, you will use the greater time. When purchasing salmon, try to ask for a center cut portion to ensure even thickness throughout the fillet; this will ensure that the salmon cooks evenly throughout. Another way to protect your salmon is by leaving the skin on, even if you are going to serve the salmon skinless. The skin will protect the salmon from drying out and give you a little cushion if you do overcook it for a minute or two. Also, use your meat thermometer! If you're really not sure if your salmon is done, you can check the internal temperature. You want the thickest part of the salmon to register at 125°F. It is also important to remember that your salmon will continue to cook after you remove it from the heat, so you need to pull it from the heat before it is completely cooked to your liking. The salmon should also flake easily when you poke it with a paring knife, and become opaque on the outside but still slightly translucent and rare in the center. Due to their less active lifestyle, farm-raised salmon has much more fat and softer flesh than wild. Because of this, it is ideal to cook farm-raised fish slightly longer than wild.

Baked Wild Salmon

SERVES 4 TO 6 · DF, GF ADAPTABLE

2 tablespoons pure Grade A maple syrup

2 tablespoons shoyu (not GF), tamari, or coconut aminos

2 tablespoons freshly squeezed orange juice

2 garlic cloves, smashed

1 (24-ounce) fillet wild salmon

1. To make the marinade, mix together all the ingredients, except the salmon, in a small bowl. Place the salmon in nonreactive dish (e.g., glass) just large enough to hold the fish and marinade. Pour the marinade over the fish and allow it to sit at room temperature for 30 minutes.

2. Preheat the oven to 425°F. Line a rimmed baking sheet with unbleached parchment paper.

3. Place the salmon, skin side down, on the baking sheet and transfer to the oven on a rack positioned in the center.

4. Roast for 4 minutes per ½-inch thickness of salmon, until the salmon flakes when you poke it with a paring knife.

Poached Wild Salmon

SERVES 4 · GF, DF

1½ cups dry white wine

Juice of ½ lemon

Juice of ½ orange

½ lemon, sliced

½ orange, sliced

A few sprigs parsley

A few sprigs dill

4 (5- to 6-ounce) fillets wild salmon

Sea salt

1. Place all the ingredients, except the salmon and salt, plus 3 cups of water, in a deep skillet, preferably one with straight sides and a lid. (I use a 10-inch.) Bring to a simmer.

2. Season the salmon with the salt. Gently transfer the salmon pieces to the pan, skin side down, beginning with the thickest pieces and ending with the thinnest. Cover the skillet and simmer over low heat until the salmon is just cooked through, 5 to 6 minutes, longer for thicker fillets. Do not allow to boil.

3. Transfer the salmon from the pan by removing the thinnest piece first and the thickest piece last. Allow to cool slightly and serve immediately, or cover and refrigerate until cold.

Slow-Roasted Wild Salmon

SERVES 4 TO 6 · GF, DF

1 (24-ounce) fillet wild salmon (I normally use skin-on)

Unrefined, cold-pressed extra-virgin olive oil

Sea salt and freshly ground black pepper

1. Preheat the oven to 250°F. Line a large rimmed baking sheet with parchment paper. Place the salmon on the prepared baking sheet and drizzle with enough olive oil to coat the top of the fish lightly. You can use your hands to oil the fish. Season with salt and pepper.

2. Bake for 25 to 35 minutes, or until the center of the salmon is rare and starting to flake when you poke it with a paring knife. The amount of time it takes to cook the salmon perfectly depends on the temperature of the fish when you place it in the oven and the thickness of the fish.

3. Serve the salmon warm, at room temperature, or cold.

Wild Salmon in Parchment

SERVES 4 · GF, DF

2 cups baby spinach leaves

4 (5- to 6-ounce) fillets of wild salmon

Sea salt and freshly ground black pepper

4 teaspoons unrefined, cold-pressed extra-virgin olive oil

8 teaspoons dry white wine

A few sprigs fresh thyme

1. Preheat the oven to 400°F. Have ready four (12-inch) squares of unbleached parchment paper.

2. Place ½ cup of the spinach leaves in the center of each piece of parchment paper. Arrange each piece of salmon on top of the spinach and sprinkle with a pinch of salt and pepper.

3. Top each fillet with 1 teaspoon of the oil, 2 teaspoons of the wine, and a sprig of thyme.

4. Bring two opposite sides of the parchment together and fold. Continue to fold all the way

down until you reach the fish. Twist both ends of the parchment so that it looks like a hard-candy wrapper. Repeat for each piece of fish. Place each packet on a baking sheet and bake for 8 to 10 minutes, based on the thickness of the salmon.

5. Transfer each packet to a plate and use caution when opening; the steam will be very hot! Do not cook the salmon until you are ready to eat it. When the salmon is removed from the oven but left in the parchment, it will continue to cook.

Grilled Wild Salmon

SERVES 4 · GF, DF

Unrefined, cold-pressed extra-virgin olive oil
4 (5- to 6-ounce) fillet wild salmon
Sea salt and freshly ground black pepper

1. Preheat a grill until hot, ideally 450°F. Make sure the grill grates are as clean as possible and then brush them with oil. This will help prevent the salmon from sticking. Drizzle each fillet with enough olive oil to coat the top of the fish lightly. You can use your hands to oil the fish. Season with salt and pepper.

2. Place the salmon on the grill, skin side down, and grill for 3 to 5 minutes per side depending on thickness, using a metal spatula (rather than tongs) to flip the salmon. Cook until the fish starts to flake but is still rare inside.

Broiled Wild Salmon

SERVES 4–6 · DF, GF

Unrefined, cold-pressed extra-virgin olive oil
1 (24-ounce) fillet wild salmon (I normally use skin-on)
Sea salt and freshly ground black pepper

1. Place an oven rack 6 inches from the heat source. This is usually the second level. Preheat the broiler to high.

2. Grease a large rimmed baking sheet with olive oil. You can use a full sheet pan or two small ones if you don't have one that will accommodate the whole side of salmon.

3. Place the fish on the prepared baking sheet. Brush with oil and season with salt and pepper.

4. Broil for 4 minutes per ½-inch thickness of the salmon, until it flakes easily when poked with a paring knife and is rare in the center.

Pan-Seared Wild Salmon

SERVES 4 · GF, DF ADAPTABLE

4 (5- to 6-ounce) fillets wild salmon
Sea salt and freshly ground black pepper
4 tablespoons ghee, unrefined virgin coconut oil, or unrefined, cold-pressed extra-virgin olive oil

1. Season the salmon with the salt and pepper. Heat a large sauté pan over medium heat for about 1 minute. Add the ghee or oil to the pan and allow to heat for 1 minute, until very warm, but not smoking.

2. Lay the salmon in the pan, seasoned side down, and cook for 3 to 4 minutes, until lightly browned. Turn the fish over, lower the heat to medium-low, and cook for a few minutes more, until it is almost cooked through. Do your best not to overcook the salmon. When it is done, the fish will begin to flake and separate a little, and the center will be slightly rare. The salmon will continue to cook a bit more while it sits.

TIPS: If you use individual fillets, adjust the cook time accordingly. Six-ounce fillets will take about 20 minutes.

   If you are using a salmon that is thicker than wild sockeye, you may need to finish it in a 350°F oven for about 6 minutes. You want the fish to get to the point where it starts to flake when prodded with the tip of a knife, but is still slightly rare in the center—it will keep cooking when removed from the heat.

Balsamic-Herb Flank Steak

SERVES 6 · GF, DF

I personally do not eat red meat, but my family loves it. I do think moderate amounts of beef can fit into a healthful diet, provided you are buying grass-fed, which I feel very strongly is a much, much healthier option over conventionally raised beef. Grass-fed beef can be tricky to cook, especially the leaner cuts, such as flank steak. Because it is leaner, it can easily dry out and become tough. Your best bet is to cook red meat to rare or medium-rare. But even if you like to cook beef all the way through, this post-marinade will help add moisture to the meat at the end, as well as flavor. A post-marinade is also great for times when you forget to plan ahead!

1. Season the flank steaks with the thyme and black pepper. Cover and refrigerate overnight or all day.

2. Prepare the post-marinade: Whisk together vinegar, olive oil, garlic, and a pinch of sea salt and set aside at room temperature.

3. Preheat a grill to medium heat, about 400°F. Brush both sides of meat with olive oil and sprinkle with sea salt.

4. Grill the meat until desired the doneness is achieved, 3 to 4 minutes on each side for medium, turning with tongs, not a fork. Transfer to a serving platter and pour the post-marinade over the meat. Cover with aluminum foil and allow to rest for 5 to 10 minutes.

5. Very important: Transfer the meat to a cutting board and slice thinly against the grain, which means you are cutting in the opposite direction of the lines in the meat. If you cut with the grain, the meat will be chewy. Place back on the platter and serve.

1½ pounds grass-fed beef flank steak or skirt steak

1 tablespoon fresh thyme leaves, chopped

Several grinds of freshly ground black pepper

Olive oil, for brushing the steak

Sea salt, for seasoning steak

POST-MARINADE:

2 tablespoons balsamic vinegar (not aged balsamic)

2 tablespoons unrefined cold-pressed extra-virgin olive oil

2 large garlic cloves, minced

Sea salt

Picadillo

SERVES 6 · GF, DF, VEGAN ADAPTABLE

2 tablespoons unrefined, cold-pressed extra-virgin olive oil

1 medium-size onion, diced

4 garlic cloves, minced

Pinch of crushed red pepper flakes

1½ pounds grass-fed ground beef

1¾ teaspoons sea salt

Freshly ground black pepper

Pinch of ground cinnamon

2 teaspoons ground cumin

Pinch of ground cloves

2 bay leaves

1 (18-ounce) jar diced tomatoes, or 1¼ pounds fresh tomatoes, skin and seeds removed, chopped

1 medium-size sweet potato, peeled and chopped

¼ cup dry white wine

2 tablespoons cider vinegar or red wine vinegar, or more if desired

½ cup unsulfured raisins

½ cup green pimiento olives, sliced (optional)

Chopped fresh cilantro, for garnish (optional)

My mother-in-law is Puerto Rican and has taught me a few of her delicious recipes, including picadillo, which is a popular dish in the Caribbean (especially Cuba) and Mexico. Picadillo reminds me of a Latin Sloppy Joe, but with a more sweet-and-sour flavor. It is a very inexpensive entrée, usually served over white rice. I have come up with my own picadillo recipe that may or may not be authentic, but it sure is flavorful. My son especially loves this and many of my students have said the same of their kids. To make this vegan, substitute an equal amount of crumbled tempeh for the beef and add a couple of drops of pure maple syrup in step 3.

1. In a large, heavy saucepan over medium heat, heat the olive oil. Add the onion and cook until tender and translucent, about 5 minutes. Add the garlic and red pepper flakes and cook for another minute, until fragrant.

2. Add the ground beef, salt, and pepper and sauté, breaking up the meat with the back of a wooden spoon. Continue to cook until all the liquid has evaporated and the meat starts to sizzle for a minute or two. This will add a lot of flavor. Add the spices and bay leaves and sauté for 30 seconds.

3. Add the tomatoes and their juices, sweet potato, wine, and vinegar. Bring to a boil, lower the heat to a simmer, cover, and cook for 15 minutes.

4. Uncover the pan and add the raisins and olives, if using. Allow the stew to cook for another 10 minutes. Garnish with chopped cilantro, if using. Delicious served over rice or Cauliflower Rice (page 251).

TIP: You can use ground turkey or chicken, but I would opt for dark meat for better flavor and more moisture. The picadillo will have a little poultry flavor.

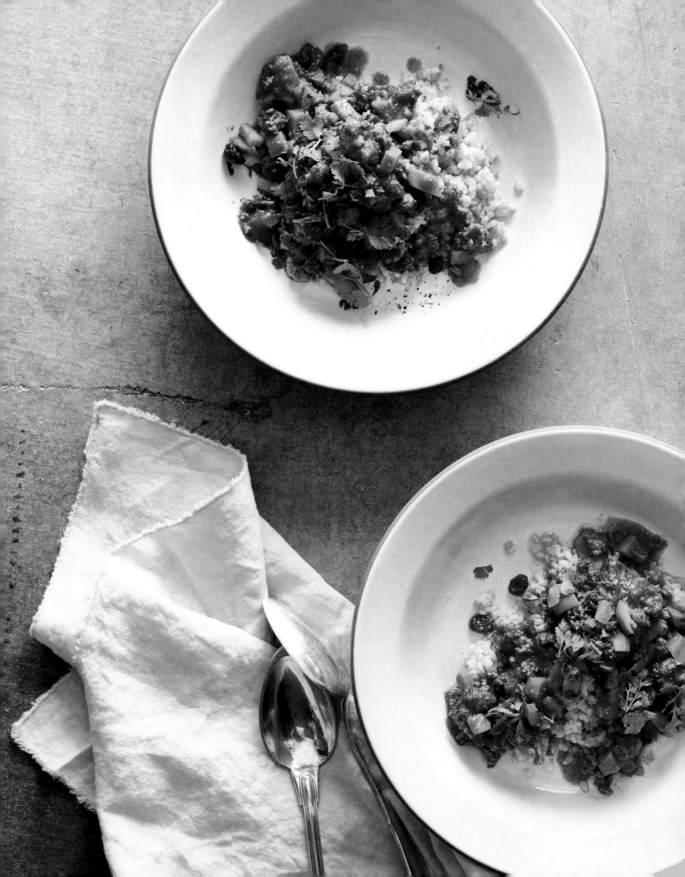

Slow Cooker Italian Pot Roast

SERVES 6 TO 8 · GF, DF

2 (2½- to 3-pound) boneless grass-fed beef chuck or bottom round roasts, tied (see tip)

Sea salt and freshly ground black pepper

1 tablespoon Italian seasoning

2 tablespoons unrefined cold-pressed extra-virgin olive oil

1 large onion, coarsely chopped

3 carrots, peeled and cut into 1-inch pieces

2 celery stalks, cut into 1-inch pieces

6 garlic cloves, crushed and chopped

¼ cup tomato paste

½ (18-ounce) jar crushed tomatoes

½ cup dry red wine, such as Barolo or cabernet

1 cup beef stock, bone broth, or chicken stock (for homemade, see pages 248–250)

2 bay leaves

1 small sprig fresh rosemary

2 tablespoons fresh flat-leaf parsley, finely chopped

ASK PAMELA: How do I "tie" a roast? *Tying a roast helps to promote even cooking. You can ask your butcher to do this for you, or you can take cotton kitchen twine, wrap it around the roast, and tie it in a basic knot. Do this in two spots, evenly spaced.*

Tough cuts of meat, such as chuck, are perfect for cooking low and slow until they become super-tender. Pot roast is the ultimate comfort food—warm, earthy, and stick-to-your-ribs. I put an Italian spin on traditional pot roast with tomatoes, red wine, and rosemary for a rich and robust flavor. This is my husband's favorite cozy Sunday dinner served over polenta or noodles. You can also make this a day in advance and refrigerate the meat and sauce separately. The next day, skim off the hardened fat from the top of the sauce and reheat in a skillet. Slice the meat and add to the skillet to heat through.

1. Pat the meat dry with paper towels and season generously on all sides with salt, pepper, and Italian seasoning.

2. Heat the oil in a large, heavy-bottomed skillet over medium heat. Sear the meat on all sides until golden brown. Transfer to a slow cooker.

3. Add the onion, carrots, celery, and garlic to the skillet, adding a little extra oil, if needed. Sauté over medium heat until the vegetables have softened and the onion is translucent, 6 to 8 minutes.

4. Add the tomato paste and crushed tomatoes and deglaze the bottom of the pan by scraping with a wooden spoon or spatula any brown bits stuck to the bottom. Pour the mixture over the meat in the slow cooker.

5. Add the wine, stock, bay leaves, and rosemary to the slow cooker and cook on low for 9 to 10 hours or high for 5 to 7 hours, until the beef is tender.

6. Transfer the pot roasts to a large cutting board, preferably with grooves to catch the juices, and tent loosely with aluminum foil.

7. Remove the bay leaves and rosemary sprig and skim any fat off the surface of the sauce. Taste for seasoning and add salt and pepper to taste.

8. If desired, blend a small amount of sauce with an immersion blender to thicken. Slice the meat, spoon the sauce over it, and sprinkle with fresh parsley.

Sweet Potato and Quinoa Veggie Burgers

MAKES 4 THIN PATTIES · VEGAN, DF, GF ADAPTABLE

I am obsessed with veggie burgers! I teach a new one in my classes every year. This one is a combo of some of my favorite ingredients, sweet potato, quinoa, and kale, which come together to make a killer burger. Don't forget the toppings, which are half the fun. I love avocado, sautéed onions, and sprouts on my veggie burger. Toppings are also my ace in the hole when I am trying to entice my son to taste something "different." It usually works! You can prep these patties the day before and keep them in the fridge or stash a few in the freezer for a quick, healthful lunch or Meatless Monday dinner.

1. Preheat the oven to 400°F. Place the sweet potato directly on a baking sheet and roast for 40 to 60 minutes, until tender. When cool enough to handle, remove the skin and mash the flesh with a fork. Set aside.

2. Heat the tablespoon of olive oil in a medium-size skillet over medium heat and add the shallot. Sauté until tender and translucent, then add the garlic and cook for 30 seconds, until fragrant, then turn off the heat and set aside.

3. Place the quinoa, oat flour, kale, vinegar, red pepper flakes, salt, pepper to taste, and the shallot mixture in a large bowl and mix to combine. Add ¾ cup of the reserved mashed sweet potato and stir to combine.

4. Form four patties and place on a parchment-lined plate or baking sheet, cover them with plastic wrap, and transfer to the refrigerator to chill for at least 30 minutes.

5. In a large skillet or on a griddle, heat ⅛ inch of oil. Add the burgers and cook over medium heat, turning once, until browned and heated through, about 3 minutes on each side. Serve with your desired accompaniments.

TIPS: If you have any mashed sweet potato leftover, save it for your next smoothie!

I like these best as thin patties, but if you'd like to bulk these up or stretch them to make more, add ¾ cup of cooked white beans, coarsely mashed plus an additional ½ teaspoon of cider vinegar.

1 sweet potato (10 to 12 ounces), scrubbed clean

1 tablespoon unrefined, extra-virgin olive oil or coconut oil, plus more for cooking patties

1 small shallot, finely diced (about 3 tablespoons)

1 garlic clove, minced

1¼ cups cooked quinoa (see page 130)

¼ cup certified-GF oat flour, or 3 tablespoons coconut flour

¼ cup finely minced kale (about 1 large leaf dinosaur kale)

1½ teaspoons cider vinegar

Pinch of crushed red pepper flakes

¾ teaspoon sea salt

Freshly ground black pepper

Sprouted-grain hamburger buns, for serving (optional; omit for GF)

Accompaniments: grilled onions, avocado, tomato, sprouts

Lentil Sloppy Joes

SERVES 6 · VEGAN, GF, DF

1 to 2 tablespoons cold-pressed, unrefined extra-virgin olive oil

¾ cup diced onion

½ green or sweet bell pepper, diced

3 garlic cloves, finely chopped

2¼ cups cooked lentils

1½ cups cooked pinto beans, or 1 (15-ounce) can, drained and rinsed

1 (18-ounce) jar crushed tomatoes or tomato puree

2 tablespoons tomato paste

2 tablespoons red wine vinegar

2 tablespoons pure Grade A or B maple syrup

4 teaspoons vegan/GF Worcester-shire sauce

2 teaspoons chili powder

1 teaspoon mustard powder

1 teaspoon sea salt

Freshly ground black pepper

Accompaniments: toasted vegan/ DF hamburger buns or cooked grains, such as brown rice, millet, or quinoa

If Sloppy Joes remind you of school lunches or camp, you're not alone. I can still visualize a pale hamburger bun with a mess of ketchup-laced ground beef on my lunch tray. But this recipe isn't the one from my childhood. I've replaced the ground beef with high-fiber, protein-rich lentils for an even better version. Lentils are a great sub for ground beef because they have a wonderful meaty flavor and perfect nubby texture. It's really the spices and seasonings that make this dish, so you'll still dig into the comforting flavors you know and love (and if you like an extra kick, add a little cayenne or hot sauce). My family enjoys these Sloppy Joes on toasted buns with dill pickles, but I'll eat mine on a scoop of millet or Cauliflower Rice (page 251). Everyone's happy!

1. Heat a large skillet over medium-high heat. Add the olive oil and sauté the onion, pepper, and garlic in the hot oil until the onion is tender and translucent.
2. Add the remaining ingredients, including black pepper to taste. Stir to combine and simmer over medium-low heat for 15 minutes. Taste for seasoning and add more salt and pepper, if needed.

TIP: If you are cooking your lentils from scratch for this recipe, start with 1 cup of dried lentils for the amount needed for the recipe.

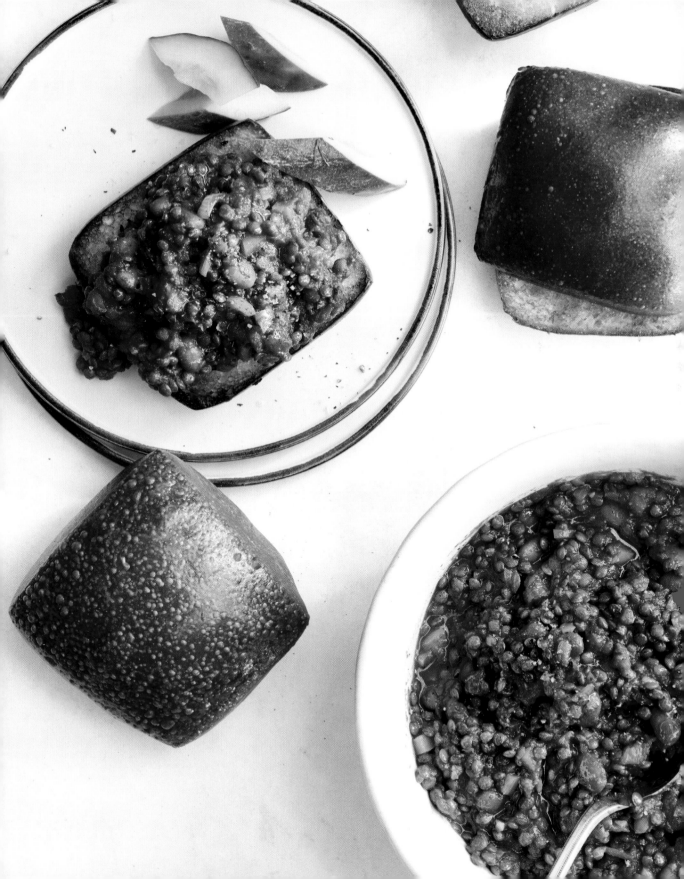

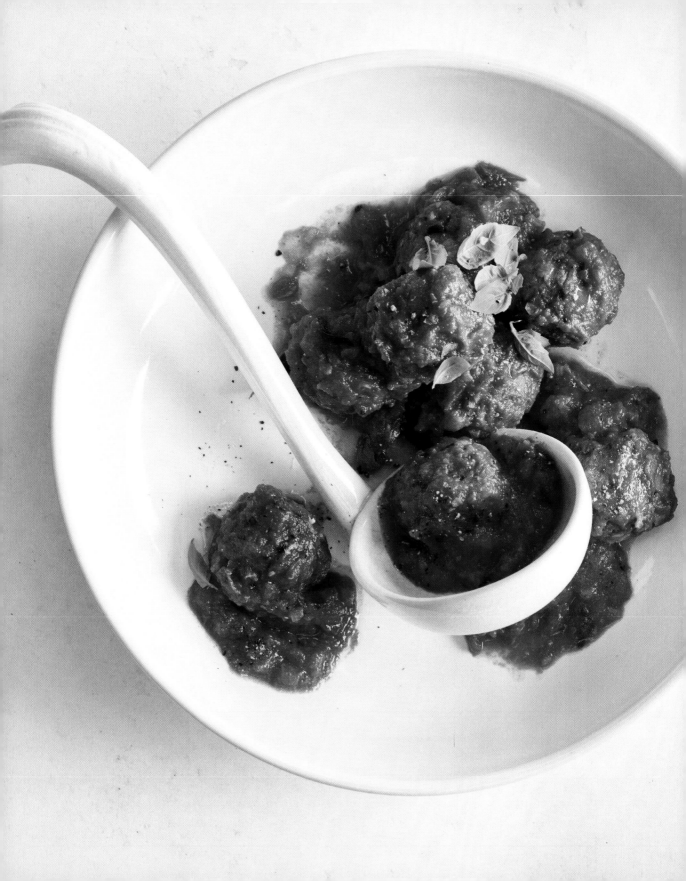

Eggplant "Meatballs"

MAKES ABOUT 24 "MEATBALLS" · VEGETARIAN, GF ADAPTABLE

I love making a vegetarian version of a traditional meat recipe. I love it even more when my family and my students go crazy for it. Meatballs are such a familiar and popular food, I was a little unsure about how everyone would react when I subbed eggplant for ground beef. But sure enough, these eggplant "meatballs" were a huge hit! I honestly think these eggplant meatballs taste incredibly similar to regular ones, especially when covered with your favorite warm marinara sauce. They are tender enough to cut with a fork and are the perfect match with spaghetti squash for a serious veggie meal.

1. Heat a large skillet over medium heat. Add the olive oil and sauté the garlic in the hot oil until just fragrant and barely starting to lightly brown, about 30 seconds. Add the eggplant and ¼ cup of water. Lower the heat to low and cover the skillet. Allow the eggplant to steam until soft, about 20 minutes. Allow to cool slightly, if you have time.

2. Meanwhile, preheat the oven to 350°F. Line a baking sheet with unbleached parchment paper.

3. Place the eggplant mixture in a food processor and pulse until well chopped, but not pureed. Or just do this on a cutting board with a knife.

4. Transfer the eggplant mixture to a large mixing bowl and add the cheese, parsley, basil, eggs, bread crumbs, salt, and pepper. Stir the mixture well to combine, using your hands or a wooden spoon. The mixture can be refrigerated at this point, covered for up to a day. It is easier to roll into meatballs when the mixture is cooled down. (If doing so, preheat the oven 30 minutes before baking the meatballs.)

5. Roll the mixture into 1½-inch balls and place on the prepared baking sheet. Bake for 25 minutes, or until firm on the outside and light brown underneath.

6. Transfer the meatballs to a large saucepan with marinara sauce and simmer for 5 to 10 minutes.

2 tablespoons unrefined, cold-pressed extra-virgin olive oil

6 garlic cloves, minced

1½ pounds eggplant, unpeeled, cut into 1-inch cubes (you should have 8 cups)

1 cup grated Parmesan or pecorino cheese

½ cup fresh flat-leaf parsley leaves and tender stems, chopped

¼ cup fresh basil leaves, chopped

4 large eggs, beaten (you can use 2 to 4 eggs, but I like to use 4 for extra protein and to hold the meatballs together better)

1½ cups regular or GF dried bread crumbs or panko bread crumbs (you can use as little as 1 cup, but the meatballs will be much softer)

⅛ teaspoon sea salt

A few grinds of black pepper

½ recipe Homemade Marinara Sauce (page 253), or about 3 cups sauce

TIPS: You can add crushed red pepper flakes to the garlic to add some heat.

You can also shape these into veggie burgers.

If fresh basil isn't available, you can add a few dashes of dried basil and dried oregano.

Vegan Mac and Cheese

SERVES 6 · VEGAN ADAPTABLE, GF ADAPTABLE, DF ADAPTABLE

2 tablespoons chopped shallot

1 cup (about 7 ounces) chopped Yukon Gold potato (you can leave the peel on)

¼ cup chopped carrot (about 1 small carrot)

⅓ cup chopped onion

1 (8-ounce) package elbow macaroni pasta (GF, if necessary); I like spelt, but any whole-grain or GF pasta will work well here

2 slices vegan/DF/GF bread, torn into large pieces (whole-grain works; sub GF, if necessary!)

6 tablespoons vegan organic butter, such as Earth Balance, or unsalted butter (not vegan/DF)

¼ teaspoon paprika

¼ cup raw cashews (soaked for 1 to 5 hours and drained if your blender is weak), or ¼ cup raw cashew butter

2 teaspoons sea salt (1¾ teaspoons if using vegan butter)

¼ teaspoon garlic, minced (about 1 medium-size clove)

¼ teaspoon Dijon mustard

1 tablespoon freshly squeezed lemon juice (optional, but add if you have it)

¼ teaspoon freshly ground black pepper

Pinch of cayenne pepper

Since this is the most-commented-on recipe on my blog, it had to go into this book. I originally found a version of this recipe on the Vegetarian News *website and my life has never been the same since. Not only is this mac and cheese amazing for a vegan version, it's better than regular mac and cheese, which can be so heavy and greasy. I really prefer to use a whole-grain pasta for the extra protein and fiber. I also like adding blanched cauliflower to the macaroni for some extra veggie power. The pureed sauce can do double duty; cook it for a few minutes on the stove and use it on Perfect Baked Potatoes (page 138) or steamed vegetables, such as broccoli and carrots. To make this nut-free, substitute ¼ cup of cooked white beans for the cashews. Or simply omit the cashews, and although the sauce won't be quite as thick, it will still be delicious and thick enough.*

1. In a medium-size saucepan, combine the chopped shallot, potato, carrot, onion, and 1 cup of water and bring to a boil. Lower the heat to a simmer and cook, covered, for 15 minutes, or until the vegetables are very soft. In the meantime, preheat the oven to 350°F.

2. Cook the pasta in salted water until al dente, drain, and put back into the pot.

3. Put the bread pieces, 1 tablespoon of the butter, and the paprika in a food processor fitted with a metal blade and process until a medium-fine texture is achieved, set aside.

4. Place the cashews, salt, garlic, remaining 5 tablespoons of butter, mustard, lemon juice, if using, black pepper, and cayenne in a blender or food processor. Add the softened vegetables and cooking water to the blender or food processor and process until perfectly smooth.

continued on page 216

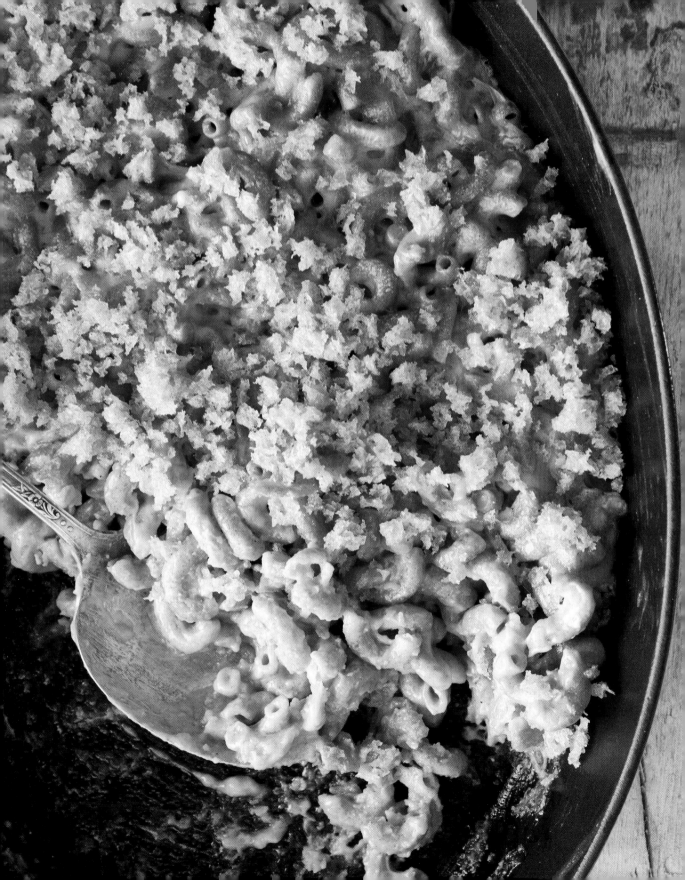

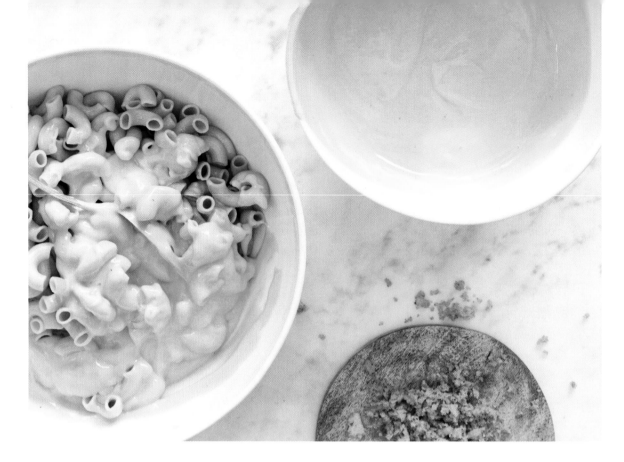

5. Pour the "cheese" sauce over the cooked pasta and combine until completely coated. Spread the mixture into an ungreased 8 x 11-inch casserole dish, sprinkle with the prepared bread crumb mixture. Bake for 30 minutes, or until the sauce is bubbling and the top is golden brown. If you add veggies (such as 1 to 2 cups of blanched cauliflower or broccoli) to the macaroni, cook in a 9 x 13-inch dish.

ASK PAMELA: Someone told me that you can eat as much gluten-free pasta as you want and not gain weight. Is that true? *Whaaaat? First of all, "eating as much as you want" could mean a lot of things, but if I assume that one would want to eat a pound of pasta in one sitting, that is a recipe for a big spike in blood sugar and probably a stomachache. Second of all, just because something is gluten-free, whether it is pasta, cookies, or bread, does not guarantee a healthful food, especially if it is processed. In fact, sometimes gluten-free products are more refined than their gluten-containing counterparts. A good rule of thumb with starches is to eat no more than 1 cup at a time.*

Mexican Millet Casserole

SERVES 6 · GF, VEGETARIAN ADAPTABLE

Millet is easy to cook, inexpensive, high in protein, alkalizing, and tastes really mild, almost like buttered corn. This casserole is a great place to start if you're just not sure what to do with millet. I liken it to a hippie version of enchiladas. It has all the flavors you love in your favorite Tex-Mex dishes, but it's really lightened up and chock-full of fiber and nutrition. Although if you need to put extra cheese on top, you have my blessing.

1. Place the millet in a medium-size saucepan with 2 cups of water and a pinch of salt (or use 2 cups of chicken or vegetable stock) and bring to a boil. Lower the heat to a simmer, cover, and cook for 30 minutes. Allow to sit for 10 minutes (or longer) off the heat and fluff with a fork.

2. Preheat the oven to 400°F. Lightly grease a 9 x 13-inch baking dish with olive oil.

3. In a large skillet, warm 2 tablespoons of the olive oil and add the onion, zucchini, and bell pepper. Sprinkle with a pinch of salt and black pepper and sauté until tender, 6 to 8 minutes. Set aside.

4. In a small saucepan, heat the remaining tablespoon of oil over medium-low heat. Add the garlic and sauté until fragrant, about 1 minute. Add the tomato puree, 6 tablespoons of stock, spices, ¼ teaspoon of salt, and pepper to taste. Simmer for 3 to 4 minutes and taste for seasoning.

5. In a large bowl, combine the cooked millet, sautéed vegetables, black beans, corn, cilantro, and ½ cup of the cheese. Mix well. Transfer to the prepared baking dish and spread in an even layer.

6. Top with the tomato mixture and the remaining cup of cheese. Cover with a lid or aluminum foil and bake until heated through and the cheese is melted, 25 to 30 minutes.

7. Garnish with diced avocado, scallion, and fresh cilantro, if desired.

TIP: Leftovers make an awesome soup! Just add good-quality veggie or chicken stock to achieve the desired consistency and reheat.

1 cup uncooked millet

2 cups (optional) + 6 tablespoons chicken stock (not vegetarian) or vegetable stock (for homemade, see pages 248–249)

3 tablespoons unrefined, cold-pressed extra-virgin olive oil, plus more for baking dish

1 onion, diced

1 zucchini, diced

1 green or sweet bell pepper, diced

½ teaspoon sea salt, plus more for seasoning

Freshly ground black pepper

1 large garlic clove, minced

12 ounces tomato puree or crushed tomatoes (not tomato paste)

2 teaspoons ground cumin

1½ teaspoons chili powder

½ teaspoon chipotle chile powder, or more if you want it spicy

¾ cup cooked black beans, or about ½ (15-ounce) can, drained and rinsed

½ cup fresh or frozen thawed organic corn kernels (fire-roasted corn is nice)

¼ cup chopped fresh cilantro, plus more for garnish (optional)

1½ cups shredded cheese, such as Mexican blend or Monterey Jack

1 medium-size avocado, diced (optional)

2 tablespoons chopped scallion (optional)

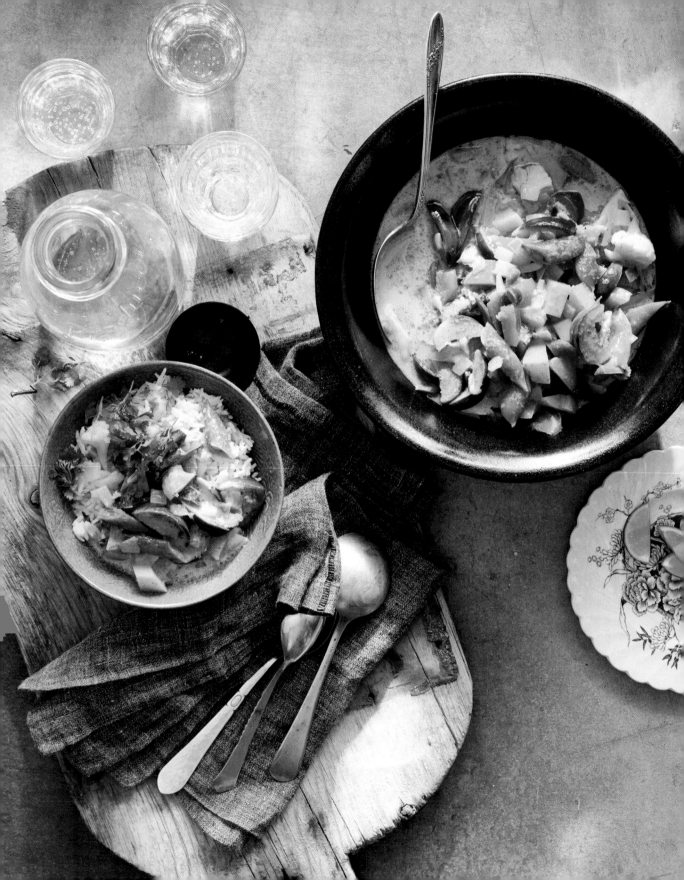

Quick Thai Yellow Vegetable Curry

SERVES 4 · VEGAN, DF, GF ADAPTABLE

My goal here is to encourage you to cook from scratch, but sometimes shortcuts are really helpful. Thai cooking is incredibly flavorful, clean, and light, but it uses a lot of ingredients that can be hard to find. That's why I always keep a container of premade yellow curry paste in the fridge so I can whip up a batch of curry for a quick dinner. Yellow curry paste (there are also red and green versions) can be made from garlic, lemongrass, shallot, red chile, salt, galangal, kaffir lime peel, and spices. In fact, Thai curry paste contains a lot of spices that are really good for you! Be sure to use paste here, not powder—they are not interchangeable. Here you can cook Thai curry quickly and according to how you prefer.

1. Melt the coconut oil in a large saucepan over medium heat. Add the onion and sauté until tender and translucent, 5 to 6 minutes.

2. Add the curry paste, break it up a bit, and sauté a minute or two, until fragrant. Stir in the turmeric.

3. Add the coconut milk, increase the heat, and bring it to a boil, whisking constantly, until smooth.

4. Add the water or vegetable stock, vegetables, and shoyu (or fish sauce, if using). Cover the pan and simmer the mixture over medium-low heat until the vegetables are tender, about 20 minutes or less, depending on the types of vegetables you use.

5. Stir in the sugar until dissolved. Taste for seasoning.

6. Serve the curry with rice and garnish with fresh cilantro leaves.

1½ tablespoons unrefined, virgin coconut oil

½ large onion, diced

2 tablespoons yellow curry paste, such as Mae Ploy or Mae Anong brand

¼ teaspoon ground turmeric

1 (14-ounce) can full-fat coconut milk (shaken so the solid and liquid is fully combined; you can also do this with an immersion blender)

1 to 1½ cups water or vegetable stock (for homemade, see page 248)

6 cups chopped vegetables (suggested: carrots, celery, cauliflower, bell pepper, peas, potatoes, sugar snap peas)

½ tablespoon shoyu (not GF) or tamari (or use Asian fish sauce for traditional flavor, although not vegan)

2 tablespoons coconut sugar

Fresh cilantro, for garnish

Freshly squeezed lime juice, to finish (optional)

Accompaniments: steamed basmati rice

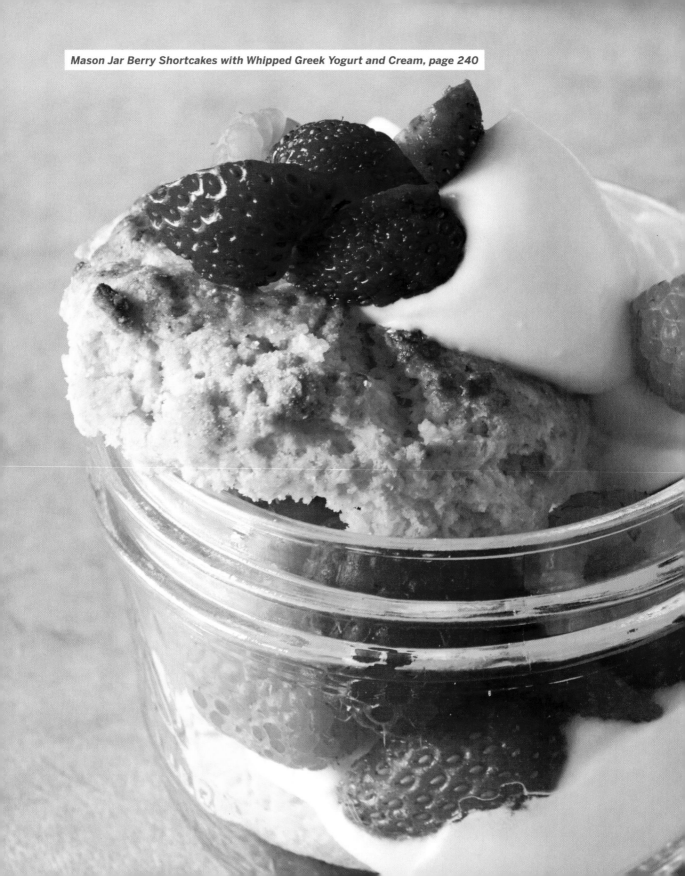

Mason Jar Berry Shortcakes with Whipped Greek Yogurt and Cream, page 240

DESSERTS

What would life be like without sweets? As a little girl, I loved baking with my friends and still to this day I enjoy making little treats for my kids and pies for the holidays. Desserts are great in moderation (by that I mean once, maybe twice a week, not every few hours). Almost all the desserts I am sharing in this section are made with unrefined sweeteners and flours. Many are fruit-based and all contain fewer concentrated sweeteners than typical desserts. I definitely notice a difference between how I feel after a commercially prepared, overly sugary dessert and one made with more natural sweeteners.

The following recipes are easy to follow and don't require any hard-to-find ingredients. They are my favorite kind of dessert— homey, wholesome, not perfect looking, but unmistakably delicious.

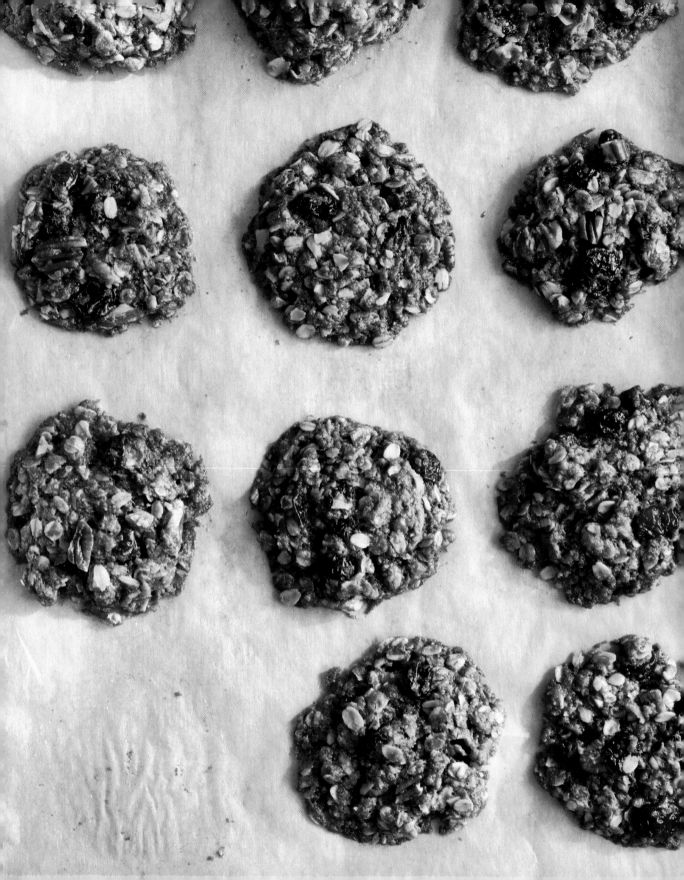

Vegan Oatmeal Cherry Pecan Cookies

MAKES ABOUT 18 COOKIES · VEGAN, GF

Who can resist a cookie studded with sweet dried cherries, crisp pecans, and chewy coconut? And what if I said these were vegan, gluten-free, and full of fiber? This cookie is the best of both worlds—delicious and a pretty clean treat, but it still tastes like a real-deal oatmeal cookie. Like most cookies, you can make the dough many days in advance and just scoop and bake as you want.

1. Preheat the oven to 350°F. Line two baking sheets with unbleached parchment paper.

2. In a small bowl, combine the chia seeds with 3 tablespoons of water and stir. Let the mixture sit, stirring it occasionally, for about 10 minutes, or until it has the consistency of a raw egg.

3. Cream the coconut oil and muscovado sugar together in a large bowl, using an electric mixer, until light and fluffy, 2 to 4 minutes. Add chia seed mixture and vanilla; cream until smooth and velvety.

4. In a small bowl, combine the oat flour, salt, cinnamon, and baking soda. Slowly add to the coconut oil mixture, stirring until well combined.

5. Stir in the oats, coconut, cherries, and pecans until evenly distributed.

6. Scoop 1½ tablespoons of cookie dough, shaping the dough with your hands to create a round ball, and place on the prepared baking sheets, with about 1 inch of space between them. Press down very slightly on each cookie to flatten just a little.

7. Bake for 12 to 14 minutes, until slightly browned on the bottom. Remove from the oven and allow to cool for 2 minutes, then transfer cookies to a cooling rack.

TIP: 1 tablespoon of chia seeds + 3 tablespoons of warm water mixed together create a "chia egg," which can be used in place of one egg where the egg is used as a binder, such as muffins, quick breads, and cookies.

1 tablespoon chia seeds

½ cup unrefined, virgin coconut oil, at room temperature

¾ cup muscovado sugar, coconut sugar, or light brown sugar

1 teaspoon pure vanilla extract

1 cup oat flour (look for certified-GF oat flour to make this a GF cookie)

½ teaspoon sea salt

½ teaspoon ground cinnamon

½ teaspoon baking soda

1½ cups certified-GF rolled oats

½ cup unsweetened shredded coconut

¾ cup dried unsulfured cherries, chopped (you don't want pieces of cherry that are too big)

½ cup pecans, chopped

Blueberry Crumble Bars

MAKES AN 8- OR 9-INCH SQUARE PAN · VEGETARIAN, VEGAN ADAPTABLE, GF ADAPTABLE, DF ADAPTABLE

Unrefined coconut oil or unsalted butter (not vegan/DF), for pan

BASE:

1¼ cups certified-GF oat flour (for GF), or whole wheat pastry flour or whole spelt flour

2½ tablespoons pure Grade A maple syrup, maple sugar, or cane sugar

⅛ teaspoon sea salt

¼ teaspoon aluminum-free baking powder

8 tablespoons (1 stick) unsalted butter (not vegan/DF) or vegan organic butter, such as Earth Balance, cut into small pieces

½ teaspoon pure vanilla extract

BLUEBERRY FILLING:

2 cups fresh or frozen blueberries, thawed

2 teaspoons arrowroot powder

3 tablespoons Grade A maple syrup or cane sugar

½ teaspoon lemon zest (optional)

CRUMBLE TOPPING:

½ cup muscovado sugar, coconut palm sugar, or light brown sugar

¾ cup certified-GF oat flour (for GF), whole wheat pastry flour, or a combo of GF oat flour and King Arthur Gluten-Free Multi-Purpose Flour

⅓ cup old-fashioned rolled oats (certified-GF if necessary)

continued on facing page

Bursting with berries and a generous crumb topping, these bars are just sweet enough to be called a dessert but not so over the top that you'll regret it afterward. The ingredients are simple and ones that you likely have in your pantry at all times. Defrosted frozen blueberries are perfectly acceptable to use when they are not in season. You can also substitute other berries (or mix and match!), if that's what you have on hand.

1. Preheat the oven to 375°F. Lightly grease an 8- or 9-inch baking pan with unsalted butter or coconut oil and line it with unbleached parchment paper.
2. Prepare the base: Pulse together all the base ingredients in a food processor until you get moist crumbs. Press firmly into the prepared pan to form a smooth even layer. If it's too sticky, you can use some plastic wrap under your fingers to help even it out. Refrigerate for 15 minutes.
3. Prepare the blueberry filling: In a medium-size bowl, toss the blueberries with arrowroot and maple syrup. Set aside.
4. Remove the base from the refrigerator and bake until just firm in the center, 12 to 15 minutes.
5. Spread the blueberry filling over the warm crust.

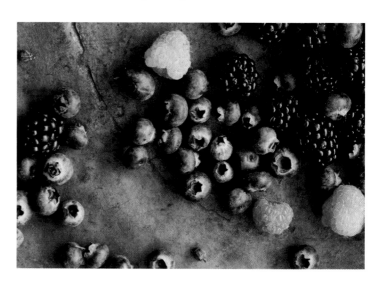

6. Make the crumble topping: In a large mixing bowl, stir together all the topping ingredients until you have made moist crumbs. Crumble over the blueberry filling.

7. Bake until the filling is bubbly and the crumble is golden brown, 25 to 30 minutes. Remove from the oven and allow to cool completely on a cooling rack before cutting. Refrigerate leftovers.

TIP: Blueberries are among the foods highest in antioxidants, which protect the cells from damage caused by free radicals. They are also rich in some very powerful phytonutrients, and have been shown to protect the brain from oxidative stress and may help mitigate the effects of age-related conditions, such as dementia. Berries, in general, have less sugar than most other fruits.

1¼ teaspoons aluminum-free baking powder

½ teaspoon ground cinnamon

Pinch of ground nutmeg

¼ teaspoon sea salt

6 tablespoons melted unsalted butter (not vegan/DF) or unrefined virgin coconut oil

Whole Wheat Peanut Butter and Jelly Thumbprint Cookies

MAKES ABOUT 25 COOKIES · VEGETARIAN, DF, VEGAN ADAPTABLE, GF ADAPTABLE

Peanut butter and jelly is a classic combo that makes me feel like a kid again. These thumbprint cookies are a one-bowl wonder that comes together in no time. They're really fun to bake with kids who, depending on their age, can probably do every step of this recipe. Peanuts, and therefore peanut butter, are very heavily sprayed, so it is well worth seeking out organic brands. I love the flavor of peanut butter and honey, but for a vegan version, go ahead and swap in maple syrup.

1. Preheat the oven to 350°F. Line a baking sheet with unbleached parchment paper.

2. Combine all the ingredients, except the jam, in a large bowl and make sure you mix well.

3. Take a tablespoon of the dough and shape into a ball. Place on the prepared baking sheet. Repeat with the remaining dough, spacing the cookies 2 inch apart.

4. Using your finger, make a dent in the center of each cookie. Fill with a small bit of jam. Bake until the cookies are very lightly browned, about 10 minutes.

2 cups whole wheat pastry flour, white whole wheat flour, whole spelt flour, or certified-GF oat flour

1½ cups whole roasted peanuts (salted or unsalted), preferably organic, pulsed in a food processor to a medium grind

½ teaspoon sea salt

½ teaspoon ground cinnamon

½ cup unrefined virgin coconut oil, melted (see Tip, page 40)

2 tablespoons smooth unsalted, unsweetened peanut butter, preferably organic

½ cup honey (swap in maple syrup for vegan)

No sugar-added jam, such as raspberry, strawberry, or blueberry

White Bean Tahini Blondies

MAKES AN 8-INCH SQUARE PAN · VEGETARIAN, GF, DF ADAPTABLE

- 4 tablespoons (½ stick) unsalted butter (not DF) or unrefined virgin coconut oil, melted, plus more for pan
- 1½ cups cooked white beans, or 1 (15-ounce) can, drained and rinsed
- ½ cup tahini, preferably raw
- 2 large eggs
- ⅔ cup muscovado sugar or light brown sugar
- 1 teaspoon pure vanilla extract
- 1 teaspoon aluminum-free baking powder
- ¼ teaspoon sea salt
- ¾ cup DF semisweet chocolate chips
- 6 tablespoons unsweetened shredded coconut
- 6 tablespoons chopped pecans

White bean blondies are the new black bean brownies! I know the ingredients seem a little bizarre, but I promise these bars taste nothing like white beans. They're dense, lightly sweet, with the perfect amount of chocolate to satisfy my sweet tooth. But these blondies have gone high protein with legumes and sesame tahini pureed into the batter. Tahini is an amazing spread made entirely from sesame seeds. Besides being rich in protein and good fat, sesame seeds boast an impressive amount of calcium, about 88 milligrams in only 1 tablespoon.

1. Preheat the oven to 350°F. Grease an 8-inch square pan with butter or coconut oil and line with unbleached parchment paper.
2. In a food processor fitted with the metal blade, combine the melted butter, white beans, tahini, eggs, muscovado sugar, vanilla, baking powder, and salt. Process until smooth. Stir in ¼ cup of the chocolate chips.
3. Pour the batter into the prepared baking pan.
4. In a medium-size bowl, mix together the remaining ½ cup of chocolate chips and the shredded coconut and chopped pecans. Spread evenly on top of the batter and press lightly into the batter.
5. Bake for 35 to 40 minutes, or until the cake springs back when pressed in the center. Remove from the oven and allow to cool completely on a wire rack before cutting. Leftovers can be refrigerated for up to 5 days. Even more delicious cold.

TIPS: You can turn this into a light and fluffy cake by adding 1 tablespoon of coconut flour.
   Creamy almond butter can also be substituted for the tahini.

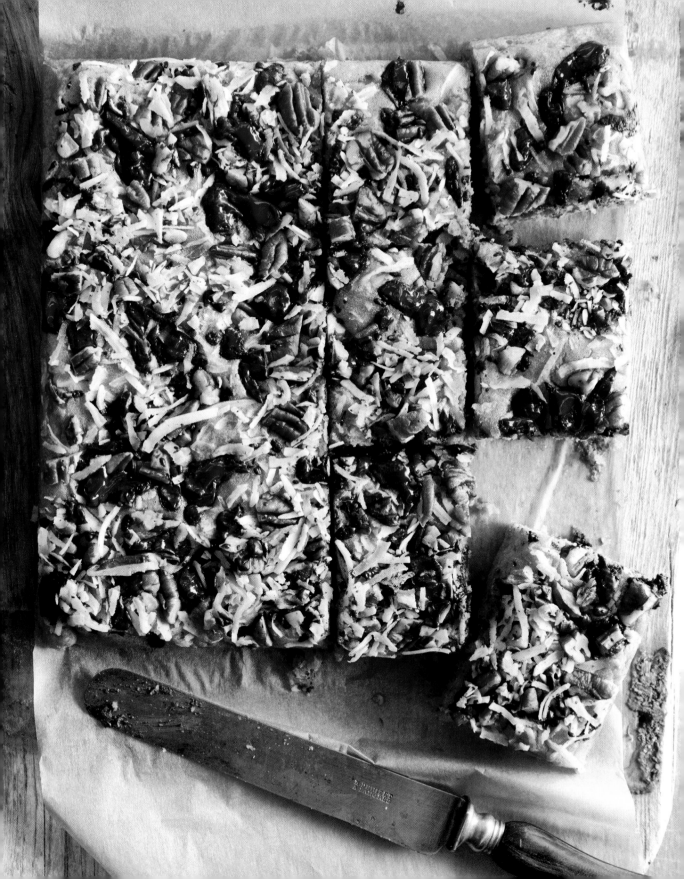

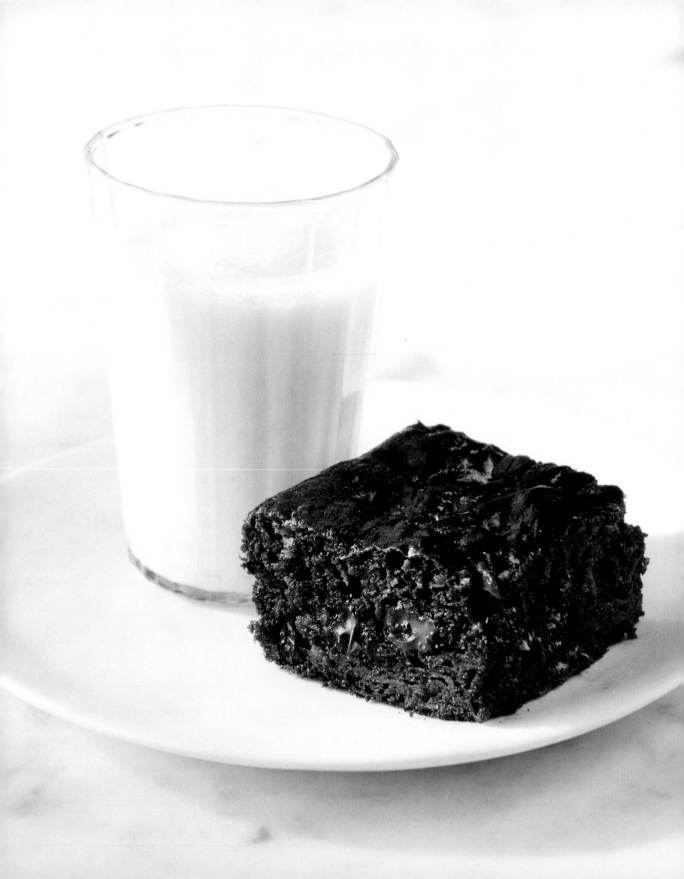

Grain-Free Chocolate Zucchini Cake

MAKES 1 8- OR 9-INCH SQUARE PAN · VEGETARIAN, GF, DF

This is probably the most popular dessert I have ever taught in a class. My students consistently report back with success stories after serving this cake to their kids, at parties, and to their friends. After telling my son that this cake contained zucchini, he inhaled another piece and, with crumbs falling out of his mouth, declared, "I don't even care." It's that good. You can also bake the batter in regular muffins tins or mini muffins tins. Just watch the time, because regular muffins will likely take 20 to 25 minutes; and minis, 7 to 12 minutes, depending on the size of your tin. These also freeze amazingly well.

1. Preheat the oven to 350°F. Grease an 8- or 9-inch square pan with coconut oil. If you want to remove the cake from the pan in one piece, line it with unbleached parchment paper as well.
2. In a large bowl, combine the almond butter, maple syrup, cacao powder, salt, coffee powder, if using, egg, vanilla, and baking soda until smooth.
3. Stir in the zucchini, chocolate chips, and nuts, if using.
4. Pour into the prepared pan and bake until just set and a toothpick inserted into the center comes out clean or with dry crumbs. Do not overbake. A 9-inch pan will take about 30 minutes; an 8-inch will take about 35 minutes. Remove from the oven and allow to cool before serving.

TIP: Instant coffee powder enhances the chocolate flavor in baked goods. It is completely optional, though. There are coffee alternatives, such as Pero, which is a chicory and barley-based product with no caffeine. Pero is not gluten-free or grain-free, due to the barley. Do not use coffee grounds in place of instant coffee powder.

Coconut oil for pan

1 cup creamy, unsweetened, unsalted almond butter, raw or roasted, or sunflower butter

1/3 cup pure Grade A maple syrup or honey

1/4 cup raw cacao powder or unsweetened cocoa powder

1/4 teaspoon sea salt

1 teaspoon instant coffee powder, regular or decaffeinated (optional)

1 large egg

1 teaspoon pure vanilla extract

1 teaspoon baking soda

1 1/2 cups shredded zucchini (about 2 small)

1 cup DF dark or semisweet chocolate chips

1/2 cup chopped walnuts or pecans (optional)

Plum Almond Galette

SERVES 6 · VEGETARIAN

DOUGH:

½ cup blanched almonds (slivered is fine)

1 cup plus 2 tablespoons all-purpose flour, plus more for dusting

1 teaspoon granulated cane sugar

½ teaspoon sea salt

¼ teaspoon ground cinnamon

8 tablespoons (1 stick) unsalted butter, cold and cut into pieces

3 to 4 tablespoons ice water

FILLING:

1 large egg

1 tablespoon whole milk, half-and-half, or heavy cream

1 tablespoon unsalted butter, melted

3 tablespoons pure Grade A maple syrup

2 teaspoons pure vanilla extract

¼ teaspoon ground cinnamon

½ cup almond flour or meal, bread crumbs, or cooked millet

1½ pounds sweet plums or pluots (about 8), quartered and pitted

⅓ cup sliced almonds

1 tablespoon granulated cane sugar

A galette is the perfect intro to making pie because it's just one free-form crust and there's no crimping required. Also called a crostata, this rustic, open tart is so beautiful and can showcase any number of seasonal fruits. Galettes are also lighter to eat because it's half the crust you would normally be getting with a standard pie. Plums and pluots come in so many varieties. Try to find ones in different colors that are sweet and not too tart. And don't stress about how you arrange the plum slices. The galette will look beautiful and taste incredible no matter what you do.

1. Prepare the dough: Preheat the oven to 350°F. Place the blanched almonds in a pie plate or small baking dish and place in the oven to toast until the almonds are fragrant and slightly golden, 13 to 15 minutes; remove from the oven and let cool.

2. Pulse the almonds in a food processor until the consistency of coarse meal. Add the flour, sugar, salt, and cinnamon and pulse until just combined. Add the butter and pulse until the mixture resembles coarse meal with a few pea-size pieces remaining.

3. Drizzle with 3 tablespoons of ice water and pulse until the dough comes together, adding up to another tablespoon of water, if needed.

4. Gently pat the dough into a 6-inch diameter disk. Wrap in plastic wrap and chill 30 to 60 minutes.

5. Increase the oven temperature to 375°F. Line a rimless baking sheet with unbleached parchment paper. If you don't have a rimless baking sheet, invert a rimmed baking sheet and line with parchment.

6. Prepare the filling: In a small bowl, beat the egg with the milk and set aside.

7. Combine the melted butter, maple syrup, vanilla, and cinnamon in a small bowl. Set aside.

8. Roll out the dough to a 12-inch-diameter round on a lightly floured surface. Carefully fold the dough in half, pick up

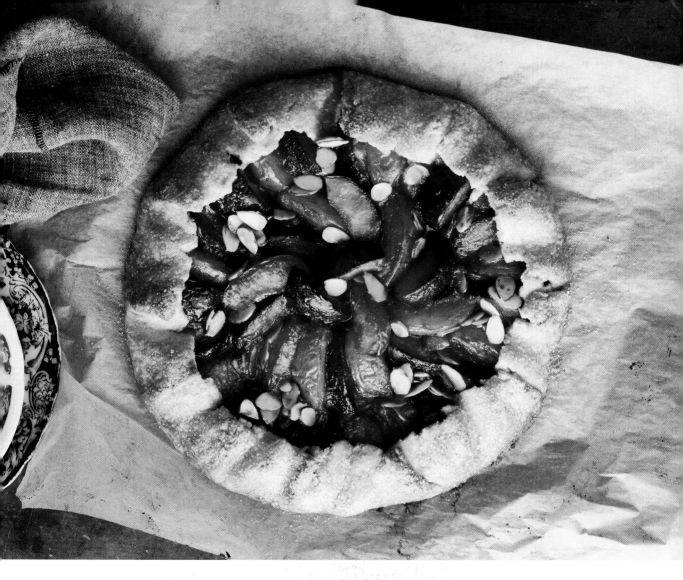

from the folded side, and transfer to prepared baking sheet. Unfold.

9. Spread the almond flour in the center of the dough, leaving a 2-inch border. Arrange the plums over the almond flour, keeping the border empty. Brush the plums with the maple syrup mixture. Sprinkle the center with sliced almonds.

10. Fold the dough edges over, overlapping slightly. Brush the folded border with egg wash. Sprinkle the whole galette, (fruit and crust) with sugar.

11. Bake the galette until the crust is golden brown and the plums are tender, 45 to 50 minutes. Remove from the oven and allow to cool slightly before serving.

TIPS: The dough can be made 2 days ahead. Keep chilled, or freeze for up to 1 month.

Save any excess egg wash for a scramble or frittata.

Spiced Pear Upside-Down Cake

MAKES A 9-INCH CAKE · VEGETARIAN

3 tablespoons unsalted butter, melted

¼ cup muscovado sugar or light brown sugar

2 firm but ripe pears (I like Bartlett and d'Anjou)

CAKE:

8 tablespoons (1 stick) unsalted butter, at room temperature

¾ cup muscovado sugar or light brown sugar

1 teaspoon pure vanilla extract

⅛ teaspoon almond extract

3 large eggs, at room temperature

⅔ cup blanched almond flour (not almond meal)

1 cup whole wheat pastry flour, white whole wheat flour, or whole spelt flour

1 teaspoon aluminum-free baking powder

¼ teaspoon sea salt

2 teaspoons ground cinnamon

2 teaspoons ground ginger

½ teaspoon ground nutmeg

½ teaspoon ground cloves

½ teaspoon orange zest (optional)

If you want to wow your friends, but you're still a novice in the kitchen, make an upside-down cake. The luscious, glossy arrangement of pear slices on top of this fragrant cake is so impressive but easy to do. I like to re-create recipes using whole-grain flours and unrefined sweeteners without sacrificing flavor or texture; this moist, rich cake does not disappoint.

1. Preheat the oven to 375°F. Using a brush, spread a small amount of butter on the bottom of a 9-inch round cake pan and line it with parchment paper. Spread the remaining melted butter evenly over bottom of prepared pan and sprinkle with the ¼ cup of muscovado sugar.

2. Quarter and core the pears. Cut the pear quarters into ¼-inch slices and arrange the slices on the bottom of the pan in a circle around the edge, with the pointed ends all turned toward the center. Use any smaller pieces to fill in the center gap if the slices did not reach all the way to the middle.

3. Make the cake: In a large bowl, cream the butter and muscovado sugar until light and fluffy, then add the vanilla and almond extracts. Beat in the eggs, one at a time, until well blended. Add the almond flour and mix just to combine. Then, add the remaining dry ingredients and orange zest, if using, and mix until just combined.

4. Spread the batter over the fruit and smooth with a spatula. Bake in the center of the oven until a toothpick inserted into the center comes out clean, 35 to 39 minutes. Remove from the oven and allow to cool in the pan for 10 minutes. Run a knife around the edges to loosen, and invert the cake onto a wire rack to cool completely.

ASK PAMELA: I tend to omit citrus zests in recipes because I don't have a zester. Is that okay? *Well, the Recipe Police are not going to come after you for omitting citrus zest. But you are leaving out a huge flavor booster. If you don't love the flavor of a particular type of citrus, then you can certainly cut back on or eliminate it. But I recommend buying an inexpensive zester or Microplane pronto, so your cooking and baking have the best results possible.*

Peach Pie with Spelt Crust

MAKES 1 PIE · VEGETARIAN

Fruit pies are my favorite thing to bake. I love how hands-on pies are, how homemade and imperfect they look. Plus I have never met anyone who didn't love a slice of homemade pie. I make my peach pies with much less sugar than most pie recipes call for, which you can do if you use ripe, naturally sweet, in-season fruit. This is the one of the few times I really prefer using refined flour because it is so much easier to roll out and doesn't taste as bitter as all whole-grain flour.

1. Prepare the pastry: Place the flour, salt, and sugar in a food processor fitted with a steel blade. Pulse once to combine.
2. Add the butter to the flour. Pulse five times. Pour the lemon juice and 4 tablespoons of ice water on top of the flour mixture. Pulse until the dough starts to cling together.
3. Scrape the dough onto a lightly floured countertop, gather into a ball, and wrap in parchment paper. Chill for 30 minutes. If you need to chill it for longer, use plastic wrap.
4. Preheat the oven to 400°F.
5. Prepare the filling: Combine the peaches, flour, sugar, cinnamon, and almond extract in a large bowl.
6. Divide the dough in half, and roll one half into an 11-inch circle. Fit the circle into a 9-inch pie plate.
7. Spoon the peach filling into the pie shell.
8. Roll the remaining dough into a 10-inch round. Cut three 2-inch slits in the center of the dough to allow steam to escape. Fit over the top of the peaches. Fold the top crust under the bottom crust and press both crusts together to seal. Crimp the edges by pushing with your thumb or using the tines of a fork. Brush the top of the pie with the egg wash and sprinkle with sugar. Place the pie on a rimmed baking sheet and place in the center of the oven.
9. Bake for 30 minutes and then lower the oven temperature to 350°F. Bake for 30 minutes more, until the top is golden brown. Remove from the oven and allow to cool for 1 hour before serving.
10. Leftovers can be kept, covered, at room temperature for up to 2 days.

PASTRY:

2½ cups unbleached white spelt flour, or half white spelt/half whole wheat spelt (or use regular unbleached flour), plus more for dusting

1 teaspoon sea salt

1 teaspoon granulated cane sugar

½ pound (2 sticks) cold unsalted butter, cut into 16 pieces

1 tablespoon freshly squeezed lemon juice

4 to 5 tablespoons ice water

FILLING:

6 cups peeled, pitted, and sliced fresh, ripe peaches (about 3 pounds or 6 large)

3 to 4 tablespoons unbleached flour (use more if the peaches are superjuicy)

6 tablespoons granulated cane sugar or muscovado sugar

½ teaspoon ground cinnamon

¼ teaspoon almond extract

1 egg yolk mixed with 1 tablespoon heavy cream or whole milk

1 tablespoon granulated cane sugar

TIP: You can definitely buy premade piecrust, but it is really not hard to make your own. The key is to keep everything cold. If you have to step away from the pastry, or if it feels as if it is getting greasy, put it in the fridge for a bit.

Mini Lemon Yogurt Cheesecakes

MAKES 14 CHEESECAKES · VEGETARIAN, GF ADAPTABLE, DF ADAPTABLE

Unsalted butter (omit for DF) or unrefined virgin coconut oil, for pan

CRUST:

12 DF graham crackers, or 2 cups DF/GF graham cracker crumbs

5 tablespoons unsalted butter (not DF) or unrefined virgin coconut oil, melted

2½ tablespoons pure Grade A or B maple syrup

Pinch of sea salt

FILLING:

1⅓ cups unsweetened whole-milk Greek yogurt (not DF) or firm tofu

6 ounces cream cheese (not DF) or vegan cream cheese, such as Kite Hill, at room temperature

⅔ cup pure Grade A maple syrup

2 large eggs

2½ tablespoons arrowroot powder

1 teaspoon lemon zest

2½ tablespoons freshly squeezed lemon juice

¾ teaspoon pure vanilla extract

Pinch of sea salt

Optional accompaniments: fresh berries or berry compote

TIP: These can be made several days ahead and kept refrigerated in the muffin cups, covered with plastic wrap.

Desserts get a bad rap but that doesn't mean a healthy lifestyle can't include a sweet treat every now and then. These little beauties are the perfect portion and are a lighter, dare I say better, version of traditional cheesecake. I usually serve these with fresh berries or the blueberry sauce from my website. You can even omit the lemon zest and juice and add mini chocolate chips for a different flavor variation.

1. Preheat the oven to 350°F. Grease 14 standard muffin cups with unsalted butter or coconut oil. Cut seven 2-inch wide, 13-inch long strips unbleached parchment paper, and then cut each in half crosswise (14 strips). Line each greased muffin cup with a parchment strip, leaving a tab on either end for easy removal.

2. Prepare the crust: In a food processor, pulse the graham crackers until they are finely ground. Add the melted butter, maple syrup, and salt to the graham crackers and pulse until moist crumbs form and the mixture is well combined.

3. Scoop about 2 tablespoons of the crumbs into each prepared muffin cup and press to form an even layer at the base, using the back of the tablespoon, if desired. Wipe out the food processor.

4. Bake the crust for 4 to 5 minutes, or until the edges are lightly golden. The crusts can be made a day ahead. Lower the oven temperature to 325°F.

5. Prepare the filling: Combine the yogurt, cream cheese, and maple syrup in the food processor and process until smooth, 1 to 2 minutes. Add the eggs, arrowroot, lemon zest and juice, vanilla, and salt and continue to process until the batter is smooth and well mixed, about a minute more.

6. Scoop ⅓ cup of the cheesecake filling onto each crust. Bake until the custard is lightly golden and set at the edges but still slightly jiggly in the center, 20 to 25 minutes.

7. Remove from the oven and allow to cool to room temperature, then refrigerate until chilled. Run a thin knife around the edge and pull up on both ends of the parchment to remove. Serve plain or with fresh berries or a berry sauce.

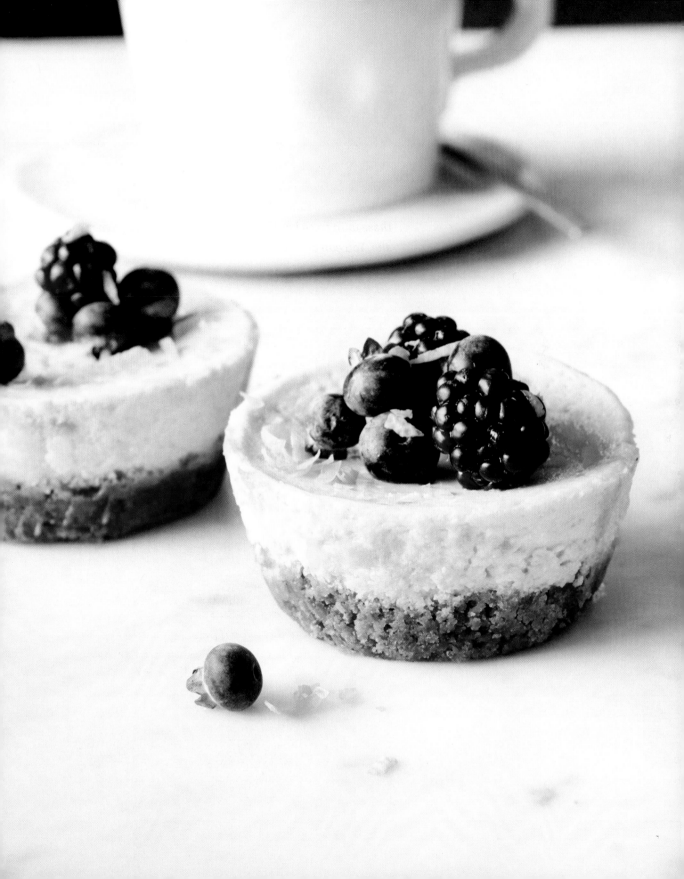

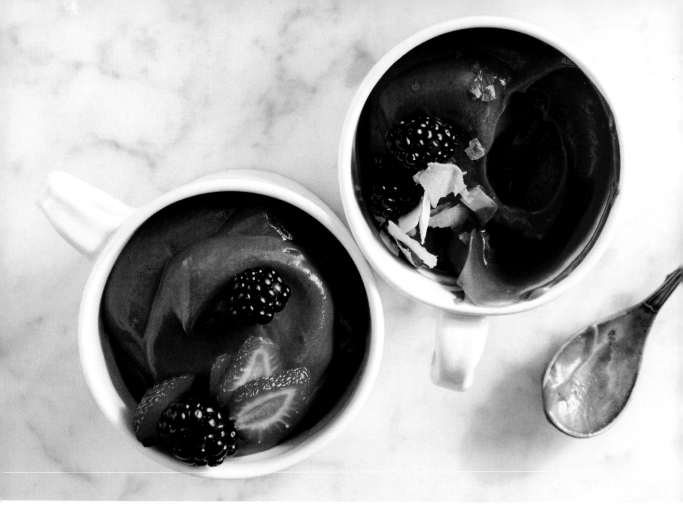

Sweet Potato Chocolate Pudding

SERVES 4 OR WORKS GREAT AS A TART FILLING · VEGAN, GF, DF

All I can say about this recipe is, don't knock it 'til you try it. Forget what you think this might taste like, because you'll never know there was even a smidge of sweet potato in here. This pudding is just light and creamy chocolaty goodness. And it happens to be the most nutritious pudding you'll probably ever love. Sweet potatoes are so good for you—high in beta-carotene, fiber, and antioxidants. I'm not going to lie, though. The best results come from using a high-powered blender, which will create an ethereally light texture.

1. Preheat the oven to 400°F and roast the sweet potatoes on a parchment-lined baking sheet until very tender. The timing depends on the size of the sweet potatoes, anywhere from 30 to 60 minutes. If there are multiple sweet potatoes, space them out on the sheet pan. Alternatively, peel the sweet potatoes, cut into chunks, and steam until tender. (This will be faster but they won't be as sweet.)

2. Remove the skin, place the cooked sweet potatoes in a food processor or high-speed blender with all the remaining ingredients, and process until perfectly smooth. A Vitamix will achieve the most puddinglike consistency. Taste and adjust the sweetness. Serve at room temperature or chill until cold. Top with your desired toppings. Can be made up to 3 days in advance.

ASK PAMELA: What's the difference between sweet potatoes and yams? *The terms sweet potato and yam are used interchangeably in the United States, but they both generally refer to sweet potatoes (which are not at all related to a regular potatoes), no matter the color. Even the dark ones labeled as "yams" are technically sweet potatoes. True yams are native to Africa and are a staple in tropical and subtropical countries. I have never actually seen one in the United States, but here's what you might find in your market if you live in the States:*

Brown- or red-skinned (often called yams) have a soft orange flesh and sweet flavor. The varieties you will likely see are Garnet, Jewel, and Christmas Beauregard.

Beige-skinned have a pale yellow flesh. Varieties include Nancy Hall and Juicy Yellow. That's what I used in the photo on the opposite page.

Purple-skinned have a white or purple flesh and are sometimes called Japanese sweet potatoes. I don't find the flesh to be quite as moist as the others discussed here.

Any of the above can be used successfully in this recipe.

1 pound sweet potatoes, preferably pale fleshed, but any variety will work

¼ cup raw cacao powder or unsweetened cocoa powder

6 tablespoons pure Grade A or B maple syrup, or more to taste

⅔ cup unsweetened almond milk, preferably homemade (page 257)

2 tablespoons unsalted, unsweetened almond butter

½ teaspoon instant coffee powder

½ teaspoon pure vanilla extract

⅜ teaspoon fine-grain sea salt

Optional toppings: toasted, shredded unsweetened coconut, flaky salt, chopped almonds, coconut whipped cream, fresh berries, and/or raw cacao nibs

TIPS: To make this nut-free, use unsweetened and unsalted sunflower butter and any milk (dairy-free if necessary).

The amount of almond milk will depend on the starchiness of the sweet potatoes and desired consistency.

Roasted Peach Sundaes with Date Caramel Sauce

SERVES 8 · VEGETARIAN, GF, VEGAN ADAPTABLE, DF ADAPTABLE

DATE-CARAMEL SAUCE:

6 Medjool dates (about ¾ cup packed dates), pitted and soaked in 1 cup warm water for 30 minutes, soaking liquid reserved

3 tablespoons unrefined virgin coconut oil, melted

3 tablespoons Grade A maple syrup

3 tablespoons brown rice syrup

¼ cup creamy, raw, unsweetened, unsalted almond butter

2 teaspoons lucuma powder (optional, but does add a nice caramel note)

½ teaspoon pure vanilla extract

½ teaspoon sea salt

PEACHES:

4 medium-size firm but ripe peaches

2 tablespoons unsalted butter (not vegan/DF) or unrefined, virgin coconut oil

2 tablespoons pure Grade A maple syrup or light brown sugar

½ teaspoon pure vanilla extract

TO SERVE:

8 scoops vanilla ice cream, frozen yogurt (not vegan/DF), or your favorite vegan frozen treat

Simple fruit desserts are my favorite kind. And while warm, caramelized juicy peaches mixed with rich, creamy ice cream would be enough, this date caramel sauce takes these sundaes over the top. Dates are an absolute miracle food that I cannot live without. They are naturally intensely sweet with a caramel undertone and they blend beautifully into a paste. I love the addition of lucuma powder, which is made from a Peruvian fruit containing, among other nutrients, iron, zinc, calcium, protein, and fiber. Its flavor profile is similar to that of maple, caramel, and custard. I use lucuma powder as a sweetener in smoothies or stirred into oatmeal, as well as adding a boost of caramel flavor in this sauce.

1. Prepare the date-caramel sauce: Combine all the sauce ingredients, including 2 tablespoons of the date-soaking liquid, in a blender or food processor and process until completely smooth. Add additional date soaking liquid, as needed, to achieve your desired consistency. Set aside.

2. Prepare the peaches: Preheat the oven to 400°F. Halve the peaches and remove the pit. Place the peach halves in a medium-size bowl.

3. In a small saucepan, melt the butter and maple syrup over medium heat. Whisk until smooth. Remove from the heat and stir in the vanilla. Pour the mixture over the peaches and gently toss to coat each peach.

4. Place the peaches, along with the butter mixture, in a 9 x 13-inch baking dish and arrange them, cut side down, in a single layer.

5. Roast the peaches for 15 to 25 minutes, or until the peaches are tender and the liquid is syrupy.

6. Create a sundae by placing a scoop of ice cream in a bowl, topping it with a roasted peach, and drizzling with date-caramel sauce. Serve immediately.

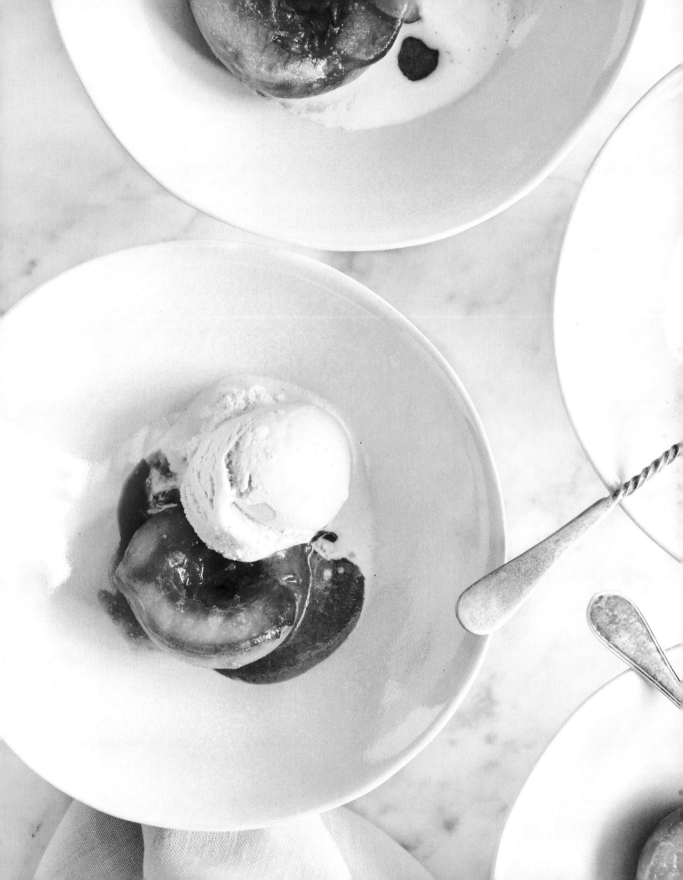

Mason Jar Berry Shortcakes with Whipped Greek Yogurt and Cream

SERVES 6 · VEGETARIAN, VEGAN-ADAPTABLE, GF-ADAPTABLE, DF-ADAPTABLE

SHORTCAKES:

1 cup flour (I like ¼ cup whole wheat pastry and ¾ cup all-purpose), plus more for dusting

⅜ teaspoon fine sea salt

2 teaspoons aluminum-free baking powder

¼ teaspoon baking soda

1½ tablespoons granulated sugar, plus more for sprinkling

4 tablespoons (½ stick) cold, unsalted butter, cut into 8 pieces

½ cup cold buttermilk (see substitutions following recipe)

Whipped Greek yogurt and cream, whipped cream, whipped coconut cream, or Sweet Cashew Cream (page 259)

4 cups fresh berries and/or sliced strawberries

WHIPPED GREEK YOGURT AND CREAM*:

1 cup organic heavy cream, preferably not ultra-pasteurized

⅓ cup plain, unsweetened whole Greek yogurt

1 tablespoon granulated sugar (optional)

½ teaspoon pure vanilla extract (optional)

not vegan/DF

I am obsessed with anything in mason jars, which I think make these shortcakes look even cuter than they normally would. Although this seems like a pint-size dessert, it packs a wallop of textures and flavors between the tender, but rough biscuits; sweet, juicy fruit; and light whipped "cream." The shortcakes can be made with a blend of whole-grain flours and come together in minutes. Any ripe, sweet seasonal fruit can be swapped for the berries. What sets these shortcakes apart from the traditional is the addition of whipped Greek yogurt and cream. Besides adding some gut-friendly probiotics, the yogurt adds such a delicious tartness that balances out the sweetness of the fruit quite nicely. Overall, this is a very low-sugar-added dessert.

1. Prepare the shortcakes: Preheat the oven to 425°F. Line a baking sheet with unbleached parchment paper. Place a large bowl and the beaters of an electric mixer in the freezer.

2. Place the flour, salt, baking powder, baking soda, and sugar in a food processor fitted with the steel blade. Pulse a couple of times to blend. Add the butter and pulse until the mixture resembles small peas or pebbles. Transfer the mixture to a medium-size bowl.

3. Add the buttermilk and blend with a fork until just combined.

4. Turn out the dough onto a lightly floured surface and knead a couple times to bring the dough together. Roll out to a 1-inch-thick disk and cut into 2¼-inch circles with a round cookie cutter or small glass dipped in flour. Do this by pressing the glass into the dough, but do not twist the glass (you will get better height in the biscuit this way.) You should be able to get four biscuits out of the first disk. Gather the scraps, pat it out gently, and cut more rounds until you have used up all the dough. Transfer the dough pieces to the prepared pan and space evenly apart.

5. This is optional, but it creates a light golden color: Remove 1 tablespoon of cream from the cup of whipped cream and use that to brush the tops of the shortcakes. Sprinkle with sugar. Bake for 12 minutes, or until puffed and lightly browned.

6. Remove from the oven and allow to cool slightly on a wire rack. Then split the shortcakes in half crosswise.

7. Prepare the whipped Greek yogurt and cream: Remove the mixing bowl and beaters from the freezer. Place the cream and yogurt in the bowl and beat on high speed. While the mixer is going, add the sugar and vanilla and beat until soft peaks form. Check the cream after 3 or 4 minutes and be sure not to overbeat.

8. Place the bottom of each shortcake in the bottom of a wide-mouth half-pint mason jar (or just use individual bowls). Top with a dollop of the cream mixture and ⅓ cup of berries. Add the top of the shortcake, plus another dollop of cream and some more berries.

TIP: For a quick and easy dessert, mix multiple types of fresh berries in a bowl and shave dark chocolate over the top. Garnish with small fresh mint leaves.

Substitutions

■ Sub ½ cup of whole milk for the buttermilk and omit the baking soda.

■ Sub 4 tablespoons of cold coconut oil for the butter and ½ cup of coconut milk for the buttermilk; omit the baking soda.

■ Sub 1 cup of King Arthur Gluten-Free Multi-Purpose Flour for the flour and add ¼ teaspoon of xanthan gum

Baked Maple Walnut Stuffed Apples

SERVES 6 · VEGETARIAN, GF, VEGAN ADAPTABLE, DF ADAPTABLE

6 large apples, such as Pink Lady, Golden Delicious, or Gala

⅔ cup raw walnuts or sunflower seeds

⅓ cup unsulfured golden raisins, chopped dates, dried cherries, or cranberries

2 tablespoons pure Grade A or B maple syrup, or honey

1 teaspoon lemon zest

1 teaspoon orange zest

½ teaspoon ground cinnamon

¼ teaspoon ground nutmeg

2 tablespoons unsalted butter, diced into 6 pieces (1-teaspoon pieces) (not vegan/DF) or unrefined, virgin coconut oil

1 cup unfiltered, unsweetened apple juice or cider

When I want something a little sweet and comforting, but without all the sugar, a baked apple is my go-to. Although a simple baked apple is perfectly delicious, the zesty filling in this recipe takes baked apples to a more interesting place. I have served these at both dinner parties and to my kids for a special after-school snack. But I always make sure there's at least one the next morning for me to eat for breakfast!

1. Preheat the oven to 375°F.

2. Core the apples, preferably with an apple corer. If any seeds still remain inside, try to cut them out. Cut a 1-inch piece off the core and "plug" the bottom of apple. This will ensure that the filling doesn't fall out. Take a vegetable peeler and peel away a bit of the apple skin around the stem (to keep the apples from bursting). Stand the apples upright in a 9 x 13-inch baking dish.

3. In a food processor fitted with the metal blade, finely chop the walnuts and dried fruit. Add the maple syrup, lemon and orange zest, and spices. Pulse until just combined. Fill the cavity of each apple with a heaping spoonful of the mixture. Dot each apple with a teaspoon of butter.

4. Pour the apple juice into the baking dish, around the apples. Cover the entire baking dish loosely with aluminum foil and bake for 30 minutes. Remove the foil and spoon some of the pan juices over the apples. Continue to bake until the apples are tender, about 30 minutes more. Bake even longer if you like your apples more falling apart. Serve with the pan juices.

5. Baked apples can be refrigerated for several days and are also delicious cold with yogurt.

Cantaloupe Granita

SERVES 6 · VEGAN, GF, DF

When it is sweltering hot in the summer, granita is one of the only things that hits the spot. It's coarse, like a shaved ice, and very light and refreshing. When I was growing up, we would make a lemon version for the kids and one with left-over espresso for the adults. In between games of bocce and badminton, my sisters and I would take turns going inside to scrape the granita. Today, I prefer granita made with sweet summer melons, which are so cooling to the body and don't need much in the way of added sugar. Although the peach liqueur is optional, it gives an incredible boost to the cantaloupe flavor in the ice. See photo on page 244.

1. Place all the ingredients in a high-powered blender or food processor. Blend until smooth.
2. Transfer the mixture to an 8-inch baking dish and place in the freezer. After 3 to 4 hours, use a fork to scrape the frozen layer so that it resembles shaved ice. Put it back in the freezer and keep taking it out to scrape every 2 hours with a fork until everything is shaved. Cover and keep frozen. Give it a scrape before serving.

ASK PAMELA: Can granitas be made all year round?
Although icy, cold beverages and treats can be refreshing in the summer, it's not a good idea to eat them every day and especially not when the weather is cold. Very cold foods weaken the digestive fire, which is responsible for converting food into energy. In addition, you don't want to bring down your internal thermometer when the temperature is cold outside.

4 cups fresh cantaloupe chunks (from a 3- to 4-pound cantaloupe)

Juice of 1 lime

2 tablespoons Grade A maple syrup or superfine cane sugar

1 tablespoon peach liqueur, such as peach schnapps (optional)

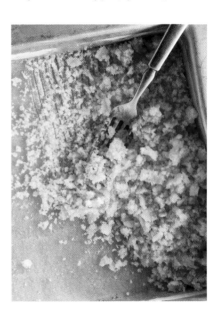

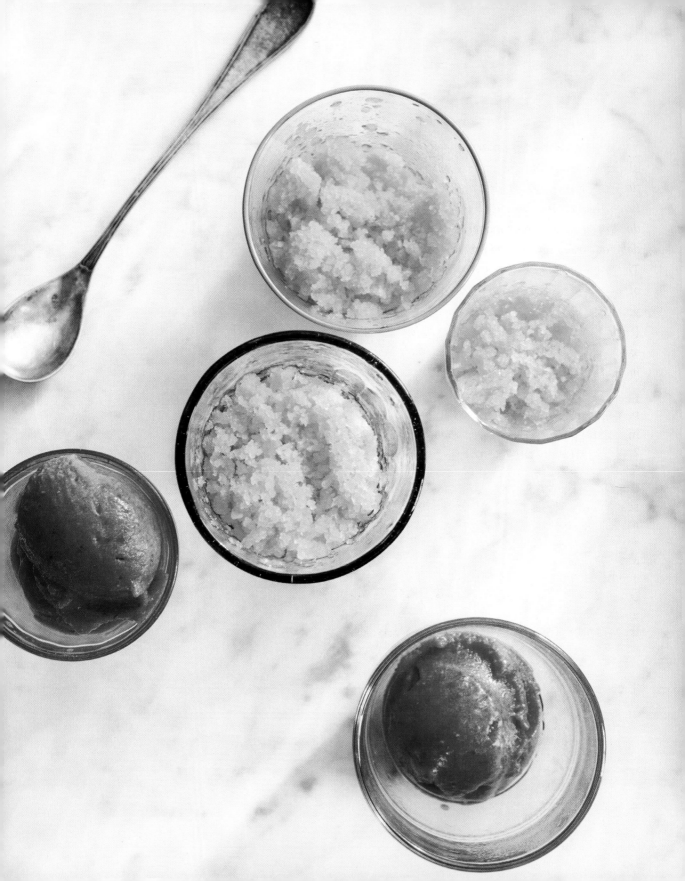

No-Churn Strawberry Gelato

MAKES 1 QUART · VEGETARIAN, GF, VEGAN ADAPTABLE, DF ADAPTABLE

Ice cream with crazy ingredient combinations seems to be all the rage right now, but I'll take a simple, but naturally flavored scoop any day. This has the creamy texture of Italian gelato, but without all the sugar and cream. Plus, you don't need an ice-cream maker to churn out this smooth and delicious treat, only a food processor and a little patience. The flavor is intensely strawberry—note that the sweetness of the gelato depends upon the sweetness of your berries. If your berries are very sweet, use the lesser amount of sugar. If they're pretty bland, use the greater. This would make an excellent sundae with toasted coconut chips and a drizzle of melted dark chocolate.

- 2 pounds strawberries, hulled and cut into ½-inch pieces
- 3 tablespoons freshly squeezed orange juice
- ½ to ⅔ cup granulated sugar or honey (not vegan), or half honey/half sugar
- ¼ cup unsweetened whole-milk Greek yogurt (not vegan/DF) or coconut yogurt

1. In a large bowl, toss the strawberries with the orange juice. Pour the mixture onto a rimmed baking sheet and spread out into one layer. Freeze until solid, about 2 hours.

2. Break up the frozen berries so you can fit the pieces into a food processor fitted with the steel blade. Add the sugar and Greek yogurt and puree the mixture, stopping a few times to scrape down the sides. This might take 4 to 5 minutes. If the mixture is not turning creamy, allow to sit in the food processor for a few minutes and then try blending again.

3. Serve immediately.

4. Store leftovers in a covered container in the freezer. It will eventually freeze solid, so to achieve a creamy consistency again, you'll have to thaw it for a few minutes and then break it up into pieces and reblend in the food processor.

No-Churn Strawberry Gelato and Canteloupe Granita (page 243)

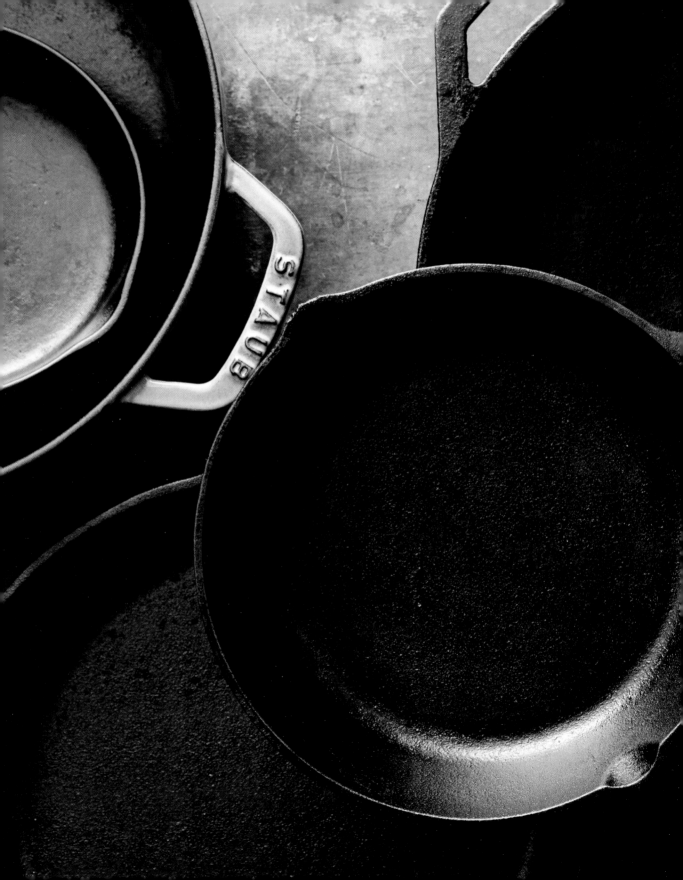

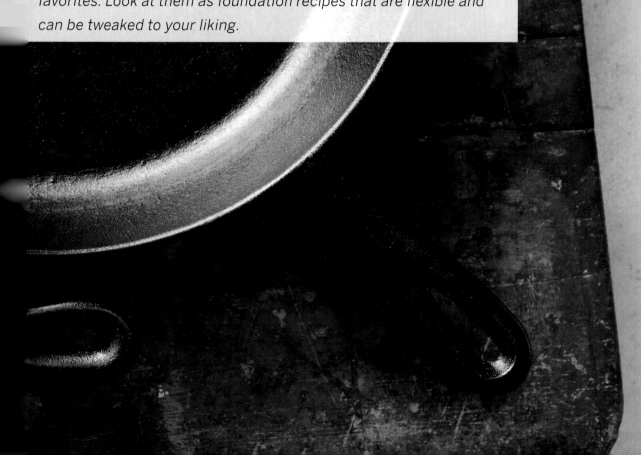

BASICS

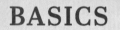

This section is exactly what it says: basics. I prepare these recipes regularly in my own kitchen. Most of these recipes have stood the test of time and I continue to rely on them after many, many years. Sure, you can replace these staple items with store-bought products, but your cooking (and your health) will benefit immensely from higher-quality, homemade foods. From stocks and sauces to cauliflower rice and even a basic foolproof pancake recipe, these basics may be used in many recipes in this book—or in your own favorites. Look at them as foundation recipes that are flexible and can be tweaked to your liking.

Hard-Boiled Eggs

VEGETARIAN, GF, DF

Eggs are a fantastic, inexpensive source of bio-available protein. Hard-boiled eggs are wonderful to have on hand in the refrigerator to add to lunchboxes or for a quick breakfast on the go. The key to avoiding a gray ring around the yolk is to not overcook the eggs and to shock them in ice water after cooking. The following method is suitable for any number of eggs; just make sure your eggs aren't crammed into the pot.

1. Place the eggs in a pot that's big enough so they won't crash into one another. Fill the pot with enough cold water to cover the eggs by an inch.

2. Over medium-high heat, bring the water to a full boil. Cover the pot, turn off the heat, and set a timer for 10 minutes.

3. In the meantime, prepare a bowl of ice water to accommodate the eggs. When the timer goes off, transfer the eggs from the pot to the ice-water bath, using a slotted spoon. Or drain them in a colander and run them under cold water if you'd like to eat them immediately.

4. Store them in the refrigerator unpeeled for up to 7 days. For a soft-boiled egg, cook for 6 minutes.

Vegetable Stock

MAKES ABOUT 3 QUARTS · VEGAN, GF, DF

Many store-bought stocks, whether meat- or vegetable-based, are full of additives and MSG; they often just don't taste fresh and clean. It's so easy to make your own, it's less expensive, and it will taste a hundred times better than anything from a box. I keep a container of washed vegetable scraps, such as mushroom stems, bottoms of asparagus, leek tops, and parsley stems in the freezer to use for this stock and just supplement with fresh vegetables. Other vegetables or scraps you can add that you might otherwise compost or discard: shiitake mushroom stems, carrot peels, ends from squashes, and so on. I usually avoid sulfur-containing vegetables, such as cabbage, broccoli and cauliflower, since their flavors can be overpowering. To increase the nutrients, you can simmer the stock with a strip of kombu.

3 large onions, cut into large chunks

2 large parsnips, unpeeled, cut into large chunks

2 large carrots, unpeeled, cut into large chunks

3 celery stalks, cut into large chunks

8 ounces white mushrooms, chopped

6 large garlic cloves, crushed

A few sprigs fresh parsley

2 sprigs fresh thyme or 2 bay leaves

1. Place all the ingredients plus 4 quarts of water in a large pot and bring to a boil over high heat. Lower the heat and simmer, uncovered, for 30 to 60 minutes.

2. Remove the pot from the heat and strain the stock into a large bowl. Push against the vegetables to extract additional liquid. Discard the vegetables.

3. Store in the refrigerator for up to 5 days, or in the freezer for up to 3 months. See page 20 for how to freeze stock.

Homemade Chicken or Turkey Stock

MAKES ABOUT 5 QUARTS · GF, DF

1 whole, organic, free-range chicken, or 4 pounds of bony chicken or turkey parts, such as backs, necks, and wings (if you can get chicken feet, use them!)

6 quarts cold water (if you have a large enough pot, use 8 quarts)

1 tablespoon cider vinegar

1 large onion, peeled and halved

2 carrots, peeled

2 celery stalks, cut if necessary

A few sprigs fresh parsley

2 teaspoons sea salt (optional—you can always leave the stock unsalted)

1. Wash the chicken and remove the gizzards from the cavity. Place the chicken and/or turkey parts in a large, stainless-steel stockpot. (You can cut the chicken into pieces if you need to, to fit in the pot.) Add the cold water and vinegar. Place over high heat and bring to a boil.

2. Immediately lower the heat to low and, using a slotted spoon, skim off any foam that rises to the surface. Try not to skim away any of the fat or you will lose a bit of flavor. At this point, it is important to keep the stock to a bare simmer and not a boil.

3. After skimming off all the foam, add all the vegetables, except the parsley. Cook, uncovered, at the gentlest possible simmer for 4 to 5 hours. (I like to go as long as 12 hours.) You want to see tiny bubbles just barely breaking the surface. If the heat from the burner does not go low enough, partially cover the pot or leave your stockpot half on the heat and half off.

4. About 10 minutes before finishing the stock, add the parsley and salt (this will impart additional mineral ions to the broth).

5. Strain the stock into a large, heatproof bowl. Remove the chicken meat from the carcass, if using a whole chicken, and discard the remaining solids. Allow to cool before refrigerating.

6. Ladle into quart-size containers or whatever size is most useful and refrigerate overnight. The next day, skim off the congealed fat at the top of each container. Refrigerate the stock for up to 5 days or freeze for up to 3 months. See page 20 for how to freeze stock.

ASK PAMELA: Does the water for the stock really have to be cold—what does it matter? *Cold water draws the flavor out of the meat and bones.*

Why do you add vinegar? *Acidic wine or cider vinegar adding during cooking helps to draw minerals, particularly calcium, magnesium and potassium, into the broth.*

Slow Cooker Chicken Bone Broth

MAKES ABOUT 4 QUARTS (BASED ON A 6½-QUART SLOW COOKER) · GF, DF

Bone broth is different from regular stock because it uses all bony parts, rather than parts with meat on the bones, and it is simmered for 18 to 36 hours (or longer), whereas traditional stock is simmered for 5 to 6 hours. The result is a rich and deeply nutritious broth that can be used in place of stock in any recipe or drunk hot out of a mug as a healing and health-supportive beverage. Bone broth is full of minerals, collagen, and amino acids, which all aid in digestion and support a healthy gut.

3½ pounds bony chicken parts, such as backs, necks, wings, and/or feet

About 5 quarts cold water (see Ask Pamela, page 249)

1 tablespoon cider vinegar (see Ask Pamela, page 249)

1 large onion, peeled and cut in half

2 carrots, cut if necessary (you can leave the peel on, just make sure they are scrubbed clean)

2 celery stalks, cut if necessary (try to use the leafy parts of celery, as they add lots of flavor)

1. Place the chicken parts and vegetables in a slow cooker and add the cold water and vinegar.
2. Set the timer to low for as long as your slow cooker will go, but a minimum of 18 hours.
3. Check periodically to skim off any foam that rises to the surface and continue to cook for 18 to 36 hours, resetting your slow cooker if the maximum time is less than 36 hours.
4. Turn off the heat and strain into a large, heat-proof bowl. You may need to use a large strainer initially and restrain it with a fine-mesh sieve to remove any smaller particles. Allow to cool before refrigerating.
5. Refrigerate, covered.
6. The next day, skim off the congealed fat at the top. If the broth is like gelatin, great job! If it's not, it's still wonderful and full of minerals.
7. Refrigerate the stock for up to 5 days or freeze for up to 3 months. See page 20 for how to freeze stock.

■ For a beef bone broth, take 3½ pounds of mixed beef bones, such as knuckles, short ribs, femur, short ribs, and neck bones. Drizzle with a little olive oil and roast at 400°F for about an hour, turning once, until the meat and bones are golden brown. Proceed with recipe as indicated above, but cook in the slow cooker for at least 24 hours. You can also mix chicken, beef, and pork bones together.

TIPS: Every time you roast a chicken, wrap the bones in aluminum foil and freeze for the next time you make stock. You can add the frozen bones directly to your stockpot.

Cold water draws the flavor out of the meat and bones. Use ice in your water if your tap water is room temperature.

ASK PAMELA: Can I make bone broth on the stove if I don't have a slow cooker? *Yes. Simmer the broth as low as possible on the stove, with the bubbles barely breaking the surface. If you have to leave the house or you are going to sleep at night, cover the pot and continue to cook in a 250°F oven.*

Cauliflower Rice

SERVES 3-4 · VEGETARIAN, GF, VEGAN ADAPTABLE, DF ADAPTABLE

1 head cauliflower (about 1¼ pounds), cut into large florets, or 3 cups premade fresh cauliflower rice or bagged frozen cauliflower rice

1 tablespoon unrefined extra-virgin olive oil

1 tablespoon unsalted butter or ghee (not vegan/DF) (or use all olive oil)

2 medium-size garlic cloves, chopped (optional)

¾ teaspoon sea salt

1. To make the cauliflower rice, place the cauliflower in a food processor fitted with a metal blade. Pulse for about 30 seconds, or until you get very small pieces (resembling snow or rice). You should have about 3 cups of cauliflower. If you are using premade cauliflower rice, fresh or frozen, skip this step.

2. Heat the oil and butter in a large sauté pan over medium heat. Add the garlic and sauté, stirring constantly, for about 30 seconds, or until fragrant. Add the cauliflower to the pan and toss to coat with the garlic mixture. Season with salt. Sauté for a couple of minutes, then cover and steam over low heat for 5 to 10 minutes, or until the desired tenderness is achieved.

TIPS: If using frozen riced cauliflower, no need to cover and steam. Continue to stir frozen cauliflower until it has defrosted and any excess water has evaporated, a couple of minutes.

If you don't have a lid, just sauté, stirring often, until the desired tenderness is achieved.

Roasted Sweet Bell Peppers

MAKES ABOUT 2 CUPS, DEPENDING ON SIZE OF PEPPERS · VEGAN, GF, DF

Roasted red peppers are silky, smoky, and a wonderful addition to salads, sandwiches, pastas, and in a frittata. You can buy jarred roasted red peppers, but I think the flavor of homemade is much better and they're very easy to make. This is the same technique I use to roast the poblano peppers in the taco recipe on page 194.

4 sweet bell peppers, any color

1. Preheat the broiler to high and position a rack 6 inches below the heat source. This is usually the second level. Place the whole peppers on a baking sheet and broil until blackened on all sides, turning every couple of minutes.
2. Set aside in a bowl and cover for at least 15 minutes, or until cool enough to handle. Remove the skin and seeds and thickly slice (about ½ inch thick). Refrigerate in an airtight container for up to 4 days.

Chimichurri Sauce

MAKES ABOUT 1¼ CUPS · VEGAN, GF, DF

Chimichurri is an amazing, healthful condiment that makes almost anything taste better. It's full of fresh green herbs and has a great tang from the vinegar. I love it over simple roasted or grilled fish, poultry or beef, as well as grilled vegetables.

¾ cup packed fresh flat-leaf parsley leaves and tender stems

½ cup packed fresh cilantro or mint leaves and tender stems, or additional parsley

2 tablespoons fresh oregano or basil leaves, or 2 teaspoons dried oregano (or omit)

3 garlic cloves

3 tablespoons unpasteurized cider vinegar or red wine vinegar

6 tablespoons unrefined cold-pressed extra-virgin olive oil

½ teaspoon fine sea salt

¼ teaspoon red pepper flakes, or more to taste

1. In a food processor fitted with the metal blade, combine all the herbs and the garlic. Process until well chopped. Or do this with a sharp knife. Transfer to a medium-size bowl. Add the remaining sauce ingredients to the herbs and mix well.
2. Serve immediately or refrigerate and use within 2 to 3 days.

Basil-Parsley Pesto

MAKES 2 CUPS · VEGETARIAN, VEGAN ADAPTABLE, GF, DF ADAPTABLE

I make pesto more than any other condiment. It is incredibly versatile, easy to prep, and stays perfectly well in the refrigerator for a few weeks or in the freezer for a couple of months. I love combining basil and parsley for a very light and fresh-tasting pesto. Pesto is obviously great on pasta, but I also serve it with grilled fish or chicken, with grilled or roasted vegetables, drizzled on raw tomatoes, as a base for pizza, swirled into cauliflower mashed potatoes, stirred into soups, and more! To make a vegan/dairy-free version, eliminate the salt and cheese and substitute ¼ cup of brown rice miso or other hearty miso. Taste for salt.

¼ cup raw walnuts (see page 25 for substitutions)

¼ cup raw pine nuts (see page 25 for substitutions)

1½ to 2 tablespoons chopped garlic

2½ cups lightly packed fresh basil leaves

2½ cups lightly packed fresh flat-leaf parsley leaves

¾ teaspoon sea salt

A couple of grinds of black pepper

1 cup unrefined, cold-pressed extra-virgin olive oil

½ cup grated Pecorino Romano or Parmesan cheese (omit for vegan/DF)

1. Place the walnuts, pine nuts, and garlic in a food processor fitted with the steel blade. Process until finely chopped.
2. Add the basil, parsley, salt, and pepper. With the motor running, slowly pour the olive oil into the bowl through the feed tube and process until the pesto is finely pureed. Add the grated cheese and puree until well blended. Store in the refrigerator for up to 2 weeks or in the freezer for up to 2 months.

Homemade Marinara Sauce

MAKES ABOUT 5 CUPS · VEGAN, GF, DF

All good Italian girls make marinara sauce from scratch and I am no exception. I don't skimp on the oil, which adds a lot of flavor. If tomatoes are not in season, I'll use organic tomatoes sold in glass jars. Good-quality marinara sauce can be tossed with pasta, as a base for pizza, poured over meatballs, and stirred into rice or polenta.

¼ cup unrefined, cold-pressed extra-virgin olive oil

1 large onion, finely diced

2 garlic cloves, finely chopped

4 pounds fresh, ripe tomatoes, peeled, seeded, and diced, or 3 (18-ounce) (I like Jovial tomatoes in glass) or 2 (28-ounce) containers crushed tomatoes

1 (7-ounce) jar tomato paste (optional, for a richer, thicker sauce)

Sea salt

A few leaves (a small handful) fresh basil, thinly sliced

1. In a medium-size saucepan, heat the olive oil over medium-low heat. Add the onion and sauté gently until softened, about 10 minutes. Add the garlic and cook for another minute.

2. Add the tomatoes and tomato paste, if using, plus two generous pinches of salt, and bring to a simmer. Cover the sauce and simmer for about 20 minutes. Taste for seasoning.

3. Puree about half of the sauce with an immersion blender or pass through a food mill. (You can also blend half the sauce in a blender or food processor.) Put the sauce back into the saucepan.

4. Add the basil and simmer for another 5 minutes. Taste and adjust the seasoning.

5. The marinara sauce can be kept refrigerated for up to 1 week and can be frozen for up to 3 months.

Taco Seasoning

MAKES ENOUGH FOR 1 POUND OF GROUND MEAT OR CRUMBLED TEMPEH · VEGAN, GF, DF

There is no need to buy prepared taco seasoning, many of which contain MSG, sugar, and (not natural) flavors. It is cheaper and perfectly simple to make your own. I mix up ten times the amount of this taco seasoning so I always have it on hand for a really quick dinner.

1 tablespoon chili powder

2 teaspoons ground cumin

½ teaspoon paprika

¼ teaspoon ground turmeric

¼ teaspoon garlic powder

¼ teaspoon onion powder

¼ teaspoon dried oregano

¾ to 1 teaspoon fine sea salt

1. Mix all the ingredients together until well blended. This will keep in a glass jar for several months.

TIP: Not all chili powders are created equal. The one I use is by Simply Organic, which has good depth of flavor with a little kick. If you don't care for any heat at all, you can cut back on the chili powder. If you like things spicy, feel free to add a few pinches of cayenne pepper.

continued on page 254

To Use the Seasoning

1 teaspoon arrowroot powder

1 pound ground meat or crumbled tempeh

Scant 3 tablespoons Taco Seasoning

Accompaniments: corn tortillas, guacamole, pico de gallo, shredded cheese, refried black beans, cilantro-lime slaw, shredded lettuce

1. Dissolve the arrowroot powder in ¾ cup of water (for meat) or 1 cup of water (for tempeh) and set aside.
2. Heat a medium-size skillet over medium heat. Place the meat or tempeh in the skillet and cook until browned. Add the spice mixture and sauté for 30 seconds. Whisk arrowroot mixture and pour into the skillet. Sauté until thickened.

Ranch Dressing

MAKES ABOUT 2 CUPS · VEGETARIAN, GF, VEGAN ADAPTABLE, DF ADAPTABLE

This is my husband's favorite dressing in the world so I had to include it here. I know how popular ranch dressing is and I think you'll love this cleaned-up version with lots of fresh herbs and tang. I prefer to use kefir in this recipe, rather than buttermilk, since kefir is loaded with incredible beneficial bacteria. This also doubles as a great dip for crudités.

½ cup soy-free Vegenaise or good-quality mayonnaise

½ cup unsweetened whole-milk Greek yogurt

½ cup unsweetened kefir or buttermilk (page 24 for substitutions)

1 tablespoon freshly squeezed lemon juice

½ teaspoon Dijon mustard

1 medium-size garlic clove, grated or minced

1 teaspoon sea salt

Freshly ground black pepper

Pinch of cayenne pepper

2 tablespoons chopped fresh chives, or 1 scallion, finely chopped

2 tablespoons fresh flat-leaf parsley leaves, finely chopped

1. Place all the ingredients, except the herbs, in a blender, adding black pepper to taste, and puree until you have a smooth mixture. Stir in the herbs.
2. Transfer to a container and refrigerate, covered, for at least an hour so that the flavors develop. The ranch dressing will last 3 days in the refrigerator. Stir before using.

TO MAKE THIS DAIRY-FREE AND VEGAN, MAKE THE FOLLOWING SUBSTITUTIONS: Combine ¼ cup of soy-free Vegenaise (instead of the ½ cup of Vegenaise or mayonnaise), 2 tablespoons of freshly squeezed lemon juice (instead of 1 tablespoon), omit the yogurt, and use a nondairy substitute for the buttermilk. Add 1 cup of water and ¾ cup raw cashews, soaked for 4 to 6 hours in water and drained. The other dressing ingredients stay the same. A high-powered blender does a good job blending the cashews until they're creamy. If you don't have one, do this in a food processor and process for at least a few minutes.

Everyday Salad Dressing

MAKES 1 CUP · VEGETARIAN, GF, DF, VEGAN ADAPTABLE

This is a bold statement, but no vinaigrette out there is better than one you can make with high-quality ingredients at home, especially a good unrefined oil. This is truly the perfect vinaigrette. It has the most delicious balance of acidity and oil, a little sharpness from the shallot, and hint of sweetness. I make a double recipe every week and use it on almost every green salad, no matter what the ingredients, as well as on any salad I am spontaneously pulling together.

1 small shallot, minced (about 2 teaspoons)

¾ to 1 teaspoon sea salt

Freshly ground black pepper

1 teaspoon Dijon mustard

2 teaspoons raw honey (omit for vegan) or pure maple syrup

2 tablespoons unpasteurized cider vinegar or red wine vinegar

2 tablespoons unseasoned rice vinegar

¾ cup unrefined, cold-pressed extra-virgin olive oil, or ½ cup olive oil + ¼ cup flax oil

1. Either whisk together all the ingredients, including black pepper to taste, in a small bowl or place them in a glass jar with a lid and shake until emulsified.
2. The dressing can be made ahead and kept in a glass jar in the refrigerator for 5 to 7 days. Because olive oil solidifies when chilled, you will need to remove it from the refrigerator well before you want to use it, for it to become pourable. Or you can leave the dressing at room temperature in a cool, dark place for a few days. If you use flax oil in the dressing, it must stay refrigerated.

Coconut Milk

MAKES ABOUT 3 CUPS · VEGAN, GF, DF

I had no idea how easy it was to make homemade coconut milk! So easy! Plus, there aren't added thickeners, sweeteners, and other junk that can be in packaged coconut milks. Coconut milk is a delicious dairy-free substitute in almost any recipe. I love it in smoothies and smoothie bowls, mixed with almond milk in porridges, combined with water to make coconut rice, in curry, and many other recipes.

2 cups unsweetened shredded coconut

4 cups warm water

1. Place the coconut in a Vitamix or blender and add the warm water.
2. Blend until it has a thick and creamy consistency.
3. Strain the mixture through a fine-mesh sieve or a nut milk bag.
4. Store in the fridge for up to 4 days. It is normal for the cream of the coconut to separate, just shake before drinking.

Homemade Coconut Yogurt

MAKES ABOUT 1¾ CUPS · VEGAN, GF, DF

My friends Stephanie and Willow from C&J Nutrition taught me this easy DIY coconut yogurt recipe. I have yet to find a great coconut yogurt in my local markets and I love having a dairy-free option in the fridge, since I try to limit the amount of dairy I eat. The flavor of this yogurt is just barely coconutty and has the slight tartness you would expect from a cultured product. Probiotics are important for gut health! Note that if you are using purchased coconut milk, you don't want the coconut beverages in the refrigerator section. Use the pure coconut milk you find in a can or, in the case of Aroy-D, small Tetra Pak boxes.

14 ounces full-fat culinary coconut milk (either homemade, page 255, or I prefer Aroy-D brand)

1 probiotic capsule (You can use whatever you like, but VSL#3 gives the best result)

1. Pour the coconut milk into a clean glass jar with a tight-fitting lid.

2. Open the probiotic capsule, using your fingers, and pour the contents into the coconut milk. Stir well. Using a fork helps break up the clumps of powder.

3. Place the lid very loosely on top of the jar. Don't screw it on at all; you want plenty of air to get to the mixture within, but you want to cover it from any dust or dirt.

4. Let sit on the countertop, out of direct sunlight, for 24 hours undisturbed.

5. After 24 hours, stir the mixture again (it should be starting to thicken) and let sit for another 24 hours, undisturbed.

6. After 48 hours total, the yogurt should be able to coat the back of a spoon. If you refrigerate it now, it will be the consistency of regular yogurt. If you let it sit for another 12 to 24 hours, it will become even thicker.

7. Store in the refrigerator with the lid tightly sealed for up to 5 days.

Almond Butter (and variations)

MAKES ABOUT 1 CUP · VEGAN, GF, DF

If you own a food processor, you can make almond butter. But the fun doesn't end there! I love adding different flavors, such as cinnamon or maple syrup, and textures, such as chia seeds, or a superfood boost, such as lucuma powder or hemp seeds. If your food processor is weak, you may need to do this in stages so you don't burn out the motor. And remember: have patience. Even if it seems as though it is not turning into nut butter, it will!

2 cups almonds, either raw, soaked and dehydrated, or roasted

Optional add-ins: a pinch of sea salt, a spoonful of pure maple syrup or raw honey (omit for vegan), ground flaxseeds, chia seeds, or a spoonful of raw cacao powder

1. Place the almonds and your desired add-ins in a food processor fitted with a steel blade. Process, scraping down the sides occasionally, until desired consistency is achieved. This can take up to 15 minutes, although roasted almonds take a little less time than raw. Keep in a covered glass container in the refrigerator for many months.

Almond Milk

MAKES ABOUT 3 CUPS · VEGAN, GF, DF

I make almond milk twice a week and we're not even dairy-free. We just love it! The flavor and consistency of homemade almond milk is so clean. It's nothing like almond milk from a carton, which tends to be loaded with thickening agents and emulsifiers. I don't bother removing the skins, but you can for a pure white almond milk. Once you've tried making homemade almond milk, you can start experimenting with other nuts and seeds, such as hazelnuts and hemp seeds.

1 cup raw almonds (or any raw nut or seed)
Filtered water, at room temperature

1. Soak the raw almonds in a bowl with plenty of room-temperature water for 6 to 8 hours. (Soaking will make the almonds softer and more digestible.)
2. Drain the almonds in a colander and rinse with fresh water. Optional: Remove the skins from the almonds by pressing them through your thumb and forefinger. Discard the skins.
3. Place the almonds in a blender or Vitamix. Add 3 cups of fresh water and blend until the nuts are pulverized.
4. Strain through a nut milk bag, fine-mesh sieve, or cheesecloth into a glass bowl. If using a sieve, use a spoon to scrape the almond meal around and allow as much liquid as possible to drain through.

5. Transfer to a glass jar and refrigerate, covered, for up to 4 days.

- Almond milk with coconut water: Soak the almonds in regular water, but use coconut water to blend with the almonds.

- Almond milk sweetened with dates: Follow the directions for basic almond milk, but blend the almonds with water plus four to eight pitted dates. You can also add a drop of pure vanilla extract and sea salt, if you like.

TIP: You can make almond milk in a pinch—with almond butter! Use a ratio of 1 cup of water to 1 tablespoon of almond butter and blend for at least 30 seconds, or until emulsified. No need to strain. Just pour into a glass jar and keep refrigerated for up to 6 days.

ASK PAMELA: What the heck should I do with this almond pulp? *Definitely make use of the leftover almond pulp, which will amount to ¾ cup from this recipe. You can add it to hot cereal and smoothies for a protein boost. I will very often substitute it for some of the flour in such recipes as pancakes, waffles, muffins, and quick breads. The key is to make sure the almond pulp makes up no more than half of the dry ingredients in the recipe. You can even freeze it for another time. Refer to my blog for more recipes in which you can use almond pulp.*

Whole-Grain Pancakes

SERVES 4 TO 5 · VEGETARIAN, VEGAN ADAPTABLE, GF ADAPTABLE, DF ADAPTABLE

This has been my default pancake recipe for the last twenty years, but ironically I never follow it to a T. I am always changing up the flours, depending on what I have and what flavor I am in the mood for. You can use oat, buckwheat, rice, millet, quinoa, sorghum and corn in any combination you want. Keep in mind that buckwheat has a more earthy flavor and a gray color and quinoa flour tastes a lot like quinoa. I also very often substitute ¾ cup of almond pulp for ¾ cup of the flour, for a great protein boost. The pancake batter can be made in advance and refrigerated for 2 to 3 days. Store in a glass container leaving very little air at the top to prevent oxidation. Another option is to make multiple batches of the dry mix and store it in the pantry. Scoop out 2 cups + 1 tablespoon of dry mix and add the wet ingredients.

2 cups whole wheat pastry flour, white whole wheat flour, or whole spelt flour (see pages 10 and 25 for GF substitutions)

1 teaspoon aluminum-free baking powder

1 teaspoon baking soda

1 teaspoon fine sea salt

2 cups buttermilk (see page 24 for DF substitutions)

2 large eggs (see page 24 for vegan substitutions)

1 tablespoon pure Grade A or B maple syrup

1 teaspoon pure vanilla extract

4 tablespoons unsalted butter (omit for vegan/ DF) or unrefined coconut oil, melted

Unrefined, virgin coconut oil, for cooking

Optional add-ins: blueberries, chocolate chips (DF, if necessary), or diced banana

1. Preheat a griddle to 400°F or medium heat.
2. Combine the flour, baking powder, baking soda, and salt in a large bowl.
3. In a medium-size bowl or a 4- to 6-cup measuring cup, whisk together the buttermilk, eggs, vanilla, maple syrup, and melted butter until well blended. (A blender can do this easily, too.)
4. Pour the wet mixture into the dry ingredients and stir until just combined.
5. Brush the griddle with coconut oil and spoon about ¼ cup of batter onto the griddle. Add blueberries, chocolate chips or diced banana to the surface, if desired. When bubbles start to form on the surface of the pancake and the edges become slightly dry, flip it over and cook until done. Maintain the heat on medium-low or 400°F to cook the remaining pancakes.

Cashew Cream

MAKES ABOUT 1¼ CUPS · VEGAN, GF, DF

Raw cashews have an incredible ability to be blended into a creamlike substance. Many people who avoid dairy use savory cashew cream instead of dolloping sour cream on soup or a baked potato, and sweet cashew cream to add an extra special (and high-protein) topping to desserts and fruit. A high-powered blender, such as Vitamix, will achieve the smoothest cream, but you can still use a food processor. I wouldn't advise using less than 1 cup of cashews since the machine won't have enough to blend. Once you get the hang of this recipe, you can have a lot of fun experimenting with other flavors. See my suggestions on the next page.

SAVORY CASHEW CREAM:

1 cup raw cashews, soaked in water for 4 to 6 hours

½ cup water, or according to desired consistency

Juice of ½ lemon

½ teaspoon sea salt

½ teaspoon cider vinegar, preferably unpasteurized

Pinch of garlic powder (optional)

Other flavors with which to experiment: chipotle powder for a chipotle cream, for tacos and grain bowls; cilantro; roasted red pepper; roasted garlic

SWEET CASHEW CREAM:

1 cup raw cashews, soaked in water for 4 to 6 hours

½ to ¾ cup water, according to desired consistency

2 to 3 tablespoons pure Grade A maple syrup or raw honey (omit for vegan), according to desired sweetness

½ teaspoon pure vanilla extract

Other flavors with which to experiment: lemon zest and ground ginger; raw cacao powder; strawberries; cinnamon

1. Drain and rinse the cashews well under fresh water. Place them in a high-powered blender or a food processor with the remaining ingredients for savory or sweet and blend on high speed for several minutes, or until very smooth. If you are using a food processor, scrape down the sides every minute or so.

2. You can use it right away, or refrigerate it for up to 4 days. It will thicken in the refrigerator. You can freeze cashew cream for up to 3 months, but you will probably need to reblend it after it has defrosted.

Raspberry Chia Seed Jam

MAKES ABOUT 1 CUP · VEGAN, GF, DF

I have friends who are into canning, but it's never something I learned to do. This a much easier way to make jam due to the key ingredient: chia seeds. When chia seeds come into contact with liquid, they become very gelatinous and bind all the fruit together. You may not even notice they're in there because they mimic the raspberry seeds. Although they're tiny, they pack a ton of protein, fiber, and omega-3 fats.

2 tablespoons + 2 teaspoons chia seeds

10 ounces frozen organic raspberries, thawed (drain the raspberries if you want a very thick jam)

2 tablespoons pure maple syrup or raw honey (omit for vegan), or more to taste

1. Place all the ingredients in a medium-size bowl. Stir to mix, making sure all the chia seeds have been moistened with the juice from the berries.

2. Cover and allow the jam to thicken in the refrigerator for at least 6 hours. Lasts for 2 to 3 weeks in the refrigerator.

TIP: This recipe also works with frozen blackberries.

METRIC CONVERSION CHARTS

The recipes in this book have not been tested with metric measurements, so some variations might occur. Remember that the weight of dry ingredients varies according to the volume or density factor: 1 cup of flour weighs far less than 1 cup of sugar, and 1 tablespoon doesn't necessarily hold 3 teaspoons.

GENERAL FORMULA FOR METRIC CONVERSION

Ounces to grams	multiply ounces by 28.35
Grams to ounces	multiply grams by 0.035
Pounds to grams	multiply pounds by 453.5
Pounds to kilograms	multiply pounds by 0.45
Cups to liters	multiply cups by 0.24
Fahrenheit to Celsius	subtract 32 from Fahrenheit temperature, multiply by 5, divide by 9
Celsius to Fahrenheit	multiply Celsius temperature by 9, divide by 5, add 32

VOLUME (LIQUID) MEASUREMENTS

1 teaspoon	= ⅙ fluid ounce	= 5 milliliters
1 tablespoon	= ½ fluid ounce	= 15 milliliters
2 tablespoons	= 1 fluid ounce	= 30 milliliters
¼ cup	= 2 fluid ounces	= 60 milliliters
⅓ cup	= 2⅔ fluid ounces	= 79 milliliters
½ cup	= 4 fluid ounces	= 118 milliliters
1 cup or ½ pint	= 8 fluid ounces	= 250 milliliters
2 cups or 1 pint	= 16 fluid ounces	= 500 milliliters
4 cups or 1 quart	= 32 fluid ounces	= 1,000 milliliters
1 gallon	= 4 liters	

WEIGHT (MASS) MEASUREMENTS

1 ounce	= 30 grams	
2 ounces	= 55 grams	
3 ounces	= 85 grams	
4 ounces	= ¼ pound	= 125 grams
8 ounces	= ½ pound	= 240 grams
12 ounces	= ¾ pound	= 375 grams
16 ounces	= 1 pound	= 454 grams

OVEN TEMPERATURE EQUIVALENTS, FAHRENHEIT (F) AND CELSIUS (C)

100°F	= 38°C
200°F	= 95°C
250°F	= 120°C
300°F	= 150°C
350°F	= 180°C
400°F	= 205°C
450°F	= 230°C

VOLUME (DRY) MEASUREMENTS

¼ teaspoon	= 1 milliliter
½ teaspoon	= 2 milliliters
¾ teaspoon	= 4 milliliters
1 teaspoon	= 5 milliliters
1 tablespoon	= 15 milliliters
¼ cup	= 59 milliliters
⅓ cup	= 79 milliliters
½ cup	= 118 milliliters
⅔ cup	= 158 milliliters
¾ cup	= 177 milliliters
1 cup	= 225 milliliters
4 cups or 1 quart	= 1 liter
½ gallon	= 2 liters
1 gallon	= 4 liters

LINEAR MEASUREMENTS

½ inch	= 1½ cm
1 inch	= 2½ cm
6 inches	= 15 cm
8 inches	= 20 cm
10 inches	= 25 cm
12 inches	= 30 cm
20 inches	= 50 cm

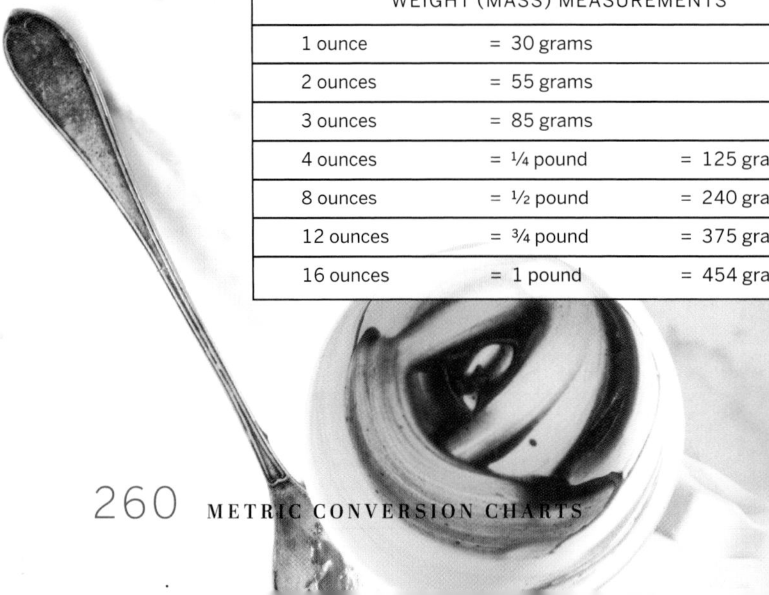

SUGGESTED MEAL PLANS FOR EACH SEASON

SPRING

MONDAY: Quick Thai Yellow Vegetable Curry (page 219) with sugar snap peas, cauliflower, carrots, and rice (make extra rice for Thursday's Not-Fried Rice)

TUESDAY: Slow-Roasted Wild Salmon, Spinach Salad with Roasted Red Onions and Shiitakes (pages 203, 174)

WEDNESDAY: Peruvian Chicken and Cilantro Soup with Quinoa (page 87), Garden Veggie Patties (page 116)

THURSDAY: Not-Fried Rice and Vegetables (page 137) (add an egg or edamame for protein)

FRIDAY: Balsamic-Herb Flank Steak (page 205), roasted carrots, sautéed peas

SUNDAY: Skillet Chicken with Asparagus, Herbed Mixed-Grain Pilaf (pages 183, 149)

MONDAY: Soft Polenta with Mushroom Ragout, Garlicky Kale (pages 144, 113)

TUESDAY: Wild Halibut Burgers, Quinoa Salad with Cherries, Almonds, Celery, and Pecorino (pages 195, 169)

WEDNESDAY: South American Roast Chicken, simple roasted potato wedges, Cauliflower Rice (pages 186, 251; pulse extra cauliflower to use in Baked Risotto the next night)

THURSDAY: Baked Cauliflower and Rice Risotto, Shaved Vegetable Salad (pages 142, 170; save the beet greens from the beets to sauté on Sunday)

FRIDAY: Chipotle Shrimp Tacos with Pineapple Slaw (page 191), refried black beans

SUNDAY: Lickety-Split Chicken, Sautéed Beet Greens (pages 184, 117), simple roasted sweet potatoes

SUMMER

MONDAY: Portobello and Poblano Tacos, Mexican Chopped Salad with Spicy Cilantro Dressing (pages 194, 166)

TUESDAY: Grilled Lemon-Herb Shrimp, Herbed Mixed-Grain Pilaf, Sautéed Zucchini with Shallots (pages 201, 149, 123)

WEDNESDAY: Grilled Summer Salad with Chicken and Spicy Cashew Dressing (page 176)

THURSDAY: Sweet Potato and Quinoa Veggie Burgers, Raw Kale Salad (pages 209, 156)

FRIDAY: Chicken Shawarma, tomato-cucumber salad, tahini sauce, Greek Nachos (pages 188, 65)

SUNDAY: Italian White Bean and Tuna Salad with Capers (page 157)

MONDAY: Pasta with Basil-Parsley Pesto, Zucchini Carpaccio (pages 252, 167)

TUESDAY: Lickety-Split Chicken, Grilled Eggplant with Pomegranate Molasses, Cauliflower Rice (pages 184, 251)

WEDNESDAY: Asian Grain Bowl with Miso-Glazed Japanese Mushrooms, Stir-Fried Baby Bok Choy (pages 133, 118, 112)

THURSDAY: Grilled Wild Salmon with Chimichurri Sauce, Arugula Salad with Nectarines, Tomatoes, and Fresh Mozzarella (pages 204, 252, 173)

FRIDAY: Green Goddess Chicken Salad (page 162), grilled seasonal vegetables

SUNDAY: Mexican Millet Casserole (page 217), green salad

FALL

MONDAY: Lentil Sloppy Joes (page 210) on toasted buns with pickles, mixed green salad

TUESDAY: Chipotle Turkey Chili with Sweet Potatoes (page 92)

WEDNESDAY: Broiled Wild Salmon, Fall Salad with Pumpkin Pie–Spiced Roasted Pears (pages 204, 179)

THURSDAY: Middle Eastern Vegetable Soup with Freekeh (page 95), grilled cheese or quesadillas

FRIDAY: Balsamic-Herb Flank Steak, Crispy Stovetop Brussels Sprouts, Herbed Mixed-Grain Pilaf (pages 205, 106, 149)

SUNDAY: Skillet Chicken with green beans subbed for asparagus, Millet and Cauliflower Mash (pages 183, 135)

MONDAY: Loaded Baked Potato Soup with topping bar, green salad with Everyday Salad Dressing (pages 85, 255)

TUESDAY: Broiled Fillet of Sole, Roasted Broccoli and Lemon with Feta, Pickled Shallots, and Pine Nuts (pages 198, 109)

WEDNESDAY: Hearty Vegetable Soup with Kale Pesto, Picadillo (pages 96, 206) with simple brown rice (page 131)

THURSDAY: Poached Wild Salmon, Braised Lentils with Brussels Sprouts and Creamy Dijon Cashew Drizzle (pages 203, 146)

FRIDAY: Spaghetti Squash with Cherry Tomatoes, Mushrooms, and Spinach, Eggplant "Meatballs" (pages 121, 213)

SUNDAY: Mexican Vegetable Soup with Rice and Beans (page 86)

WINTER

MONDAY: Kitchari (page 98), avocado toasts

TUESDAY: Lickety-Split Chicken, Turmeric Roasted Cauliflower with Raisins, Capers, and Crispy Quinoa (pages 184–185, 110–111)

WEDNESDAY: Slow Cooker Chicken Tacos, Saturday Chopped Salad (pages 190, 155)

THURSDAY: Pasta with Kale, Walnuts, and Ricotta (page 150), green salad

FRIDAY: Wild Salmon in Parchment, One-Pot Barley with Melted Cabbage (pages 203–204, 139)

SUNDAY: Cauliflower and Roasted Red Pepper Frittata, Braised Fennel with Tomatoes and Thyme (pages 59, 115)

MONDAY: Vegan Mac and Cheese, green salad with red cabbage, sunflower seeds, and avocado and Everyday Salad Dressing (pages 214, 255) (double the sauce and save some for Baked Potato Night)

TUESDAY: Baked potato night

WEDNESDAY: Italian Wedding Soup, Pizza Muffins (pages 90, 66)

THURSDAY: Baked Wild Salmon, Winter Vegetable Slaw with Ginger and Lime, Moroccan Spiced Butternut Squash (pages 203, 161, 141)

FRIDAY: Thai Coconut Chicken Soup, Asian Green Salad with Avocado and Oranges, simple roasted sweet potato wedges (pages 91, 165)

SUNDAY: Slow Cooker Italian Pot Roast (freeze half for another time), simple polenta, Garlicky Kale (pages 208, 113)

RESOURCES

Because I cook so much, I really put products to the test. If you see a brand listed here, it is because I love it, not because I have a relationship with a particular company. In fact, I have not received any compensation by any brand for being listed here.

Most of these products can be found at your local Whole Foods Market or health food store, but everything can be ordered online from either Amazon or ThriveMarket.com. I have provided the manufacturer's website if you would like more information about the products or to see if they may be found at a retail store close to where you live.

GRAINS AND FLOURS

Alter Eco, www.alterecofoods.com: Organic rainbow quinoa

Arrowhead Mills, www.arrowheadmills.com: Organic whole-grain flours, barley

Bob's Red Mill, www.bobsredmill.com: Organic whole-grain flours, coconut flour, certified gluten-free oat flour, certified gluten-free steel-cut and old-fashioned rolled oats, quinoa, freekeh, arrowroot powder, buckwheat groats and buckwheat cereal, xanthan gum, barley, spelt, and farro

De la Estancia, www.delaestancia.com: Organic, quick-cooking polenta (not precooked or processed)

Eden Foods, www.edenfoods.com: Organic millet

King Arthur Flour, www.kingarthur.com: Gluten-free Multi-Purpose Flour

Lotus Foods, www.lotusfoods.com: Forbidden/ black rice

Lundberg, www.lundberg.com: Whole-grain rices

To Your Health Sprouted Flour Company, www.organicsproutedflour.net: Sprouted organic whole-grain flours in every variety

BEANS AND LEGUMES

Banyan Botanicals, www.banyanbotanicals.com: Organic split yellow mung dal (for kitchari)

Eden Foods, www.edenfoods.com: Organic cooked beans with kombu in BPA-free cans

Farmer Direct Co-op, www.farmerdirectcoop.com: Organic French lentils

Jovial Foods, www.jovialfoods.com: Organic cooked chickpeas and cannellini beans in glass jars

Rancho Gordo, www.ranchogordo.com: The best-quality heirloom and traditional dried beans, as well as hominy

Trader Joe's, www.traderjoes.com: Organic cooked beans in BPA-free cans

NUTS, SEEDS, NUT AND SEED BUTTERS, AND ALMOND FLOUR

Bob's Red Mill, www.bobsredmill.com: Unsweetened flaked and shredded coconut, whole flaxseeds, blanched almond flour and meal

Digestive Wellness, www.digestivewellnessbook.com: Blanched almond flour

Honeyville, www.honeyville.com: Blanched almond flour

Living Nutz, www.livingnutz.com: High-quality organic nuts and seeds, including truly raw almonds

Living Tree Community Foods, www.livingtreecommunity.com: Organic nut butters and tahini in glass jars

Nuttzo, www.nuttzo.com: Organic spreads made from nuts and seeds in glass jars

Once Again, www.onceagainnutbutter.com: Organic raw almond butter and sunflower seed butters in glass jars

Santa Cruz Organic, www.santacruzorganic.com: Organic peanut butter in glass jars

Solstice Canyon, www.solsticecanyon.com: Small-batch almond butters sweetened with coconut sugar in glass jars

DAIRY AND DAIRY ALTERNATIVES

Fourth and Heart, www.fourthandheart.com: 100 percent grass-fed flavor-infused ghee

Kite Hill, www.kite-hill.com: Almond milk cream cheese, ricotta and yogurt

Organic Pastures, www.organicpastures.com: Raw organic milk, butter, and cream

Organic Valley, www.organicvalley.coop: Organic buttermilk, ghee

Straus Family Farms, www.strausfamilycreamery.com: Organic cultured butter, Greek yogurt

White Mountain, www.whitemountainfoods.com: Organic Bulgarian yogurt in glass jars

BREADS, BREAD CRUMBS, CRACKERS, TORTILLAS, AND PASTA

Annie's, www.annies.com: Whole wheat graham crackers

Baia, www.baiapasta.com: High-quality pastas made from heirloom grains

Food for Life Baking Company, www.foodforlife.com: Ezekiel bread, sprouted breads, English muffins, hamburger buns and tortillas, gluten-free breads

Ian's, www.iansnaturalfoods.com: Organic bread crumbs, panko crumbs, including gluten-free

Jovial, www.jovialfoods.com: Organic, whole-grain and gluten-free pastas

Nature's Legacy, www.natureslegacyforlife.com: Organic spelt pasta

Trader Joe's, www.traderjoes.com: Organic brown rice and quinoa pasta, black bean pasta

SUPERFOODS

Do Matcha, www.domatcha.com: Matcha powder

Honey Pacifica, www.honeypacifica.com: Bee pollen

Nativas Naturals, www.navitasnaturals.com: Organic raw cacao powder and nibs, maca powder, lucuma powder, dried mulberries, chia seeds

Nutiva, www.nutiva.com: Organic coconut manna (butter), shelled hempseed, chia seeds,

Sun Potion, www.sunpotion.com: He shou wu powder, Ashwagandha ayurvedic antioxidant, chlorella

JARRED FRUIT AND VEGETABLE PRODUCTS

Bionaturae, www.bionaturae.com: Organic tomato paste in glass jars

Jovial, www.jovialfoods.com: Organic tomatoes in glass jars

St. Dalfour, www.stdalfour.us: No-sugar-added fruit preserves in glass jars

OILS AND VINEGARS

Al Wadi Natural, www.olivenation.com: Pomegranate molasses made from 100 percent pomegranate juice.

Bariani, www.barianioliveoil.com: Unrefined olive oil—peppery and grassy, great for finishing a dish

Barleans, www.barleans.com: Cold-pressed flax oil

Bella Vado, www.bellavado.com: Unrefined, extra-virgin avocado oil

Bragg, www.bragg.com: Organic, unpasteurized cider vinegar and organic, unrefined olive oil

Follow Your Heart, www.followyourheart.com: Soy-free Vegenaise

Gourmet Blends, www.gourmetblends.us: Aged balsamic vinegars

Marukan, www.marukan-usa.com: Organic, unseasoned rice vinegar

Napa Valley Naturals, www.napavalleynaturals .com: Organic, unrefined, organic, extra-virgin olive oil, red wine, white wine and balsamic vinegars

Nutiva, www.nutiva.com: Organic, unrefined virgin coconut oil

Primal Kitchen, www.primalkitchen.com: Organic unrefined avocado oil

Spectrum, www.spectrumorganics.com: Organic, unrefined toasted sesame oil

Whole Foods 365, www.wholefoodsmarket.com: Organic, unrefined, virgin coconut oil

ASIAN PRODUCTS

Eden Foods, www.edenfoods.com: Sea vegetables, bonito flakes, wasabi powder, gomasio, mirin

Gimme Organic, www.gimmehealth.com: Roasted Seaweed Snacks

Lightlife, www.lightlife.com: Organic tempeh products

Mae Ploy: Thai yellow curry paste

Miso Masters, www.great-eastern-sun.com: Non-GMO miso

Ohsawa: www.mikuniwildharvest.com: Traditionally brewed, organic shoyu and gluten-free tamari

Red Boat, www.redboatfishsauce.com: Preservative-free fish sauce

San-J, www.san-j.com: Organic shoyu and gluten-free tamari

Thai Kitchen, www.thaikitchen.com: Red curry paste

Vermont Maple Sriracha, www.vermontmaple sriracha.com: Sriracha sweetened with maple instead of sugar

Wildwood Organics, www.wildwoodfoods.com: Organic, sprouted tofu

SALT, HERBS AND SPICES, EXTRACTS, CONDIMENTS

Chiquilin, www.worldmarket.com: Smoked paprika

Diamond Crystal, www.diamondcrystalsalt.com: Additive-free kosher salt

Edward & Sons, www.edwardandsons.com: The Wizard's vegan, gluten-free Worcestershire sauce

Maldon, www.maldonsalt.co.uk: Flaky sea salt

Mountain Rose Herbs, www.mountainroseherbs .com: Organic and sustainable herbs and spices

Oaktown Spice Shop, www.oaktownspiceshop .com: Amazing and fresh spice blends, including pumpkin pie spice

Pacific Foods, www.pacificfoods.com: Mushroom stock

Rumford, www.clabbergirl.com: Aluminum-free baking powder with non-GMO cornstarch

Selina Naturally Celtic Sea Salt, www.selina naturally.com: Finely ground gray Celtic sea salt

Simply Organic, www.simplyorganic.com: Organic pure vanilla and almond extracts

SWEETENERS

Alter-Eco, www.altereco.com: Organic muscovado sugar

Big Tree Farms, bigtreefarms.com: Organic coconut palm sugar

Coombs Family Farms, www.coombsfamilyfarms .com: Organic maple sugar, pure maple syrup

Enjoy Life, www.enjoylifefoods.com: Allergen-free chocolate chips

Lundberg, www.lundberg.com: Organic brown rice syrup

Omica Organics, www.omicaorganics.com: Pure stevia

Trader Joe's, www.traderjoes.com: 100 percent pure organic maple syrup in glass bottles

FISH AND SEAFOOD PRODUCTS

Tonnino, www.tonnino.com: Wild-caught tuna in olive oil in glass jars

Vital Choice Seafood, www.vitalchoice.com: Low-mercury albacore tuna and wild salmon in BPA-free cans, frozen wild Alaskan seafood

EQUIPMENT

All-Clad 6.5 quart Slow Cooker with ceramic insert: I have used this slow cooker with consistently good results. The insert is ceramic and not nonstick. I use it for slow cooking, making bone broth, beans, oatmeal, and even keeping foods warm on the warm setting.

Breville Sous Chef food processor, Breville.com: Powerful and easy to use. I am obsessed with the adjustable slicing disk and the reversible shredding disk. I also like that the buttons are metal and not thin plastic, which gets worn down quickly.

Breville immersion blender, Breville.com: This handheld blender goes right into the pot to puree beautifully. I appreciate the nonscratch guard on the bottom to protect my stainless-steel pots. It is very easy to clean.

Global carbon stainless knives, Global-knife.com: These knives feel good in my hands and work well for me as a solid set of everyday knives. I get them professionally sharpened when they start to lose their edge.

Instant Pot, Instantpot.com: Slightly smaller than my All-Clad slow cooker, this appliance is a slow cooker, pressure cooker, rice cooker, yogurt maker, and more. The insert is stainless steel and it even has a sauté feature for browning vegetables and meats.

Kyocera ceramic knives, Kyocera.com: Lightweight and stay really sharp for a long time. They are not indestructible, though, but if you send your chipped or broken knife to the manufacturer with $10 for shipping, the company will send you a brand-new knife.

Kikuichi knives, Kikuichi.net: I have one Kikuichi knife which I call my "serious" knife. It is very high quality and razor sharp.

Oster Duraceramic Flip Waffle Maker, Oster.com: This is coated in nonstick, but nontoxic, lead-free ceramic and is very reasonably priced. I use it to make traditional waffles, but also Hash Brown Waffles (page 46) and waffled sandwiches, to name a few.

Silpat baking sheets, Silpat.com: I prefer to line my nonstick and aluminum baking sheets with either unbleached parchment paper or reusable Silpat silicone mats. Silicone is an inert material that doesn't leach. Refrain from using these mats with foods that have a strong odor (e.g., fish).

STORAGE

Ambatalia, www.ambatalia.green: Linen bowl covers

Glasslock, www.glasslockusa.com: Glass storage containers

If You Care, www.ifyoucare.com: Unbleached parchment paper rolls, sandwich bags, and muffin liners

Neat-os, www.neat-os.com: Reusable canvas storage bags

Pyrex, www.pyrexware.com: Glass bowl and storage containers

Weck Jars, www.weckjars.com: Glass storage containers

GENERAL WEBSITES

Amazon, www.amazon.com
Environmental Working Group, Ewg.com
Thrive Market, Thrivemarket.com
Vitacost, Vitacost.com
Wildnerness Family Naturals, www.wildernessfamilynaturals.com

ACKNOWLEDGMENTS

Sometimes we get to where we want not by design, but by a confluence of events. Although twenty years ago I did not see this book or teaching cooking classes in my future, I always asked the universe to point me in the direction of personal fulfillment and meaningful societal contribution. Nothing could make me happier than empowering others to nourish themselves and their families. Writing this book was both exciting and challenging, and I have many people to thank for steering me through the process.

To my husband, Daniel, the love of my life, my best friend, and my biggest cheerleader. Thank you for encouraging me every step of the way, for tasting beet greens and quinoa and date-sweetened muffins for the last twenty-plus years, and allowing me to do what I love.

To my three precious jewels, Emma, Anna, and Andrew (a.k.a. Mr. Picky), for giving me my favorite job in the world—being your mom. You have inspired me to be more patient, challenged me to make better food and filled my heart with an infinite amount of love.

To my parents, Lois and Mario, who taught me everything I know about hard work and putting family first, and who made a lot of sacrifices for me to have the opportunities I did. An extra special thank-you to my father, who allowed us to live a life with organic vegetable gardens, compost heaps, and an understanding of why eating whole foods matters.

To my Aunt Maria, my soul sister in the kitchen and whom I credit with encouraging my love of food and cooking from the time I was a wee one. You are the most talented cook I know and my best teacher.

To my mother-in-law and father-in-law, Sonia and David, who have been West Coast parents to me for almost twenty-eight years. Thank you for your unconditional support, for treating me like your daughter, and (Sonia) for buying me every new kitchen gadget you thought I had to have.

To Brandi Bowles, my incredible book agent, for peeling back the layers and seeing what I had to share in this book. Thank you for your guidance and believing in me. I know you always had my back.

To my cookbook editor, Renée Sedliar, who patiently and deftly helped guide me through this process of my first book. Thank you for going to bat for me when I needed it and for never making me feel that too many questions were too many questions. To the rest of the team at Da Capo: John Radziewicz, Kevin Hanover, Raquel Hitt, Miriam Riad, Lisa Diercks, and Christine Marra, thank you for your enthusiasm for this cookbook and for helping me share the message of good food.

To Amy Neunsinger, my most incredible photographer. You are so gifted and perfectly understood my philosophy and translated it through your lens. Not only were your images beautiful, you were the leader I needed for this book's shoot.

To Vivian Lui, whom I trusted to cook my recipes for this book. You were flawless, a joy to work with, and I learned so much from you.

To Brian Boone for helping me pick the perfect props, which is definitely not my forte, and making it fun.

To my friend Hillary Hartman, for insisting I teach that first cooking class. You started it all! Thank you for not taking no for an answer! To all my girlfriends, but especially Andrea Stanford, Lori Goler, Melissa Bomes, Nancy Paul, and Nina Kotick. I couldn't ask for a better crew. Thank you for always being available for an opinion, a taste, advice, or a shoulder to lean on. And thank you for encouraging me not to sell myself short. I love you dearly.

To Jenni Kayne, for inviting me into your beautiful kitchen every month for the last seven and half years, and for always inspiring me to take my recipes to the next level. I have loved our collaborations and our friendship that has developed.

And to Nicole Hirshberg, my most dedicated cooking class student over the last decade, my sounding board, and my friend. Thank you for showing up every month with your amazing group of gals and for all your valuable feedback. You have made me a better teacher.

To Peggy Curry and the entire Growing Great organization. You are pioneers in the farm-to-table, whole foods movement. Thank you for allowing me to help educate children and their parents about the value of eating higher-quality food. The work you do has made a difference in so many lives and has inspired me to pay it forward.

To my cooking class assistants, Elizabeth Lim, Lauren O'Neil, Leslie Scheid, Danielle Wolfe, and my summer interns, Hannah Geiser and Sydney Navid. Thank you for making me look good every single every day with your professionalism, attention to detail, and positive energy. Thank you for putting up with me when I wanted to test the squash recipe for the twelfth time or when I couldn't remember how many tablespoons of vinegar I added to that dressing we tested last week. I adore each of you and I couldn't have done any of this without you.

To all my cooking class students, who inspire me to create the best recipes possible and who push me to keep learning. I continue to do what I do because of you. Thank you for showing up to my classes every day with your open hearts and open minds. You have taught me so much and you have influenced the pages of this book more than you know. I love you all.

Last, but certainly not least, to the readers of my blog, all of whom I wish I could meet in my kitchen, this book is for you.

INDEX

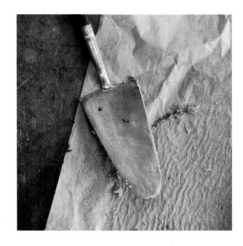